Diagnostic or Therapeutic Strategies for Pregnancy Complications

Diagnostic or Therapeutic Strategies for Pregnancy Complications

Editors

Alexander Heazell
Sylvie Girard

MDPI • Basel • Beijing • Wuhan • Barcelona • Belgrade • Manchester • Tokyo • Cluj • Tianjin

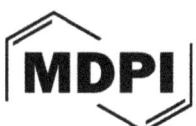

Editors
Alexander Heazell
Manchester Academic Health
Science Centre
UK

Sylvie Girard
Mayo Clinic College of Medicine
and Science
USA

Editorial Office
MDPI
St. Alban-Anlage 66
4052 Basel, Switzerland

This is a reprint of articles from the Special Issue published online in the open access journal *Journal of Clinical Medicine* (ISSN 2077-0383) (available at: https://www.mdpi.com/journal/jcm/special_issues/High-Risk_Pregnancies_Pregnancy_Complications).

For citation purposes, cite each article independently as indicated on the article page online and as indicated below:

LastName, A.A.; LastName, B.B.; LastName, C.C. Article Title. *Journal Name* **Year**, *Volume Number*, Page Range.

ISBN 978-3-0365-4877-7 (Hbk)
ISBN 978-3-0365-4878-4 (PDF)

© 2022 by the authors. Articles in this book are Open Access and distributed under the Creative Commons Attribution (CC BY) license, which allows users to download, copy and build upon published articles, as long as the author and publisher are properly credited, which ensures maximum dissemination and a wider impact of our publications.

The book as a whole is distributed by MDPI under the terms and conditions of the Creative Commons license CC BY-NC-ND.

Contents

About the Editors vii

Camille Couture and Sylvie Girard
Diagnostic or Therapeutic Strategies for Pregnancy Complications
Reprinted from: *J. Clin. Med.* **2022**, *11*, 3144, doi:10.3390/jcm11113144 1

Samantha J. Benton, Erika E. Mery, David Grynspan, Laura M. Gaudet, Graeme N. Smith and Shannon A. Bainbridge
Placental Pathology as a Tool to Identify Women for Postpartum Cardiovascular Risk Screening following Preeclampsia: A Preliminary Investigation
Reprinted from: *J. Clin. Med.* **2022**, *11*, 1576, doi:10.3390/jcm11061576 5

Ciara N. Murphy, Catherine A. Cluver, Susan P. Walker, Emerson Keenan, Roxanne Hastie, Teresa M. MacDonald, Natalie J. Hannan, Fiona C. Brownfoot, Ping Cannon, Stephen Tong and Tu'uhevaha J. Kaitu'u-Lino
Circulating SPINT1 Is Reduced in a Preeclamptic Cohort with Co-Existing Fetal Growth Restriction
Reprinted from: *J. Clin. Med.* **2022**, *11*, 901, doi:10.3390/jcm11040901 19

Dorsa Mavedatnia, Jason Tran, Irina Oltean, Vid Bijelić, Felipe Moretti, Sarah Lawrence and Dina El Demellawy
Impact of Co-Existing Placental Pathologies in Pregnancies Complicated by Placental Abruption and Acute Neonatal Outcomes
Reprinted from: *J. Clin. Med.* **2021**, *10*, 5693, doi:10.3390/jcm10235693 29

Julja Burchard, Ashoka D. Polpitiya, Angela C. Fox, Todd L. Randolph, Tracey C. Fleischer, Max T. Dufford, Thomas J. Garite, Gregory C. Critchfield, J. Jay Boniface, George R. Saade and Paul E. Kearney
Clinical Validation of a Proteomic Biomarker Threshold for Increased Risk of Spontaneous Preterm Birth and Associated Clinical Outcomes: A Replication Study
Reprinted from: *J. Clin. Med.* **2021**, *10*, 5088, doi:10.3390/jcm10215088 39

Monika Kniotek, Aleksander Roszczyk, Michał Zych, Małgorzata Wrzosek, Monika Szafarowska, Radosław Zagożdżon and Małgorzata Jerzak
Sildenafil Citrate Downregulates PDE5A mRNA Expression in Women with Recurrent Pregnancy Loss without Altering Angiogenic Factors—A Preliminary Study
Reprinted from: *J. Clin. Med.* **2021**, *10*, 5086, doi:10.3390/jcm10215086 49

Emmanuel Bujold, Alexandre Fillion, Florence Roux-Dalvai, Marie Pier Scott-Boyer, Yves Giguère, Jean-Claude Forest, Clarisse Gotti, Geneviève Laforest, Paul Guerby and Arnaud Droit
Proteomic Analysis of Maternal Urine for the Early Detection of Preeclampsia and Fetal Growth Restriction
Reprinted from: *J. Clin. Med.* **2021**, *10*, 4679, doi:10.3390/jcm10204679 61

Michelle A. Wyatt, Sarah C. Baumgarten, Amy L. Weaver, Chelsie C. Van Oort, Bohdana Fedyshyn, Rodrigo Ruano, Chandra C. Shenoy and Elizabeth Ann L. Enninga
Evaluating Markers of Immune Tolerance and Angiogenesis in Maternal Blood for an Association with Risk of Pregnancy Loss
Reprinted from: *J. Clin. Med.* **2021**, *10*, 3579, doi:10.3390/jcm10163579 75

Natalie K. Binder, Teresa M. MacDonald, Sally A. Beard, Natasha de Alwis, Stephen Tong, Tu'uhevaha J. Kaitu'u-Lino and Natalie J. Hannan
Pre-Clinical Investigation of Cardioprotective Beta-Blockers as a Therapeutic Strategy for Preeclampsia
Reprinted from: *J. Clin. Med.* **2021**, *10*, 3384, doi:10.3390/jcm10153384 87

Joon Hyung Lee, Chan-Wook Park, Kyung Chul Moon, Joong Shin Park and Jong Kwan Jun
The Inflammatory Milieu of Amniotic Fluid Increases with Chorio-Deciduitis Grade in Inflammation-Restricted to Choriodecidua, but Not Amnionitis, of Extra-Placental Membranes
Reprinted from: *J. Clin. Med.* **2021**, *10*, 3041, doi:10.3390/jcm10143041 105

Marwa Ben Ali Gannoun, Nozha Raguema, Hedia Zitouni, Meriem Mehdi, Ondrej Seda, Touhami Mahjoub and Julie L. Lavoie
MMP-2 and MMP-9 Polymorphisms and Preeclampsia Risk in Tunisian Arabs:
A Case-Control Study
Reprinted from: *J. Clin. Med.* **2021**, *10*, 2647, doi:10.3390/jcm10122647 119

Hyun Soo Park, Hayan Kwon, Ja-Young Kwon, Yun Ji Jung, Hyun-Joo Seol, Won Joon Seong, Hyun Mi Kim, Han-Sung Hwang, Ji-Hee Sung and Soo-young Oh
Uterine Cervical Change at Term Examined Using Ultrasound Elastography:
A Longitudinal Study
Reprinted from: *J. Clin. Med.* **2021**, *10*, 75, doi:10.3390/jcm10010075 129

Amy M. Inkster, Icíar Fernández-Boyano and Wendy P. Robinson
Sex Differences Are Here to Stay: Relevance to Prenatal Care
Reprinted from: *J. Clin. Med.* **2021**, *10*, 3000, doi:10.3390/jcm10133000 141

Brahm Seymour Coler, Oksana Shynlova, Adam Boros-Rausch, Stephen Lye, Stephen McCartney, Kelycia B. Leimert, Wendy Xu, Sylvain Chemtob, David Olson, Miranda Li, Emily Huebner, Anna Curtin, Alisa Kachikis, Leah Savitsky, Jonathan W. Paul, Roger Smith and Kristina M. Adams Waldorf
Landscape of Preterm Birth Therapeutics and a Path Forward
Reprinted from: *J. Clin. Med.* **2021**, *10*, 2912, doi:10.3390/jcm10132912 163

Marie-Eve Brien, Virginie Gaudreault, Katia Hughes, Dexter J. L. Hayes, Alexander E. P. Heazell and Sylvie Girard
A Systematic Review of the Safety of Blocking the IL-1 System in Human Pregnancy
Reprinted from: *J. Clin. Med.* **2022**, *11*, 225, doi:10.3390/jcm11010225 197

About the Editors

Alexander Heazell

Alexander Heazell is a Professor of Obstetrics and Director of the Tommy's Stillbirth Research Centre, University of Manchester, UK. His research portfolio includes basic science and clinical and qualitative research studies to gain better understanding of the causes of placental dysfunction, to prevent stillbirth, and to improve care for parents after stillbirth or perinatal death. He has received over GBP 3.7M of grant income and has published over 240 research papers. He was the lead investigator for the MiNESS case–control study and the national evaluation of Saving Babies Lives Care Bundle (SBLCB). He is currently leading a follow-up evaluation of Version 2 of the SBLCB. He is part of the national steering group of the Perinatal Mortality Review Tool.

Sylvie Girard

Sylvie Girard holds a PhD in Immunology (focused on perinatal inflammation and brain development) and a postdoctoral fellowship in neuroimmunology in Manchester, UK. She continued with her postdoctoral studies focused on reproductive immunology both in Manchester, UK and at Yale University, USA. She began her independent research career within the Department of Obstetrics & Gynecology at the Universite de Montreal in Quebec, Canada, in late 2014 and recently (Oct 2021) moved to the Mayo Clinic in Rochester, Minnesota, USA. She is currently an Associate Professor in Obstetrics & Gynecology and part of the Department of Obstetrics & Gynecology with joint appointment in the Department of Immunology. Her overall body of work is dedicated to studying the short- and long-term impact of pregnancy complications on maternal health as well as on neonates exposed to a sub-optimal in utero environment. The primary interest of her laboratory is inflammation and immune modulation in the maternal, placental, and foetal compartment and the interplay between all three in order to understand the mediators and mechanisms involved. Through this work, Dr Girard and her team's main goal is to develop novel diagnostic and therapeutic strategies to protect the placenta and subsequently decrease negative health impacts on mother and child.

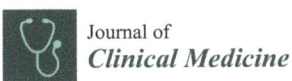

Editorial

Diagnostic or Therapeutic Strategies for Pregnancy Complications

Camille Couture [1] and Sylvie Girard [2,*]

[1] Ste-Justine Hospital Research Center, Department of Microbiology, Infectiology and Immunology, Universite de Montreal, Montreal, QC H3T 1C5, Canada; camille.couture.2@umontreal.ca
[2] Department of Obstetrics & Gynecology, Department of Immunology, Mayo Clinic College of Medicine and Science, Rochester, MN 55905, USA
* Correspondence: girard.sylvie@mayo.edu

Pregnancy complications including preeclampsia, preterm birth, recurrent pregnancy loss, and fetal growth restriction affect over 12% of all pregnancies worldwide. However, the risks of suffering from pregnancy loss or developing pregnancy complications could be detectable at an earlier stage giving opportunity for meaningful interventions. For example, fetal sex differences, which arise very early in development due to differential gene expression from the X and Y chromosomes, could be integrated into the development of risk prediction tools for certain complications [1]. On the other hand, once a pregnancy is closer to term, uterine cervical changes can be detected using ultrasound elastography, which could in turn also improve the management of delivery [2].

Pregnancy complications have negative short- and long-term impacts on both maternal and neonatal health such as the increased risk of neurodevelopmental and cardiovascular diseases (CVD). There are currently limited ways for the early identification of such long-term health outcomes. However, the examination of the placenta and extra-placental membranes offers new opportunities, which could optimize the care given to mothers and babies who are at greater risk of neurodevelopmental and cardiovascular consequences. Women who had more severe placental lesions of maternal vascular malperfusion after preeclampsia had a three-fold increased risk of screening as high-risk for CVD compared to women without these lesions [3]. Interestingly, fetal health can also be investigated through placental pathology, where the odds of neonatal intensive care unit (NICU) admission were twice as high in pregnancies with placental pathologies in addition to placental abruption [4]. Furthermore, inflammation in the extra-placental membranes showed that the inflammatory milieu of amniotic fluid increases with chorio-deciduitis grade, but not amnionitis of these membranes [5].

Advances in the early detection of women at risk of pregnancy complications have increased in the last decade, in part due to bioinformatic improvements, making it much easier to access and analyze large amounts of data and identify novel biomarkers. Indeed, proteomic biomarkers in maternal urine have proven promising as a non-invasive way of identifying women at risk of preeclampsia and fetal growth restriction [6]. Proteomic biomarkers, this time in maternal serum samples, were also investigated in a replication study looking at the ratio of IBP4/SHBG proteins as a predictive biomarker for spontaneous preterm birth [7]. Maternal blood has additionally been used to identify markers of immune tolerance and angiogenesis, showing decreased galactin-9 and VEGF-A in patients with prior miscarriage [8].

Potential novel therapeutic targets have also been uncovered using other techniques, where for example, a polymorphism in MMP-9, correlated with high MMP-9 production, has been associated with preeclampsia [9]. Of course, identifying biomarkers and women who are at risk of pregnancy complications is not an end-all-be-all solution. Novel therapeutic strategies must also be developed in parallel to optimize the health of both mother and baby. By identifying proteins, we can then hope to target them, as has been performed by Kniotek et al., where sildenafil citrate was used to downregulate *PDE5A* expression

Citation: Couture, C.; Girard, S. Diagnostic or Therapeutic Strategies for Pregnancy Complications. *J. Clin. Med.* **2022**, *11*, 3144. https://doi.org/10.3390/jcm11113144

Received: 20 May 2022
Accepted: 30 May 2022
Published: 31 May 2022

Publisher's Note: MDPI stays neutral with regard to jurisdictional claims in published maps and institutional affiliations.

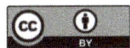

Copyright: © 2022 by the authors. Licensee MDPI, Basel, Switzerland. This article is an open access article distributed under the terms and conditions of the Creative Commons Attribution (CC BY) license (https://creativecommons.org/licenses/by/4.0/).

in vitro in immune cells from patients with recurrent pregnancy loss [10]. This process could also potentially be applied to the protein SPINT1, which is reduced in preeclamptic pregnancies with co-existing fetal growth restriction, to help promote adequate blood flow and nutrient delivery to the placenta to facilitate fetal growth [11]. Similarly, another in vitro study showed that cardioprotective beta-blockers could promote the secretion of pro-angiogenic mediators in endothelial cells and mitigate inflammation, offering potential novel therapeutic strategies in preeclampsia [12].

Since we know that inflammatory pathways are dysregulated in pregnancy complications and that they can even aggravate cardiovascular disorders, they have become key targets for therapeutic strategies and drug delivery. A great example of this is IL-1, which is known to be increased in pregnancy complications and is thus a promising target in clinical settings. The therapeutic potential of blocking IL-1 in human pregnancies, as used for several inflammatory pathologies such as arthritis, was investigated in a review by Brien et al., which most importantly showed that there was no association with adverse perinatal outcomes [13]. To better understand the designs and hurdles in therapeutics for pregnancy complications, Coler et al., present possible steps to expedite drug development to better meet the growing need for effective therapeutics in preterm birth [14].

Over the past decade, numerous groups have investigated how to mitigate these effects, promote healthier pregnancies and optimize neonatal health, however, this has been difficult to translate into clinical settings due to difficulties related to early diagnostic, drug delivery, specificity, and importantly, the lack of novel therapeutic strategies. This series of fourteen articles shed light on current advances in prenatal diagnostics, knowledge gaps in the development of novel therapeutic strategies, uses of artificial intelligence to understand the placental impact of pregnancy complications, as well as recent advances in targeted drug delivery to optimize the health of both mothers and their babies.

Funding: This research received no external funding.

Conflicts of Interest: The authors declare no conflict of interest.

References

1. Inkster, A.M.; Fernández-Boyano, I.; Robinson, W.P. Sex differences are here to stay: Relevance to prenatal care. *J. Clin. Med.* **2021**, *10*, 3000. [CrossRef] [PubMed]
2. Park, H.S.; Kwon, H.; Kwon, J.-Y.; Jung, Y.J.; Seol, H.-J.; Seong, W.J.; Kim, H.M.; Hwang, H.-S.; Sung, J.-H.; Oh, S.-Y. Uterine cervical change at term examined using ultrasound elastography: A longitudinal study. *J. Clin. Med.* **2020**, *10*, 75. [CrossRef] [PubMed]
3. Benton, S.J.; Mery, E.E.; Grynspan, D.; Gaudet, L.M.; Smith, G.N.; Bainbridge, S.A. Placental pathology as a tool to identify women for postpartum cardiovascular risk screening following preeclampsia: A preliminary investigation. *J. Clin. Med.* **2022**, *11*, 1576. [CrossRef] [PubMed]
4. Mavedatnia, D.; Tran, J.; Oltean, I.; Bijelić, V.; Moretti, F.; Lawrence, S.; El Demellawy, D. Impact of co-existing placental pathologies in pregnancies complicated by placental abruption and acute neonatal outcomes. *J. Clin. Med.* **2021**, *10*, 5693. [CrossRef] [PubMed]
5. Lee, J.H.; Park, C.-W.; Moon, K.C.; Park, J.S.; Jun, J.K. The inflammatory milieu of amniotic fluid increases with chorio-deciduitis grade in inflammation-restricted to choriodecidua, but not amnionitis, of extra-placental membranes. *J. Clin. Med.* **2021**, *10*, 3041. [CrossRef] [PubMed]
6. Bujold, E.; Fillion, A.; Roux-Dalvai, F.; Scott-Boyer, M.P.; Giguère, Y.; Forest, J.-C.; Gotti, C.; Laforest, G.; Guerby, P.; Droit, A. Proteomic analysis of maternal urine for the early detection of preeclampsia and fetal growth restriction. *J. Clin. Med.* **2021**, *10*, 4679. [CrossRef] [PubMed]
7. Burchard, J.; Polpitiya, A.D.; Fox, A.C.; Randolph, T.L.; Fleischer, T.C.; Dufford, M.T.; Garite, T.J.; Critchfield, G.C.; Boniface, J.J.; Saade, G.R.; et al. Clinical validation of a proteomic biomarker threshold for increased risk of spontaneous preterm birth and associated clinical outcomes: A replication study. *J. Clin. Med.* **2021**, *10*, 5088. [CrossRef] [PubMed]
8. Wyatt, M.A.; Baumgarten, S.C.; Weaver, A.L.; Van Oort, C.C.; Fedyshyn, B.; Ruano, R.; Shenoy, C.C.; Enninga, E.A.L. Evaluating markers of immune tolerance and angiogenesis in maternal blood for an association with risk of pregnancy loss. *J. Clin. Med.* **2021**, *10*, 3579. [CrossRef] [PubMed]
9. Gannoun, M.B.A.; Raguema, N.; Zitouni, H.; Mehdi, M.; Seda, O.; Mahjoub, T.; Lavoie, J. MMP-2 and MMP-9 polymorphisms and preeclampsia risk in Tunisian Arabs: A case-control study. *J. Clin. Med.* **2021**, *10*, 2647. [CrossRef] [PubMed]

10. Kniotek, M.; Roszczyk, A.; Zych, M.; Wrzosek, M.; Szafarowska, M.; Zagożdżon, R.; Jerzak, M. Sildenafil citrate downregulates PDE5A mRNA expression in women with recurrent pregnancy loss without altering angiogenic factors—A preliminary study. *J. Clin. Med.* **2021**, *10*, 5086. [CrossRef] [PubMed]
11. Murphy, C.N.; Cluver, C.A.; Walker, S.P.; Keenan, E.; Hastie, R.; MacDonald, T.M.; Hannan, N.J.; Brownfoot, F.C.; Cannon, P.; Tong, S.; et al. Circulating SPINT1 is reduced in a preeclamptic cohort with co-existing fetal growth restriction. *J. Clin. Med.* **2022**, *11*, 901. [CrossRef] [PubMed]
12. Binder, N.K.; MacDonald, T.M.; Beard, S.A.; de Alwis, N.; Tong, S.; Kaitu'U-Lino, T.; Hannan, N. Pre-clinical investigation of cardioprotective beta-blockers as a therapeutic strategy for preeclampsia. *J. Clin. Med.* **2021**, *10*, 3384. [CrossRef] [PubMed]
13. Brien, M.-E.; Gaudreault, V.; Hughes, K.; Hayes, D.J.L.; Heazell, A.E.P.; Girard, S. A systematic review of the safety of blocking the IL-1 system in human pregnancy. *J. Clin. Med.* **2021**, *11*, 225. [CrossRef] [PubMed]
14. Coler, B.S.; Shynlova, O.; Boros-Rausch, A.; Lye, S.; McCartney, S.; Leimert, K.; Xu, W.; Chemtob, S.; Olson, D.; Li, M.; et al. Landscape of preterm birth therapeutics and a path forward. *J. Clin. Med.* **2021**, *10*, 2912. [CrossRef]

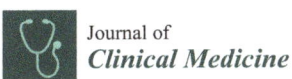

Article

Placental Pathology as a Tool to Identify Women for Postpartum Cardiovascular Risk Screening following Preeclampsia: A Preliminary Investigation

Samantha J. Benton [1,†], Erika E. Mery [2,†], David Grynspan [3], Laura M. Gaudet [4], Graeme N. Smith [4] and Shannon A. Bainbridge [2,*]

1. Department of Health Sciences, Carleton University, Ottawa, ON K1S 5B6, Canada; samanthabenton@cunet.carleton.ca
2. School of Interdisciplinary Health Sciences, University of Ottawa, Ottawa, ON K1H 8L1, Canada; emery103@uottawa.ca
3. Department of Pathology and Laboratory Medicine, University of British Columbia, Vancouver, BC V6T 1Z7, Canada; david.grynspan@interiorhealth.ca
4. Department of Obstetrics and Gynaecology, Queen's University, Kingston, ON K7L 2V7, Canada; laura.gaudet@kingstonhsc.ca (L.M.G.); gns@queensu.ca (G.N.S.)
* Correspondence: shannon.bainbridge@uottawa.ca
† These authors contributed equally to this work.

Abstract: Preeclampsia (PE) is associated with an increased risk of cardiovascular disease (CVD) in later life. Postpartum cardiovascular risk screening could identify patients who would benefit most from early intervention and lifestyle modification. However, there are no readily available methods to identify these high-risk women. We propose that placental lesions may be useful in this regard. Here, we determine the association between placental lesions and lifetime CVD risk assessed 6 months following PE. Placentas from 85 PE women were evaluated for histopathological lesions. At 6 months postpartum, a lifetime cardiovascular risk score was calculated. Placental lesions were compared between CVD risk groups and the association was assessed using odds ratios. Multivariable logistic regression was used to develop prediction models for CVD risk with placental pathology. Placentas from high-risk women had more severe lesions of maternal vascular malperfusion (MVM) and resulted in a 3-fold increased risk of screening as high-risk for CVD (OR 3.10 (1.20–7.92)) compared to women without these lesions. MVM lesion severity was moderately predictive of high-risk screening (AUC 0.63 (0.51, 0.75); sensitivity 71.8% (54.6, 84.4); specificity 54.7% (41.5, 67.3)). When clinical parameters were added, the model's predictive performance improved (AUC 0.73 (0.62, 0.84); sensitivity 78.4% (65.4, 87.5); specificity 51.6% (34.8, 68.0)). The results suggest that placenta pathology may provide a unique modality to identify women for cardiovascular screening.

Keywords: preeclampsia; placenta; histopathology; cardiovascular disease; cardiovascular risk; postpartum screening

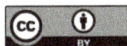

1. Introduction

Preeclampsia (PE) is a life-threatening hypertensive disorder of pregnancy, affecting 5–7% of pregnancies worldwide [1]. Importantly, PE is a significant risk indicator for cardiovascular disease (CVD) in later life. Women diagnosed with PE have a ~4-fold increased risk of hypertension and a ~2-fold increased risk of ischemic heart disease and stroke compared to women with uncomplicated pregnancies [2–5]. Moreover, evidence suggests that women who develop severe PE during pregnancy are at the highest risk of these outcomes [4,6–8]. Alarmingly, studies show that the onset of CVD and CVD-related death occur at much younger ages than the general female population [6–9]. The link(s) between PE and cardiovascular risk are not fully understood, but PE may indicate the presence of underlying, often undiagnosed, cardiovascular risk factors (CVRs) [10,11].

Moreover, underlying CVRs may directly contribute to placental dysfunction associated with PE; however, this relationship has yet to be fully elucidated [12,13].

Histopathological lesions of maternal vascular malperfusion (MVM) are commonly observed in placentas from PE pregnancies, particularly in cases of severe, early-onset disease [14–16]. These lesions, including increased syncytial knots and accelerated villous maturation, are believed to reflect placental hypoxia and oxidative stress arising from incomplete uterine artery modeling and abnormal uteroplacental blood flow [1,17,18]. Although common, MVM lesions are not observed in all PE cases, and a proportion of PE placentas are histologically normal or exhibit other pathology such as chronic inflammation [19,20]. Recent population-based studies have shown an association between placental lesions and future maternal health [21–26]. Catov et al. observed altered cardiometabolic profiles in women with preterm birth and lesions of MVM compared to women with term deliveries [21,26]. Additionally, women with preterm birth and co-morbid placental pathologies (MVM, inflammatory lesions) had the most severe atherogenic profiles [21]. More recently, Catov et al. demonstrated that MVM lesions are associated with vascular impairments 8–10 years after pregnancy [26]. While the mechanisms underlying these associations have yet to be fully elucidated, collectively, these studies provide strong evidence that the placenta and its pathology may provide a snapshot into future maternal cardio-metabolic health [26,27].

To reduce the burden of CVD on PE women, specialized postpartum cardiovascular health clinics are being established across North America to screen women for CVRs and initiate postpartum CVD prevention, including pharmaceutical and lifestyle interventions [28–30]. However, these clinics are resource-intensive, and, thus, follow-up of all PE women is prohibitive. Moreover, a proportion of PE women will remain at low risk for CVD postpartum and not require follow-up. As placental pathology is inexpensive and readily available, it may offer a unique modality to identify PE women for CVR screening. Here, we investigate the association between placental pathology and lifetime CVD risk in postpartum women following PE.

2. Materials and Methods

In this study, a cohort of women diagnosed with PE who underwent cardiovascular health screening at 6 months postpartum was assembled from two study sites (Kingston and Ottawa, ON, Canada).

2.1. Recruitment at the Kingston Site

In Kingston, women who develop a pregnancy complication are referred to the Maternal Health Clinic (Kingston General Hospital, Kingston, ON, Canada) for postpartum cardiovascular health screening at 6 months postpartum as part of routine standard of care. Assessments and evaluations, including the calculation of a lifetime cardiovascular risk score conducted at the Maternal Health Clinic, have been previously described [29]. From this clinic, we recruited eligible study participants at the time of their 6-month postpartum visit (between 2011 and 2017). Women diagnosed with PE who had placenta pathology performed at delivery of the index pregnancy (PE diagnosis) were approached to participate in the study.

2.2. Recruitment at the Ottawa Site

In Ottawa, women were recruited to participate in the study as part of the DREAM Study research protocol designed to emulate the Maternal Health Clinic. Women diagnosed with PE prior to delivery were recruited from inpatient services at the Ottawa Hospital General Campus (Ottawa, ON, Canada) between 2013 and 2018. Placentas from each participant were sent to Anatomical Pathology at the Children's Hospital of Eastern Ontario (Ottawa, ON, Canada). Six months after delivery, participants returned to the Ottawa Hospital for cardiovascular health screening performed by the research study nurse. The assessments performed at this study visit were identical to those performed at the Maternal

Health Clinic, and a lifetime cardiovascular risk score was calculated for each participant, as described previously [29]. At both sites, all women provided written informed consent to participate in the study.

2.3. Inclusion and Exclusion Criteria

PE was defined according to the contemporaneous Society of Obstetricians and Gynaecologists of Canada criteria, including hypertension (blood pressure $\geq$140/90 mmHg, on at least two occasions >15 min apart after 20 weeks' gestation) with new proteinuria ($\geq$0.3 g/day by 24 h urine collection, $\geq$30 mg/mmol by protein:creatinine ratio, or $\geq$1+ by urinary dipstick) or one or more adverse conditions (e.g., headache/visual symptoms, chest pain/dyspnea, nausea or vomiting, right upper quadrant pain, elevated WBC count) or one or more severe complications (e.g., eclampsia, uncontrolled severe hypertension, platelet count <50 $\times$ 10^9/L, acute kidney injury) [31]. Women with chronic hypertension, known CVD prior to pregnancy, known kidney disease prior to pregnancy, or diabetes (type I, type II, gestational) were excluded. Small-for-gestational age (SGA) status was used as a proxy for fetal growth restriction and was defined conservatively as infant birth weight <5th percentile for gestational age at delivery and sex [32]. Clinical data, including medical and family history, pregnancy outcome, and postpartum cardiovascular health results, were collected by chart review following 6 months postpartum cardiovascular screening.

2.4. Placenta Pathology

For study participants in Ottawa, placentas were collected at the time of delivery and sent to the Pathology department. Trimmed placental weight was recorded, and gross pathology was recorded by an experienced pathology assistant. Four full-thickness tissue biopsies were randomly excised from each quadrant of the placenta, between the cord insertion site and the placental margins. Areas of visible pathology were sampled separately and not used for the full-thickness sections. Tissue was fixed in 4% neutral buffered formalin and paraffin-embedded. Following sectioning (5 µm), the tissue was stained with hematoxylin and eosin (H&E) using standard protocol [33] and stored for examination. In Kingston, archived H&E-stained tissue slides (4–5 slides/participant) were accessed from the Pathology archives for each participant. Sampling procedures were similar to those followed in Ottawa in that full-thickness biopsies were excised from each quadrant of the placenta, between the margin and cord insertion site.

At both study sites, trimmed placenta weight and gross pathology were collected from the accompanying placental pathology reports. A single, experienced placental pathologist examined the stained slides from all study participants, blinded to all clinical information apart from gestational age at delivery. Placental lesions were evaluated according to a standardized placental pathology data collection form, with pre-specified severity criteria derived from clinical practice guidelines and published literature [34]. Within the evaluation scheme, each lesion has a severity score to achieve a quantitative output for the severity of pathology. Lesions were either given a binary score of 0 (absent) or 1 (present) or a graded score according to a linear scale (i.e., 0 = absent, 1 = focal, 2 = patchy, 3 = diffuse). Individual lesions are grouped according to broad etiological categories, with a maximum severity score calculated for each category. Lesion categories and maximum severity score for each category are as follows: MVM (max score 14), implantation site abnormalities (max score 4), histological chorioamnionitis (max score 11), placental villous maldevelopment (max score 5), fetal vascular malperfusion (max score 6), maternal-fetal interface disturbance (max score 5), and chronic inflammation (max score 6). Gross anatomy (e.g., placental weight, umbilical cord length) was obtained from the corresponding historical placental pathology reports, in addition to several microscopic lesions (e.g., placental infarction, chronic deciduitis), as the tissue biopsies were collected from areas that appeared grossly normal and only included villous parenchyma (i.e., maternal decidua was not sampled).

2.5. Cardiovascular Risk Assessment

At 6 months postpartum, all women underwent physical and biochemical CVR screening in the Maternal Health Clinic (Kingston General Hospital) or at the Ottawa Hospital (Ottawa) according to published protocol [29]. A full medical history was taken and included information on family history, breastfeeding, and lifestyle such as smoking status and alcohol intake. A physical examination, specifically focusing on cardiovascular-related clinical predictors, was performed and collected information on weight, height, and blood pressure. A maternal blood sample was collected, and total cholesterol, LDL cholesterol, HDL cholesterol, triglycerides, glucose, and high sensitivity C-reactive protein were quantified for each participant. Physical and biochemical CVR findings were integrated to calculate a lifetime risk score for CVD, according to the previously published protocol [29]. Calculations for lifetime cardiovascular risk are based on the following risk factors: total cholesterol, systolic blood pressure, diastolic blood pressure, use of anti-hypertensive medication(s), fasting blood glucose, diagnosis of diabetes, and current smoking status. Risk stratification for each risk factor was based on predetermined measurement thresholds (optimal, not optimal, elevated, major). Lifetime cardiovascular risk estimates are also categorical and based on the total number of optimal, not optimal, elevated, and major risk factors of each individual (8%, all risk factors are optimal; 27%, $\geq$1 risk factor is not optimal; 39%, $\geq$1 risk factor is elevated; 39%, 1 risk factor is major; 50%, $\geq$2 risk factors are major). Lifetime cardiovascular risk estimates were simplified to categorize the women as low risk (<39% risk) or high risk ($\geq$39% risk) for lifetime CVD. This threshold corresponds to the baseline lifetime CVD risk attributed to healthy women enrolled in the Framingham Heart Study [35].

2.6. Statistical Analysis

Data were analyzed using SPSS 26.0 (SPSS Inc., Chicago, IL, USA). Descriptive data were expressed as means and standard deviations for normally distributed data or medians with interquartile ranges for non-normally distributed data. Chi-square tests were used for the comparison of categorical variables, while Student's *t*-test or Mann–Whitney U-tests were used for continuous variables. Placental lesions (frequencies and severity scores) were compared between the low CVD risk and high CVD risk groups. The association between individual placental lesions and lifetime CVD risk was assessed using odds ratios (OR) with 95% confidence intervals. Multivariable logistic regression was used to develop prediction models for lifetime CVD risk with placental data alone or in combination with clinical data. The performance of the models was assessed using area under the receiver operator characteristic (AUC ROC) curve analysis. Statistical significance was defined as $p < 0.05$.

3. Results

3.1. Clinical Characteristics

A total of 85 women were included in this study (35 from Ottawa and 50 from Kingston). The clinical characteristics of the participants, as a combined cohort and by each study site, are shown in Tables 1 and 2. The demographic characteristics of the women between the two study sites were not significantly different, apart from maternal age and pre-pregnancy BMI. Although the average age of women in Kingston was 2 years younger than the women in Ottawa ($p = 0.015$), the mean age of participants at both sites was <34 years (31.9 $\pm$ 6.0 vs. 33.9 $\pm$ 5.6), and this was not deemed to be of high clinical relevance. Although women in Ottawa had significantly higher pre-pregnancy BMIs than women in Kingston ($p = 0.024$), the gestational weight gain for the index pregnancy was similar between the two sites (13.2 $\pm$ 7.1 vs. 14.6 $\pm$ 7.1, $p = 0.393$).

Table 1. Maternal characteristics of the study participants as a combined cohort and by individual study site.

	Combined (n = 85)	Ottawa (n = 35)	Kingston (n = 50)	p-Value [§] (t-Test, KW, X²)
Maternal Characteristics				
Maternal age at delivery (y)	31.9 ± 6.0	33.9 ± 5.6	30.7 ± 5.9	0.015
Postsecondary education (%)	74 (88.1) [a]	31 (91.2) [a]	43 (86.0)	0.520
Married or common law	80 (95.2) [a]	35 (100)	45 (91.8) [a]	0.137
Nulliparous (%)	59 (69.4)	22 (62.9)	37 (74.0)	0.341
Pre-pregnancy BMI	24.5 (22.1, 31.0)	28.2 (23.0, 35.5)	24.4 (21.9, 28.5)	0.024
Smoking (%)	6 (7.1)	1 (2.9)	5 (10.0)	0.393
Previous history of HDPs (%)	11 (12.9)	7 (20.0)	4 (8.0)	0.187
Family history of CVD * (%)	44 (52.4) [a]	16 (47.1) [a]	28 (56.0)	0.506
Family history of PE (%)	12 (15.0) (n = 80)	6 (20.0) (n = 30)	6 (12.0)	0.520

Data presented as mean ± SD, median (IQR) or n (%). BMI: body mass index; CVD: cardiovascular disease; HDP: hypertensive disorders of pregnancy; IQR: interquartile range; PE: preeclampsia; SD: standard deviation. [§] Comparison between participants in Ottawa and Kingston. * Includes coronary artery disease and cerebral vascular disease. [a] Data missing for one participant.

Table 2. Delivery and postpartum characteristics of the study participants as a combined cohort and by individual study site.

	Combined (n = 85)	Ottawa (n = 35)	Kingston (n = 50)	p-Value [§] (t-Test, KW, X²)
At delivery				
Systolic BP * (mmHg)	152 ± 25	136 ± 17	164 ± 22	<0.0001
Diastolic BP * (mmHg)	93 ± 13	85 ± 10	98 ± 13	<0.0001
Antihypertensive medication ** (%)	38 (44.7)	28 (80.0)	6 (12.0)	<0.0001
Pregnancy weight gain (kg)	14.0 ± 7.1	13.2 ± 7.1	14.6 ± 7.1	0.393
Gestational age delivery	36.0 (32.2, 38.0)	37.5 (34.4, 39.4)	34.0 (31.0, 38.0)	<0.001
Delivery before 37 weeks gestation (%)	48 (56.5)	11 (31.4)	37 (74.0)	<0.001
Cesarean section (%)	44 (51.8)	14 (40.0)	30 (60.0)	0.081
Female infant (%)	42 (49.4)	13 (37.1)	29 (58.0)	0.078
Birth weight (g)	2200 (1495, 3098)	2655 (2075, 3280)	1920 (1285, 2351)	0.0003
Small for gestational age (<5th percentile)	15 (17.6)	5 (14.3)	10 (20.0)	0.573
Admission to NICU (%)	59 (69.4)	15 (42.9)	44 (88.0)	<0.001
Placental weight (g)	334 (274, 443)	382 (326, 516)	312 (236, 431)	0.057
At 6 months postpartum				
Systolic BP (mmHg)	119 ± 18	116 ± 23	121 ± 13	0.164
Diastolic BP (mmHg)	81 ± 10	78 ± 9	82 ± 10	0.081
Antihypertensive medication use (%)	13 (15.3)	5 (14.3)	8 (16.0)	1.00
Breastfeeding (%)	44 (52.4)	22 (64.7)	22 (44.0)	0.077
Total cholesterol	4.8 ± 1.0	4.9 ± 1.0	4.7 ± 1.0	0.292
Fasting glucose	4.8 ± 0.5	4.7 ± 0.5	4.8 ± 0.5	0.397
HDL	1.5 ± 0.4	1.5 ± 0.4	1.5 ± 0.4	0.541
LDL	2.8 (2.2, 3.4)	3.0 (2.2, 3.5)	2.6 (2.1, 3.3)	0.231
hsCRP	2.6 (1.0, 7.4)	2.6 (0.9, 8.4)	2.0 (0.98, 5.9)	0.443
Triglycerides	0.98 (0.67, 1.69)	0.98 (0.72, 1.88)	0.96 (0.65, 1.60)	0.500
Screen high-risk for lifetime CVD (%)	53 (62.4)	18 (51.4)	35 (70.0)	0.112

Data presented as mean ± SD, median (IQR) or n (%). BP: blood pressure; hsCRP: high sensitivity C-reactive protein; CVD: cardiovascular disease; HDL: high density lipoprotein; IQR: interquartile range; LDL: low density lipoprotein; NICU: neonatal intensive care unit; PE: preeclampsia; SD: standard deviation. [§] Comparison between participants in Ottawa and Kingston. * Highest BP measurement following admission before delivery. ** Medication started during index pregnancy or postpartum prior to discharge from hospital.

As for pregnancy outcomes, women in Kingston had significantly higher blood pressures at delivery, increased use of anti-hypertensive medication in pregnancy, and delivered at earlier gestational ages compared to women in Ottawa (34.0 (31.0, 38.0) weeks vs. 37.5 (34.4, 39.4), $p < 0.0001$) and had more SGA infants compared with women in Ottawa. At 6 months postpartum, there were no significant differences in cardiometabolic parameters between the participants at the study sites. Of the 85 women included in the analysis, 53 (62.4%) women screened high-risk for lifetime CVD at 6 months postpartum.

3.2. Histopathology Findings in Low- and High-Risk Women

The frequency of placenta lesions between women who screened as low- and high-risk for lifetime CVD are shown in Table 3. A total of 5 placentas (15.6%) in the low-risk group and 6 placentas (11.3%) in the high-risk group had no observed pathology ($p = 0.74$). The mean cumulative severity score (sum of scores for all categories) for the low-risk group was 3.1 ± 2.2 and 3.6 ± 2.4 for the high-risk group ($p = 0.374$). By etiological category, women who screened as high-risk for lifetime CVD had placentas with more severe lesions of MVM (score ≥ 2: 54.7% vs. 28.1%, $p = 0.017$); however, the frequency of individual lesions belonging to the MVM category was not found to be significantly different between the groups. There were no differences in the frequencies of placental lesions between high and low-risk groups when stratified by individual study site (data not shown).

Table 3. Frequency of placental lesions by cardiovascular risk group.

Placental Lesion	High CVD Risk ($n = 53$)	Low CVD Risk ($n = 32$)	p-Value (Pearson X^2)
Evidence of maternal vascular malperfusion			
Placental infarction	16 (30.2)	7 (21.9)	0.403
Distal villous hypoplasia	15 (28.3)	8 (25.0)	0.740
Accelerated villous maturation	31 (58.5)	12 (37.5)	0.061
Syncytial knots	34 (64.2)	17 (53.1)	0.315
Perivillous fibrin deposition	5 (9.4)	6 (18.8)	0.215
Villous agglutination	7 (13.2)	1 (3.1)	0.123
Presence of retroplacental hematoma	0 (0)	2 (6.3)	0.066
MVM Score of 0	8 (15.1)	9 (28.1)	0.146
MVM Score 2 or more	29 (54.7)	9 (28.1)	**0.017**
Evidence of maternal decidual arteriopathy			
Insufficient vessel remodeling	7 (13.2)	2 (6.3)	0.312
Fibrinoid necrosis	4 (7.5)	2 (6.3)	0.821
Decidual arteriopathy present	9 (17.0)	3 (10.3)	0.416
Evidence of ascending intrauterine infection			
Maternal inflammatory response	2 (3.8)	4 (4.7)	0.128
Fetal inflammatory response	2 (3.8)	2 (6.3)	0.601
Ascending intrauterine infection present	3 (5.7)	5 (15.6)	0.127
Evidence of placenta villous maldevelopment			
Chorangiosis	0 (0)	0 (0)	–
Chorangiomas	0 (0)	0 (0)	–
Delayed villous maturation	1 (1.9)	2 (6.3)	0.291
Evidence of fetal vascular malperfusion			
Avascular fibrotic villi	2 (3.8)	0 (0)	0.266
Thrombosis	1 (1.9)	1 (3.1)	0.715
Intramural fibrin deposition	0 (0)	3 (9.4)	**0.023**
Karyorrhexis	0 (0)	0 (0)	–
High-grade fetal vascular malperfusion	2 (3.8)	0 (0)	0.266
Fetal vascular malperfusion present	4 (7.5)	5 (15.6)	0.241

Table 3. Cont.

Placental Lesion	High CVD Risk (n = 53)	Low CVD Risk (n = 32)	p-Value (Pearson X^2)
Fibrinoid			
Massive Perivillous fibrin deposition pattern	1 (1.9)	0 (0)	0.434
Maternal floor infarction pattern	0 (0)	0 (0)	–
Intervillous thrombi			
Intervillous thrombi	5 (9.4)	1 (3.1)	0.271
Evidence of chronic inflammation			
Villitis of unknown etiology	5 (9.4)	3 (9.4)	0.993
Chronic intervillositis	0 (0)	0 (0)	–
Chronic plasma cell deciduitis	5 (9.4)	3 (9.4)	0.993
Chronic inflammation present	7 (13.2)	6 (18.8)	0.492

Data presented as n (%). MVM: maternal vascular malperfusion.

3.3. Association of Placental Lesions and CVD Risk

Individually, no placental lesions were found to be significantly associated with high-risk CVD screening at 6 months postpartum. However, PE women with lesions of MVM with a severity score of 2 or more were more likely to screen high-risk for lifetime CVD than PE women without severe MVM lesions (severity score <2) (OR 3.10 (1.20–7.92)). Clinical data in the absence of placenta pathology findings (maternal age, gestational weight gain, blood pressure at delivery, gestational age at delivery) was moderately predictive of high-risk screening at 6 months postpartum AUC 0.68 (0.55, 0.81); sensitivity: 86.5% (74.7, 93.3); specificity: 29.0% (16.1, 46.6)) (Figure 1a). Severity of MVM lesions alone (score 2 or more) was similarly predictive of high-risk screening at 6 months postpartum (AUC 0.63 (0.51, 0.75); sensitivity: 71.8% (54.6, 84.4); specificity: 54.7% (41.5, 67.3)) (Figure 1b). However, when clinical data and MVM lesion severity were combined, the model's predictive performance improved (AUC 0.73 (0.62, 0.84) sensitivity 78.4% (65.4, 87.5); specificity 51.6% (34.8, 68.0)) (Figure 1c).

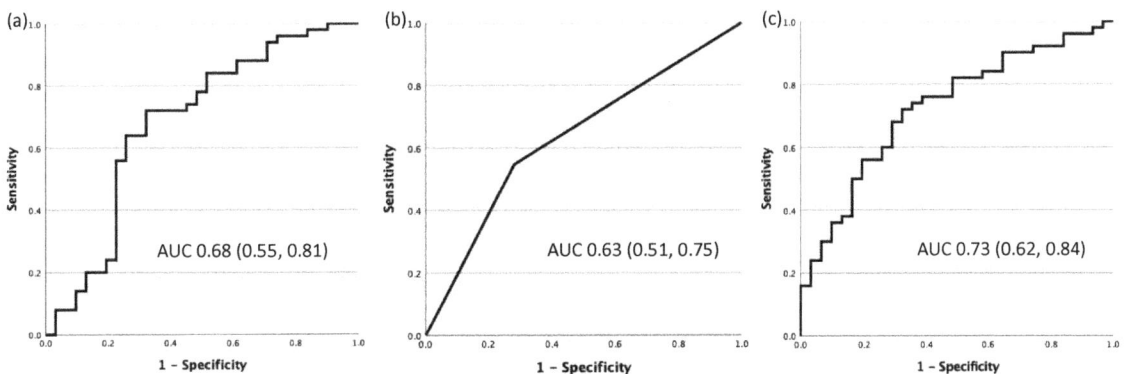

Figure 1. Area under the receiver operator characteristic curves for the prediction of screening high-risk for lifetime cardiovascular disease at 6 months postpartum by (**a**) maternal age, gestational weight gain, blood pressure at delivery, and gestational age at delivery, (**b**) maternal vascular malperfusion severity score, and (**c**) maternal vascular malperfusion severity score, maternal age, gestational weight gain, blood pressure at delivery, and gestational age at delivery.

4. Discussion

4.1. Main Findings

In this study, we observed an increase in placental histopathological lesions in women who screened high risk for lifetime CVD at 6 months postpartum following a PE pregnancy. Specifically, high-risk women had more severe lesions of MVM, the placental pathology traditionally associated with PE. MVM lesions with a severity score >2 resulted in a 3-fold increased risk of screening high risk for lifetime CVD at 6 months postpartum. The cumulative severity of MVM lesions was important in this association, suggesting that there may be critical thresholds of placental damage that reflect increased lifetime cardiovascular risk.

4.2. Interpretation

Previous studies have demonstrated an association between placental pathology and increased postpartum maternal cardiovascular health risk [21–26]. One study found that in normotensive women who experienced placental abruption during pregnancy, CVRs were significantly altered 6–9 months postpartum compared to women without uncomplicated pregnancies [25]. Lesions of maternal vascular maldevelopment (defined as mural hyperplasia, unaltered decidual vessels, and decidual atherosis) are associated with maternal hypertension 7 to 15 years after pregnancy [36]. Catov et al. reported that in normotensive women who delivered preterm without fetal growth restriction, those who had placental lesions of MVM and inflammation had significantly elevated atherogenic profiles assessed 4–12 years after delivery [21]. Our findings are in line with this study in which the cumulative severity of placental lesions may be important for identifying women at the highest cardiovascular risk following pregnancy. Together with our current findings, significant placental pathology may be indicative of a greater risk for CVD postpartum.

The mechanisms linking PE and postpartum maternal cardiovascular risk have yet to be fully elucidated. The most commonly held hypothesis to explain this link proposes that pre-pregnancy maternal CVRs, including both clinically diagnosed and subclinical risk factors, may contribute to the development of PE, including abnormal placental development, and predispose women to CVD after pregnancy. Placentation requires the invasion of fetal trophoblast cells into the maternal decidua, resulting in the conversion of the maternal uterine spiral arteries to high capacity, venous-like conduits to increase blood flow into the uteroplacental unit to support fetal growth and development [37]. This physiological remodeling of the uterine spiral arteries is known to be defective in PE, and the two-stage model of pathogenesis proposes that this failed remodeling leads to placental ischemia, oxidative stress, and placental dysfunction, which stimulates the release of angiogenic factors, pro-inflammatory cytokines, syncytiotrophoblast vesicles, and other factors from the placenta [1]. These processes result in characteristic histopathological lesions observed in placentas from pregnancies complicated by PE, particularly lesions of MVM [38]. Placenta-derived circulating factors interact with the maternal endothelium at the systemic level, leading to the end-organ dysfunction observed in the clinical manifestation of the disorder. The maternal environment, including subclinical CVRs common to PE and CVD, may directly contribute to impaired trophoblast invasion and defective spiral artery conversion and its downstream effects. Dyslipidemia, including elevated pre-pregnancy levels of serum triglycerides, cholesterol, LDL, and non-HDL cholesterol, have been associated with increased risk of developing PE and are known contributors to CVD [39]. Studies have shown that lipids modulate human trophoblast invasion, and alterations in maternal lipid profiles could potentially contribute to abnormal trophoblast invasion and spiral artery remodeling [40,41]. Systemic (often subclinical) inflammation, common in obesity and other cardiometabolic conditions, may also play a role in limited trophoblast invasion and spiral artery conversion during placentation in PE [42,43]. Pro-inflammatory cytokines are known to inhibit trophoblast invasion by increasing apoptosis and decreasing proliferation [44]. Cytokine imbalance prior to pregnancy may alter the maternal inflammatory milieu over and above the physiological immune/inflammatory changes that occur in pregnancy; however, exactly how this imbalance contributes to altered placentation is unknown.

PE and placental dysfunction, reflected as MVM lesions in the placenta, may also cause lasting damage to the maternal cardiovascular system that results in altered cardiovascular health trajectories. Circulating levels of inflammatory cytokines such as tumor necrosis factor-a (TNF-a) and interleukin-6 (IL-6) are elevated in PE and interfere with the maternal endothelium to produce systemic endothelial dysfunction. Women diagnosed with PE have been found to have chronically altered circulating levels of these cytokines >20 years after pregnancy, suggesting that PE may program the maternal cardiovasculature such that there is persistent cardiovascular dysregulation, precipitating CVD in later life [45]. Other maternal cardiometabolic pathways, including the renin–angiotensin system, may also contribute to abnormal placentation and reduced uteroplacental exchange, the two main features of PE [46]. While yet to be fully elucidated, dysregulation of these cardio-regulatory pathways in the mother after pregnancy may contribute to the increased risk for CVD after PE [47]. Additionally, anti-angiogenic imbalance in the maternal circulation, including elevated soluble Fms-like tyrosine kinase-1 (sFlt-1) and reduced placental growth factor (PlGF), may contribute to lasting cardiovascular dysfunction after PE. Alternations in circulating angiogenic factors during pregnancy are associated with cardiovascular changes, including increased blood pressure 6 to 12 years after pregnancy [48,49]. Although angiogenic factor levels significantly drop following delivery, a recent study suggests that angiogenic imbalance may be persistent in the postpartum period [50]. While the mechanisms of angiogenic factors on cardiovascular health are not fully known, sFlt-1 and PlGF have been shown to influence vasodilatory function in preclinical models [51,52].

It is plausible that a combination of the pre-pregnancy maternal environment and persistent alterations to the maternal cardiovascular system from placental dysfunction contributes to future CVD risk. Placental pathology, particularly lesions of MVM, may reflect both abnormalities in the maternal milieu as well as the significant cardiovascular burden from abnormal placentation, thereby identifying patients at particularly increased risk of postpartum CVD. As such, placental lesions identified at the time of delivery could provide a modality to triage PE women for cardiovascular health screening postpartum. Future studies are required to confirm the utility of placental pathology in this capacity; it may offer a unique opportunity to extend the clinical benefits of the placenta pathology exam while targeting postpartum resource-intensive cardiovascular screening to the most vulnerable patients.

4.3. Strengths and Limitations

The limitations of our study need to be considered. First, we did observe a significant difference in several important pregnancy parameters between our study sites, including blood pressure at delivery, anti-hypertensive use at delivery, and gestational age at delivery—indicative of a more severe form of maternal disease in our Kingston cohort. We believe these differences are likely the result of sampling bias introduced by the different study designs used across the two sites. In Kingston, a retrospective analysis was performed on placentas originally submitted to pathology based on the clinical judgment of the treating physician. Despite a PE diagnosis being identified as an indicator for placenta pathology submission, only 53% of placentas were submitted for evaluation at this site during the study period (unpublished internal audit data), in line with previous literature on the topic of suboptimal placenta pathology submission practices [53]. On the other hand, a prospective study design was employed at the Ottawa site, with 100% placental pathology submission for recruited PE study participants, irrespective of the severity of their clinical characteristics. As cardiovascular parameters were similar between our cohorts at the 6-month postpartum clinic visit, we do not feel these delivery parameters influenced our findings. Due to our small sample size, we may be underpowered to detect differences between low and high-risk groups for less common pathology, such as chronic inflammation. However, for MVM lesions, we found that a sample size of 48 was needed to detect differences between MVM scores greater than 2 within the high- and low-risk groups at the confidence level of 95% and power of 80%. Confirming our results in an adequately powered prospective study may identify a predictive combination of placental lesions that robustly identifies high-priority women for postpartum CVD screening at the time of delivery. Our study is strengthened by the standardized placental evaluations we conducted using our evidence-based synoptic data collection [34]. Variability in placenta pathology examination is a known challenge, and the use of this synoptic collection form ensures each placenta was evaluated in a reproducible manner. Moreover, our cohort study design reflects routine clinical practice in which only placentas from complicated pregnancies are submitted for histopathological examination. While placentas from uncomplicated pregnancies exhibit placental lesions with varying degrees of prevalence and severity [54], these placentas are not routinely sent for examination and the use of placental pathology in this population is limited.

5. Conclusions

Women with PE and severe lesions of MVM are more likely to screen as high-risk for lifetime CVD at 6 months postpartum compared to women without these lesions. Placenta pathology may provide a unique modality to identify women for postpartum cardiovascular screening. Triaging at the time of delivery would allow for targeted screening and resource allocation to the truly at-risk PE women.

Author Contributions: Conceptualization, S.A.B., S.J.B. and G.N.S.; methodology, D.G., S.A.B., S.J.B. and G.N.S.; formal analysis, S.J.B. and E.E.M.; writing—original draft preparation, S.J.B. and E.E.M.; writing—review and editing, S.A.B., G.N.S., D.G. and L.M.G.; supervision, S.A.B., S.J.B., G.N.S., L.M.G. and D.G.; funding acquisition, L.M.G. and S.A.B. All authors have read and agreed to the published version of the manuscript.

Funding: This research was funded by a Canadian Institutes of Health Research (CIHR) operating grant (grant number 130548) and an innovation grant from The Ottawa Hospital Academic Medical Organization.

Institutional Review Board Statement: The study was conducted in accordance with the Declaration of Helsinki and approved by the Institutional Review Boards (or Ethics Committees) of Ottawa Health Science Network (protocol code 20140799-01H; 22 April 2015), Children's Hospital of Eastern Ontario (protocol code 14/210X; 23 March 2015), University of Ottawa (A04-15-01; 1 April 2014), and Queen's University Health Science (OBGY-295-16; 13 January 2017).

Informed Consent Statement: Informed consent was obtained from all participants involved in the study.

Data Availability Statement: Reasonable requests for data will be considered.

Acknowledgments: The authors thank the staff and patients and the Maternal Health Clinic at Kinston Hospital for their participation in this study, particularly Jessica Pudwell for her help in extracting clinical chart data and helping with the identification of archived placental samples. Likewise, the authors would like to thank the staff and patients that participated in the DREAM study at the Ottawa Hospital. Special thanks to Alysha Harvey and members of Obstetrics and Maternal Newborn Investigations (OMNI, the Ottawa Hospital) for their help in the coordination of patient recruitment and the collection of clinical chart data for the DREAM study participants.

Conflicts of Interest: The authors declare no conflict of interest.

References

1. Rana, S.; Lemoine, E.; Granger, J.P.; Karumanchi, S.A. Preeclampsia. *Circ. Res.* **2019**, *124*, 1094–1112. [CrossRef]
2. Bellamy, L.; Casas, J.-P.; Hingorani, A.D.; Williams, D.J. Pre-eclampsia and risk of cardiovascular disease and cancer in later life: Systematic review and meta-analysis. *BMJ* **2007**, *335*, 974. [CrossRef]

3. Okoth, K.; Chandan, J.S.; Marshall, T.; Thangaratinam, S.; Thomas, G.N.; Nirantharakumar, K.; Adderley, N.J. Association between the re-productive health of young women and cardiovascular disease in later life: Umbrella review. *BMJ* **2020**, *371*, m3502. [CrossRef]
4. Brown, M.C.; Best, K.E.; Pearce, M.S.; Waugh, J.; Robson, S.C.; Bell, R. Cardiovascular disease risk in women with pre-eclampsia: Systematic review and meta-analysis. *Eur. J. Epidemiol.* **2013**, *28*, 1–19. [CrossRef] [PubMed]
5. Smith, G.N.; Pudwell, J.; Walker, M.; Wen, S.-W. Ten-Year, Thirty-Year, and Lifetime Cardiovascular Disease Risk Estimates Following a Pregnancy Complicated by Preeclampsia. *J. Obstet. Gynaecol. Can.* **2012**, *34*, 830–835. [CrossRef]
6. McDonald, S.D.; Malinowski, A.; Zhou, Q.; Yusuf, S.; Devereaux, P.J. Cardiovascular sequelae of preeclampsia/eclampsia: A systematic review and meta-analyses. *Am. Heart J.* **2008**, *156*, 918–930. [CrossRef]
7. Mongraw-Chaffin, M.L.; Cirillo, P.M.; Cohn, B.A. Preeclampsia and cardiovascular disease death: Prospective evidence from the child health and development studies cohort. *Hypertension* **2010**, *56*, 166–171. [CrossRef]
8. Ray, J.G.; Vermeulen, M.J.; Schull, M.; Redelmeier, D.A. Cardiovascular health after maternal placental syndromes (CHAMPS): Population-based retrospective cohort study. *Lancet* **2005**, *366*, 1797–1803. [CrossRef]
9. Smith, G.C.; Pell, J.; Walsh, D. Pregnancy complications and maternal risk of ischaemic heart disease: A retrospective cohort study of 129 290 births. *Lancet* **2001**, *357*, 2002–2006. [CrossRef]
10. Smith, G.N.; Walker, M.C.; Liu, A.; Wen, S.W.; Swansburg, M.; Ramshaw, H.; White, R.R.; Roddy, M.; Hladunewich, M.; Pre-Eclampsia New Emerging Team (PE-NET). A history of preeclampsia identifies women who have underlying cardiovascular risk factors. *Am. J. Obstet. Gynecol.* **2009**, *200*, 58.e1–58.e8. [CrossRef]
11. Heidema, W.M.; Scholten, R.R.; Lotgering, F.K.; Spaanderman, M.E. History of preeclampsia is more predictive of cardiometabolic and cardiovascular risk factors than obesity. *Eur. J. Obstet. Gynecol. Reprod. Biol.* **2015**, *194*, 189–193. [CrossRef]
12. Yinon, Y.; Kingdom, J.C.P.; Odutayo, A.; Moineddin, R.; Drewlo, S.; Lai, V.; Cherney, D.Z.I.; Hladunewich, M.A. Vascular dysfunction in women with a history of preeclampsia and intrauterine growth restriction: Insights into future vascular risk. *Circulation* **2010**, *122*, 1846–1853. [CrossRef] [PubMed]
13. Kvehaugen, A.S.; Dechend, R.; Ramstad, H.B.; Troisi, R.; Fugelseth, D.; Staff, A.C. Endothelial Function and Circulating Biomarkers Are Disturbed in Women and Children After Preeclampsia. *Hypertension* **2011**, *58*, 63–69. [CrossRef] [PubMed]
14. Fillion, A.; Guerby, P.; Menzies, D.; Lachance, C.; Comeau, M.-P.; Bussières, M.-C.; Doucet-Gingras, F.-A.; Zérounian, S.; Bujold, E. Pathological investigation of placentas in preeclampsia (the PEARL study). *Hypertens. Pregnancy* **2021**, *40*, 56–62. [CrossRef] [PubMed]
15. Weiner, E.; Feldstein, O.; Tamayev, L.; Grinstein, E.; Barber, E.; Bar, J.; Schreiber, L.; Kovo, M. Placental histopathological lesions in correlation with neonatal outcome in preeclampsia with and without severe features. *Pregnancy Hypertens.* **2018**, *12*, 6–10. [CrossRef] [PubMed]
16. Kovo, M.; Schreiber, L.; Ben-Haroush, A.; Gold, E.; Golan, A.; Bar, J. The placental component in early-onset and late-onset preeclampsia in relation to fetal growth restriction. *Prenat. Diagn.* **2012**, *32*, 632–637. [CrossRef]
17. Burton, G.J.; Redman, C.W.; Roberts, J.M.; Moffett, A. Pre-eclampsia: Pathophysiology and clinical implications. *BMJ* **2019**, *366*, l2381. [CrossRef] [PubMed]
18. Schneider, H. Placental Dysfunction as a Key Element in the Pathogenesis of Preeclampsia. *Dev. Period Med.* **2018**, *21*, 309–316.
19. Benton, S.J.; Leavey, K.; Grynspan, D.; Cox, B.J.; Bainbridge, S.A. The clinical heterogeneity of preeclampsia is related to both placental gene expression and placental histopathology. *Am. J. Obstet. Gynecol.* **2018**, *219*, 604.e1. [CrossRef]
20. Falco, M.L.; Sivanathan, J.; Laoreti, A.; Thilaganathan, B.; Khalil, A. Placental histopathology associated with pre-eclampsia: Systematic review and meta-analysis. *Ultrasound Obstet. Gynecol.* **2017**, *50*, 295–301. [CrossRef]
21. Catov, J.M.; Muldoon, M.F.; Reis, S.; Ness, R.B.; Nguyen, L.; Yamal, J.-M.; Hwang, H.; Parks, W.T. Preterm birth with placental evidence of malperfusion is associated with cardiovascular risk factors after pregnancy: A prospective cohort study. *BJOG* **2018**, *125*, 1009–1017. [CrossRef] [PubMed]
22. Brosens, I.; Benagiano, M.; Puttemans, P.; D'Elios, M.M.; Benagiano, G. The placental bed vascular pathology revisited: A risk indicator for cardiovascular disease. *J. Matern. Fetal Neonatal Med.* **2019**, *32*, 1556–1564. [CrossRef] [PubMed]
23. Stevens, D.U.; Smits, M.P.; Bulten, J.; Spaanderman, M.E.A.; Van Vugt, J.M.G.; Al-Nasiry, S. Prevalence of hypertensive disorders in women after preeclamptic pregnancy associated with decidual vasculopathy. *Hypertens. Pregnancy* **2015**, *34*, 332–341. [CrossRef] [PubMed]
24. Stevens, D.U.; Al-Nasiry, S.; Fajta, M.M.; Bulten, J.; van Dijk, A.P.; van der Vlugt, M.J.; Oyen, W.J.; van Vugt, J.M.; Spaanderman, M.E. Cardiovascular and thrombogenic risk of decidual vasculopathy in preeclampsia. *Am. J. Obstet. Gynecol.* **2014**, *210*, 545.e1. [CrossRef] [PubMed]
25. Veerbeek, J.H.W.; Smit, J.G.; Koster, M.P.; Uiterweer, E.D.P.; Van Rijn, B.B.; Koenen, S.V.; Franx, A. Maternal Cardiovascular Risk Profile After Placental Abruption. *Hypertension* **2013**, *61*, 1297–1301. [CrossRef] [PubMed]
26. Catov, J.M.; Muldoon, M.F.; Gandley, R.E.; Brands, J.; Hauspurg, A.; Hubel, C.A.; Tuft, M.; Schmella, M.; Tang, G.; Parks, W.T. Maternal Vascular Lesions in the Placenta Predict Vascular Impairments a Decade After Delivery. *Hypertension* **2022**, *79*, 424–434. [CrossRef]
27. Parks, W.T.; Catov, J.M. The Placenta as a Window to Maternal Vascular Health. *Obstet. Gynecol. Clin. N. Am.* **2020**, *47*, 17–28. [CrossRef] [PubMed]

28. Park, K.; Minissian, M.B.; Wei, J.; Saade, G.R.; Smith, G.N. Contemporary clinical updates on the prevention of future cardiovascular disease in women who experience adverse pregnancy outcomes. *Clin. Cardiol.* **2020**, *43*, 553–559. [CrossRef]
29. Cusimano, M.; Pudwell, J.; Roddy, M.; Cho, C.-K.J.; Smith, G. The maternal health clinic: An initiative for cardiovascular risk identification in women with pregnancy-related complications. *Am. J. Obstet. Gynecol.* **2014**, *210*, 438.e1. [CrossRef] [PubMed]
30. Smith, G.N. The Maternal Health Clinic: Improving women's cardiovascular health. *Semin. Perinatol.* **2015**, *39*, 316–319. [CrossRef] [PubMed]
31. Magee, L.A.; Pels, A.; Helewa, M.; Rey, E.; von Dadelszen, P.; Audibert, F.; Bujold, E.; Côté, A.-M.; Douglas, M.J.; Eastabrook, G.; et al. Diagnosis, Evaluation, and Management of the Hypertensive Disorders of Pregnancy: Executive Summary. *J. Obstet. Gynaecol. Can.* **2014**, *36*, 416–438. [CrossRef]
32. Kramer, M.S.; Platt, R.W.; Wen, S.W.; Joseph, K.S.; Allen, A.; Abrahamowicz, M.; Blondel, B.; Breart, G.; for the Fetal/Infant Health Study Group of the Canadian Perinatal Surveillance System. A New and Improved Population-Based Canadian Reference for Birth Weight for Gestational Age. *Pediatrics* **2001**, *108*, e35. [CrossRef]
33. Warrander, L.; Batra, G.; Bernatavicius, G.; Greenwood, S.; Dutton, P.; Jones, R.; Sibley, C.P.; Heazell, A.E.P. Maternal Perception of Reduced Fetal Movements Is Associated with Altered Placental Structure and Function. *PLoS ONE* **2012**, *7*, e34851. [CrossRef]
34. Benton, S.J.; Lafreniere, A.J.; Grynspan, D.; Bainbridge, S.A. A synoptic framework and future directions for placental pathology reporting. *Placenta* **2019**, *77*, 46–57. [CrossRef] [PubMed]
35. Lloyd-Jones, D.M.; Leip, E.P.; Larson, M.; D'Agostino, R.B.; Beiser, A.; Wilson, P.W.; Wolf, P.A.; Levy, D. Prediction of Lifetime Risk for Cardiovascular Disease by Risk Factor Burden at 50 Years of Age. *Circulation* **2006**, *113*, 791–798. [CrossRef] [PubMed]
36. Holzman, C.B.; Senagore, P.; Xu, J.; Dunietz, G.L.; Strutz, K.L.; Tian, Y.; Bullen, B.L.; Eagle, M.; Catov, J.M. Maternal risk of hypertension 7–15 years after pregnancy: Clues from the placenta. *BJOG* **2021**, *128*, 827–836. [CrossRef] [PubMed]
37. Pijnenborg, R.; Vercruysse, L.; Hanssens, M. The Uterine Spiral Arteries in Human Pregnancy: Facts and Controversies. *Placenta* **2006**, *27*, 939–958. [CrossRef] [PubMed]
38. Bustamante Helfrich, B.; Chilukuri, N.; He, H.; Cerda, S.R.; Hong, X.; Wang, G.; Pearson, C.; Burd, I.; Wang, X. Maternal vascular malperfusion of the placental bed associated with hypertensive disorders in the Boston Birth Cohort. *Placenta* **2017**, *52*, 106–113. [CrossRef] [PubMed]
39. Magnussen, E.B.; Vatten, L.J.; Lund-Nilsen, T.I.; Salvesen, K.Å.; Smith, G.D.; Romundstad, P.R. Prepregnancy cardiovascular risk factors as predictors of pre-eclampsia: Population based cohort study. *BMJ* **2007**, *335*, 978. [CrossRef]
40. Pavan, L.; Tsatsaris, V.; Hermouet, A.; Therond, P.; Evain-Brion, D.; Fournier, T. Oxidized low-density lipoproteins inhibit trophoblastic cell invasion. *J. Clin. Endocrinol. Metab.* **2004**, *89*, 1969–1972. [CrossRef]
41. Pavan, L.; Hermouet, A.; Tsatsaris, V.; Thérond, P.; Sawamura, T.; Evain-Brion, D.; Fournier, T. Lipids from Oxidized Low-Density Lipoprotein Modulate Human Trophoblast Invasion: Involvement of Nuclear Liver X Receptors. *Endocrinology* **2004**, *145*, 4583–4591. [CrossRef]
42. Wolf, M.; Kettyle, E.; Sandler, L.; Ecker, J.L.; Roberts, J.; Thadhani, R. Obesity and preeclampsia: The potential role of inflammation. *Obstet. Gynecol.* **2001**, *98 Pt 1*, 757–762. [CrossRef] [PubMed]
43. Bodnar, L.M.; Ness, R.B.; Harger, G.F.; Roberts, J.M. Inflammation and Triglycerides Partially Mediate the Effect of Prepregnancy Body Mass Index on the Risk of Preeclampsia. *Am. J. Epidemiol.* **2005**, *162*, 1198–1206. [CrossRef]
44. Otun, H.A.; Lash, G.E.; Innes, B.A.; Bulmer, J.N.; Naruse, K.; Hannon, T.; Searle, R.F.; Robson, S.C. Effect of tumour necrosis factor-α in combination with interferon-γ on first trimester extravillous trophoblast invasion. *J. Reprod. Immunol.* **2011**, *88*, 1–11. [CrossRef] [PubMed]
45. Freeman, D.J.; McManus, F.; Brown, E.A.; Cherry, L.; Norrie, J.; Ramsay, J.E.; Clark, P.; Walker, I.D.; Sattar, N.; Greer, I.A. Short- and long-term changes in plasma inflam-matory markers associated with preeclampsia. *Hypertension* **2004**, *44*, 708–714. [CrossRef] [PubMed]
46. Lumbers, E.R.; Delforce, S.J.; Arthurs, A.; Pringle, K. Causes and Consequences of the Dysregulated Maternal Renin-Angiotensin System in Preeclampsia. *Front. Endocrinol.* **2019**, *10*, 563. [CrossRef]
47. Spaan, J.J.; Brown, M.A. Renin-angiotensin system in pre-eclampsia: Everything old is new again. *Obstet. Med.* **2012**, *5*, 147–153. [CrossRef] [PubMed]
48. Garrido-Gimenez, C.; Mendoza, M.; Cruz-Lemini, M.; Galian-Gay, L.; Sanchez-Garcia, O.; Granato, C.; Rodriguez-Sureda, V.; Rodriguez-Palomares, J.; Carreras-Moratonas, E.; Cabero-Roura, L.; et al. Angiogenic Factors and Long-Term Cardiovascular Risk in Women That Developed Preeclampsia During Pregnancy. *Hypertension* **2020**, *76*, 1808–1816. [CrossRef]
49. Benschop, L.; Schalekamp-Timmermans, S.; Broere-Brown, Z.A.; Roeters van Lennep, J.E.; Jaddoe, V.W.V.; Roos-Hesselink, J.W.; Ikram, M.K.; Steegers, E.A.P.; Roberts, J.M.; Gandley, R.E. Placental growth factor as an indicator of maternal cardiovascular risk after pregnancy. *Circulation* **2019**, *139*, 1698–1709. [CrossRef] [PubMed]
50. Akhter, T.; Wikström, A.; Larsson, M.; Larsson, A.; Wikström, G.; Naessen, T. Association between angiogenic factors and signs of arterial aging in women with pre-eclampsia. *Ultrasound Obstet. Gynecol.* **2017**, *50*, 93–99. [CrossRef]
51. Osol, G.; Celia, G.; Gokina, N.; Barron, C.; Chien, E.; Mandala, M.; Luksha, L.; Kublickiene, K. Placental growth factor is a potent vasodilator of rat and human resistance arteries. *Am. J. Physiol. Circ. Physiol.* **2008**, *294*, H1381–H1387. [CrossRef] [PubMed]
52. Amraoui, F.; Spijkers, L.; Lahsinoui, H.H.; Vogt, L.; Van Der Post, J.; Peters, S.; Afink, G.; Ris-Stalpers, C.; Born, B.-J.V.D. SFlt-1 Elevates Blood Pressure by Augmenting Endothelin-1-Mediated Vasoconstriction in Mice. *PLoS ONE* **2014**, *9*, e91897. [CrossRef] [PubMed]

53. Magann, E.; Sills, A.; Steigman, C.; Ounpraseuth, S.T.; Odibo, I.; Sandlin, A. Pathologic examination of the placenta: Recommended versus observed practice in a university hospital. *Int. J. Women's Health* **2013**, *5*, 309–312. [CrossRef] [PubMed]
54. Romero, R.; Kim, Y.M.; Pacora, P.; Kim, C.J.; Benshalom-Tirosh, N.; Jaiman, S.; Bhatti, G.; Kim, J.S.; Qureshi, F.; Jacques, S.M.; et al. The frequency and type of placental histologic lesions in term pregnancies with normal outcome. *J. Perinat. Med.* **2018**, *46*, 613–630. [CrossRef] [PubMed]

Article

Circulating SPINT1 Is Reduced in a Preeclamptic Cohort with Co-Existing Fetal Growth Restriction

Ciara N. Murphy [1,2,*], Catherine A. Cluver [2,3], Susan P. Walker [1,2], Emerson Keenan [1,2], Roxanne Hastie [1,2], Teresa M. MacDonald [1,2], Natalie J. Hannan [1,2], Fiona C. Brownfoot [1,2], Ping Cannon [1,2], Stephen Tong [1,2,†] and Tu'uhevaha J. Kaitu'u-Lino [1,2,†]

1. Department of Obstetrics & Gynaecology, Mercy Hospital for Women, The University of Melbourne, Heidelberg, VIC 3084, Australia; spwalker@unimelb.edu.au (S.P.W.); emerson.keenan@unimelb.edu.au (E.K.); hastie.r@unimelb.edu.au (R.H.); teresa.mary.macdonald@gmail.com (T.M.M.); nhannan@unimelb.edu.au (N.J.H.); fiona.brownfoot@unimelb.edu.au (F.C.B.); ping.cannon@unimelb.edu.au (P.C.); stong@unimelb.edu.au (S.T.); t.klino@unimelb.edu.au (T.J.K.-L.)
2. Mercy Perinatal, Mercy Hospital for Women, Heidelberg, VIC 3084, Australia; cathycluver@hotmail.com
3. Department of Obstetrics & Gynaecology, Stellenbosch University and Tygerberg Hospital, Cape Town 7505, South Africa
* Correspondence: ciaram1@student.unimelb.edu.au
† These authors contributed equally to this work.

Abstract: Fetal growth restriction (FGR), when undetected antenatally, is the biggest risk factor for preventable stillbirth. Maternal circulating SPINT1 is reduced in pregnancies, which ultimately deliver small for gestational age (SGA) infants at term (birthweight < 10th centile), compared to appropriate for gestational age (AGA) infants (birthweight ≥ 10th centile). SPINT1 is also reduced in FGR diagnosed before 34 weeks' gestation. We hypothesised that circulating SPINT1 would be decreased in co-existing preterm preeclampsia and FGR. Plasma SPINT1 was measured in samples obtained from two double-blind, randomised therapeutic trials. In the Preeclampsia Intervention with Esomeprazole trial, circulating SPINT1 was decreased in women with preeclampsia who delivered SGA infants ($n = 75$, median = 18,857 pg/mL, IQR 10,782–29,890 pg/mL, $p < 0.0001$), relative to those delivering AGA ($n = 22$, median = 40,168 pg/mL, IQR 22,342–75,172 pg/mL). This was confirmed in the Preeclampsia Intervention 2 with metformin trial where levels of SPINT1 in maternal circulation were reduced in SGA pregnancies ($n = 95$, median = 57,764 pg/mL, IQR 42,212–91,356 pg/mL, $p < 0.0001$) compared to AGA controls ($n = 40$, median = 107,062 pg/mL, IQR 70,183–176,532 pg/mL). Placental Growth Factor (PlGF) and sFlt-1 were also measured. PlGF was significantly reduced in the SGA pregnancies, while ratios of sFlt-1/SPINT1 and sFlt1/PlGF were significantly increased. This is the first study to demonstrate significantly reduced SPINT1 in co-existing FGR and preeclamptic pregnancies.

Keywords: fetal growth restriction (FGR); intra-uterine growth restriction (IUGR); preeclampsia; SPINT1; HAI-1; stillbirth; placental insufficiency

1. Introduction

Fetal Growth Restriction (FGR), particularly when undetected antenatally, is the single largest risk factor for preventable stillbirth in singleton pregnancies without congenital abnormalities [1]. Despite this, the current means of detecting FGR are inadequate [2], leaving many pregnancies vulnerable to the increased risk of perinatal morbidity and mortality associated with FGR. In many cases, FGR arises due to placental insufficiency, whereby a suboptimal placenta fails to sustain fetal growth. Since placental insufficiency is also implicated in preeclampsia, these pregnancy complications often occur in tandem, as the poorly perfused placenta struggles to maintain the pregnancy with advancing gestation. Identifying biomarkers of placental insufficiency to facilitate improved diagnosis of FGR is therefore of great interest. The current clinical approach is to detect small for gestational age (SGA) fetuses (birthweight < 10th centile), which will likely include most growth-restricted infants and some constitutionally, but not pathologically, small infants.

Serine protease inhibitor, Kunitz type 1 (SPINT1, also known as HAI-1), is a biomarker that we have shown to be deranged in the maternal circulation preceding a diagnosis of SGA at term gestations [3]. Circulating SPINT1 levels were markedly decreased at 36 weeks' gestation in those women who ultimately delivered an SGA infant, relative to appropriate for gestational age (AGA) counterparts with birthweights >10th centile. Importantly, in addition to being reduced in the maternal circulation, our prior report demonstrated that reduced circulating SPINT1 is associated with key indicators of placental insufficiency. It is most significantly reduced in the circulation of women carrying the smallest babies (birthweight < 3rd centile) and is associated with increased vascular resistance in the uterine artery and reduced placental weight and neonatal body mass index. While marked changes in SPINT1 are apparent close to term gestations, we have also identified reduced circulating levels in pregnancies carrying fetuses destined to deliver SGA infants as early as 24–26 weeks' gestation [4].

Both preeclampsia and poor fetal growth (indicated by an SGA infant) are believed to originate from placental insufficiency. SPINT1 is a highly expressed placental protein, expressed largely on placental cytotrophoblast cell surfaces [5], which has been demonstrated in murine models to be critical to placentation through its inhibition of its peptide substrates, matriptase and prostasin [6,7]. These results were also recently confirmed in a porcine model [8]. Although our prior work demonstrates reductions in SPINT1 are associated with poor fetal growth, no studies have found its expression to be deranged in preeclampsia.

It was therefore hypothesised that SPINT1 perturbations associated with FGR might also be observed in those with a primary diagnosis of preeclampsia. If confirmed, it means that it could be a biomarker of FGR even among women with preeclampsia. At the biological level it would imply FGR in preeclampsia has a distinct molecular pathogenesis to preeclampsia without FGR. In this study, we therefore measured circulating SPINT1 protein levels in women with pregnancies complicated by preterm preeclampsia, to assess whether SPINT1 was differentially expressed among those with and without an SGA infant at birth.

2. Materials and Methods

Blood samples from two clinical trials testing novel therapeutics for preeclampsia, provided a unique opportunity to examine SPINT1 in women with concomitant preeclampsia and FGR, as indicated by delivery of a small for gestational age (SGA) infant. Both trials included women with early-onset preeclampsia who had varying degrees of disease severity. As such, this study was able to assess whether, in the context of placental insufficiency manifesting as preterm preeclampsia, SPINT1 is still decreased in pregnancies complicated by growth restriction as previously established. Both trials assessed prolongation of pregnancy following randomisation and collected maternal plasma samples at randomisation and twice weekly until delivery.

2.1. PIE Trial

The Preeclampsia Intervention with Esomeprazole (PIE) trial was a randomised, double-blind, placebo-controlled clinical trial assessing esomeprazole as a treatment of preterm preeclampsia in women undergoing expectant management. Women with preterm preeclampsia, diagnosed between 26 + 0– and 31 + 6–weeks' gestation, were randomised to a daily 40 mg dose of either esomeprazole or placebo. Specific eligibility and exclusion criteria have previously been described in detail [9,10]. Participant characteristics are detailed in Supplementary Table S1. This study had ethical approval from Stellenbosch University Health Research Ethics Committee (M14/09/038, Federal Wide Assurance Number (FWAN) 00001372, Institutional Review Board (IRB) number 0005239).

2.2. PI-2 Trial

The Preeclampsia Intervention 2 (PI-2) trial was a randomised, double-blind, placebo-controlled trial of metformin to treat preterm preeclampsia in women undergoing expectant management. Women with preterm preeclampsia, diagnosed between 26 + 0– and 31 + 6–weeks' gestation, were randomised to 3 g of either metformin or an identical placebo, administered in divided daily doses. Specific eligibility and exclusion criteria have previously been described in detail [11,12]. Patient characteristics are detailed in Supplementary Table S2. The trial had ethical approval from Stellenbosch University Health Research Ethics Committee (M16/09/037, FWAN00001372, IRB0005239).

2.3. Classification of Samples

Plasma samples were classified as either Appropriate for Gestational Age (AGA) or SGA according to customised infant birthweight centile above or below the 10th centile (respectively), determined post-partum using the Gestation-Related Optimal Weight (GROW) Bulk Centile calculator (v8.0.4, 2019).

2.4. Measurement of Plasma Protein Levels

SPINT1 protein levels in maternal plasma samples were ascertained using a SPINT1 ELISA kit (Sigma-Aldrich, St. Louis, MO, USA), following the manufacturer's specifications. A dilution of 1:5 was deemed optimal and used for both cohorts. Plasma placental growth factor (PlGF) and soluble FMS-like tyrosine kinase-1 (sFlt-1) was measured using a commercial electrochemiluminescence immunoassay platform (Roche Diagnostics).

2.5. Statistical Analysis

Statistical analyses were performed using GraphPad Prism 9 (GraphPad Software, Inc., San Diego, CA, USA), with all data first assessed for Gaussian distribution and subsequently analysed using appropriate statistical tests. No data points were excluded as outliers. Maternal characteristics and birth-outcome data (Supplementary Tables S1 and S2) of FGR pregnancies relative to AGA "controls" were compared using Mann–Whitney U, unpaired t-, Fisher's exact, or Chi square tests. For linear regression analysis, the natural logarithm of each biomarker value (lnSPINT1 or lnPlGF) was used for fitting. For all biomarker data, when two groups were compared, a Mann–Whiney U-test was used. For more than two groups (i.e., >10th v. 3rd–10th v. <3rd), a Kruskal–Wallis test was used and post-hoc analyses ascertained by Dunn's multiple comparisons test.

3. Results

3.1. Circulating SPINT1 Is Reduced in Women with Preterm Preeclampsia Complicated by SGA–PIE Trial

SPINT1 levels were first measured in all samples to determine the effect of esomeprazole treatment on the concentration of circulating SPINT1 (Figure 1a). Compared to placebo-treated participants, women in the esomeprazole group did not have significantly altered SPINT1 levels. Therefore, we utilised all available samples from trial participants (n = 97 of a total 120 participants), regardless of the treatment received, for further analyses of SPINT1, sFlt-1, and PlGF. Having selected the samples collected closest to delivery, the median gestation at sampling across all samples was 29 + 3 weeks (Table S1). In preeclampsia cases who delivered an SGA infant, the gestation at delivery and the interval between sampling and delivery were significantly decreased with a median value of 219 days (IQR 204–230 days, $p < 0.01$) and 14 days (IQR 6–21 days, $p < 0.05$), respectively, compared to 236 days (IQR 215–239 days) and 20 days (IQR 12–33 days) in preeclamptic patients delivering an AGA infant (Table S1).

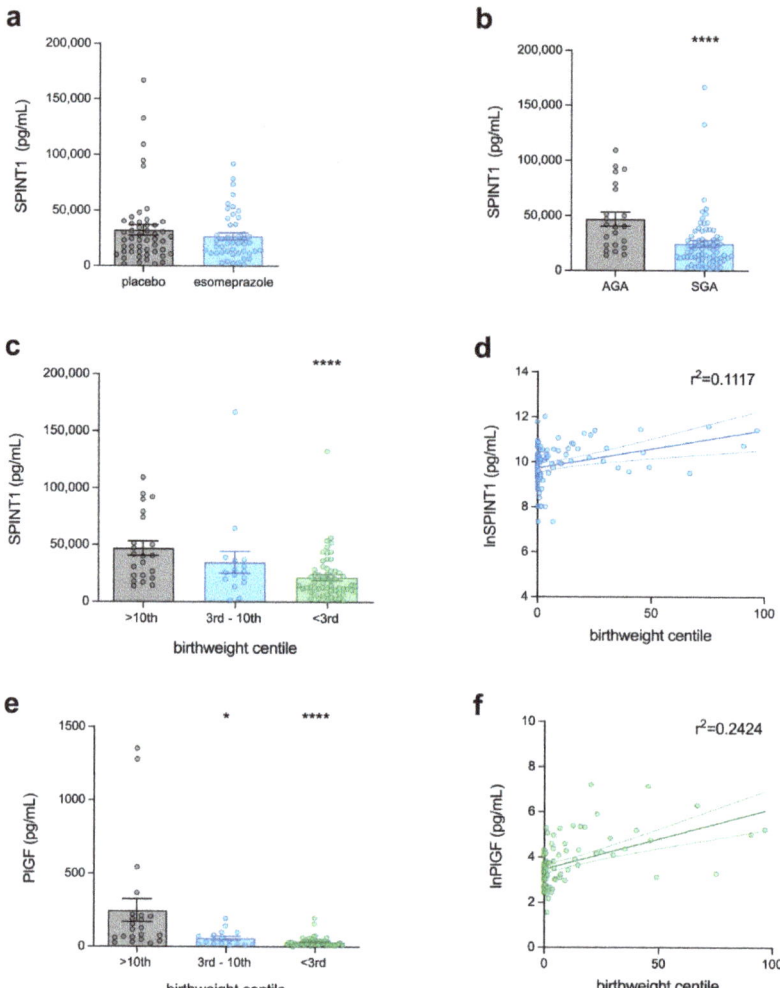

Figure 1. Circulating SPINT1 levels relative to infant birthweight centile in preeclamptic patients (PIE trial samples). (**a**) Esomeprazole intervention ($n = 47$) had no significant influence ($p = 0.63$) on SPINT1 levels compared to placebo ($n = 50$); (**b**) SPINT1 levels were decreased in small for gestational age (SGA) pregnancies ($n = 75$), relative to appropriate for gestational age (AGA) controls ($n = 22$); (**c**) this difference was most marked in severe SGA (birthweight <3rd centile, $n = 59$), with no significant decrease in moderately SGA pregnancies (birthweight centile 3rd–10th, $n = 16$) relative to AGA controls (birthweight ≥ 10th centile, $n = 22$); (**d**) lnSPINT1 levels also increased with higher birthweight centile ($r^2 = 0.1117$, $p = 0.0008$); (**e**) PlGF levels were significantly decreased in severe ($n = 59$) and moderately ($n = 16$) SGA pregnancies, again most markedly in severe cases, relative to AGA controls ($n = 22$); (**f**) lnPlGF levels increased with birthweight centile ($r^2 = 0.2424$, $p < 0.0001$). Each data point represents a single patient; $n = 97$ total, * $p < 0.05$, **** $p < 0.0001$.

In the PIE cohort, SPINT1 levels were significantly decreased in preeclamptic patients who subsequently delivered an SGA infant (Figure 1b, $n = 75$) with a median SPINT1 concentration of 18,857 pg/mL (IQR 10,782–29,890 pg/mL, $p < 0.0001$), relative to preeclamptic participants who delivered an AGA infant ($n = 22$, median = 40,168 pg/mL, IQR 22,342–75,172 pg/mL). Our previous study confirmed that circulating SPINT1 at

36 weeks' gestation was most deranged in women with infants who ultimately had a birthweight <3rd centile [3], so we next divided the <10th centile group into those <3rd centile ($n = 59$) and those between 3rd and 10th centiles ($n = 16$). In doing so, we found that the change in SPINT1 associated with SGA pregnancies was driven by the most severe cases of growth restriction (those SGA infants with a birthweight <3rd centile). In these severe instances of SGA (Figure 1c), SPINT1 was significantly reduced with a median SPINT1 concentration of 14,516 pg/mL (IQR 9967–27,627 pg/mL, $p < 0.0001$) relative to the AGA group (median = 40,168 pg/mL, IQR 22,342–75,172 pg/mL), The SGA pregnancies delivering between 3rd and 10th birthweight centiles, however, were not accompanied by any significant changes in SPINT1 (median = 26,416 pg/mL, IQR 17,911–36,975 pg/mL, $p = 0.2$). The relationship between lnSPINT1 expression in maternal plasma and birthweight centile was then assessed (Figure 1d), and a significant association was identified using linear regression ($r^2 = 0.1117$, $p = 0.0008$).

Having established these differences in SPINT1 levels, we next assessed Placental Growth Factor (PlGF) in the same samples (Figure 1e). As expected, PlGF levels were significantly reduced, in both <3rd (median = 27.94 pg/mL, IQR 15.65–40.67 pg/mL, $p < 0.0001$) and 3rd–10th samples (median = 39.47 pg/mL, IQR 20.42–93.51 pg/mL, $p = 0.01$) relative to AGA controls (median = 121.7 pg/mL, IQR 57.67–214.1 pg/mL). The association between PlGF and birthweight centile (Figure 1f) was also significant ($r^2 = 0.2424$, $p < 0.0001$).

3.2. Validation That SPINT1 Is Reduced in Women with Preterm Preeclampsia Complicated by SGA–PI-2 Trial

Given that circulating SPINT1 was significantly reduced in SGA pregnancies in PIE, we next sought to validate this observation in the PI-2 cohort. We initially confirmed that metformin did not significantly alter circulating SPINT1 relative to the placebo-treated cohort (Figure 2a). This again allowed us to combine data from all available samples for further analyses ($n = 135$ of 180 participants), with a median gestation of 34 + 1 weeks (AGA) and 32 + 2 weeks (SGA; Table S2). In preeclampsia cases who delivered an SGA infant, the gestation at delivery and interval between sampling and delivery was significantly decreased, with a median value of 227 days (IQR 212–239 days, $p < 0.0001$) and 5 days (IQR 3–7 days, $p < 0.001$), respectively, compared to 239 days (IQR 237–240 days) and 8 days (IQR 6–11 days) in preeclamptic patients delivering an AGA infant (Table S2).

As observed in PIE, SPINT1 was significantly reduced in the plasma of preeclamptic pregnancies complicated by SGA ($n = 95$, median = 57,764 pg/mL, IQR 42,212–91,356 pg/mL, $p < 0.0001$), relative to those who delivered an AGA infant ($n = 40$, median = 107,062 pg/mL, IQR 70,183–176,532 pg/mL, Figure 2b). Analysis of this second cohort reflected the findings of PIE, with significantly decreased SPINT1 levels in only the most severely growth-restricted pregnancies (<3rd birthweight centile; $n = 77$, median = 54,871 pg/mL, IQR 42,037–78,771 pg/mL, Figure 2c, $p < 0.0001$) compared to AGA controls (median = 107,062 pg/mL, IQR 70,183–176,532 pg/mL), whereas there was no significant decrease in those pregnancies delivering an infant in the 3rd–10th birthweight centile ($n = 18$, median = 84,542 pg/mL, IQR 41,280–118,013 pg/mL, $p = 0.1$). A similar association between lnSPINT1 levels and birthweight centile, as seen in PIE, was also observed in PI-2 (Figure 2d, $r^2 = 0.1520$, $p < 0.0001$). Absolute differences in SPINT1 between cohorts likely reflect differences in assay kit batches associated with research-grade ELISAs. Importantly, each cohort was run using ELISAs from the same manufactured batch.

Again, we also measured PlGF concentrations in the PI-2 samples. We found that relative to AGA controls (median = 321.2 pg/mL, IQR 97.6–550.4 pg/mL), there was a reduction in PlGF concentration in the 3rd–10th cohort ($n = 18$, median = 35.9 pg/mL, IQR 17.4–228.0 pg/mL, $p = 0.001$) and the <3rd cohort ($n = 77$, median = 29.7 pg/mL, IQR 21.4–47.1 pg/mL, $p < 0.0001$). The association of lnPlGF concentration with birthweight centile (Figure 2f) was also verified ($r^2 = 0.3822$, $p < 0.0001$).

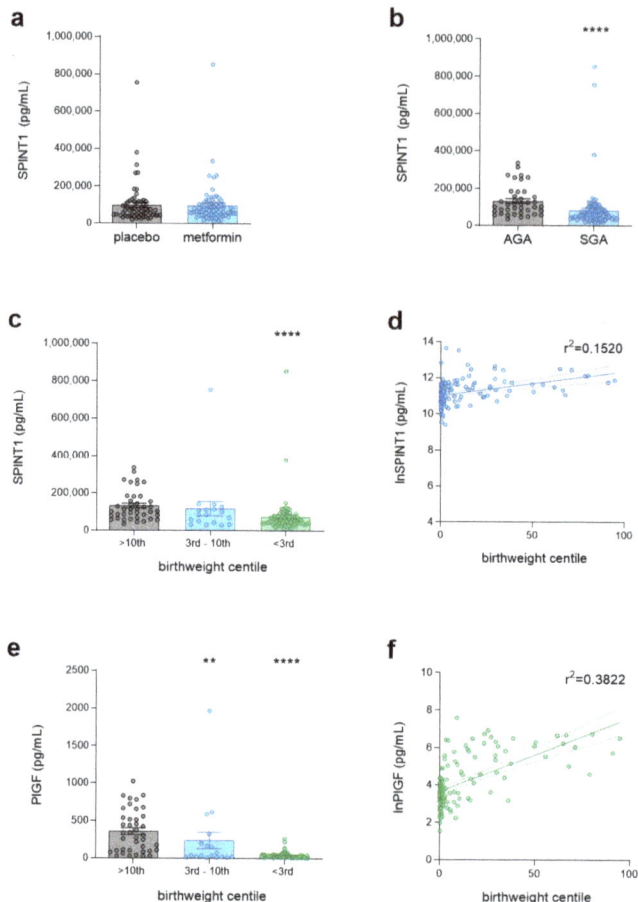

Figure 2. Validation of circulating SPINT1 levels relative to infant birthweight centile in preeclamptic patients (PI-2 trial samples). (**a**) Metformin intervention ($n = 72$) had no significant influence ($p = 0.63$) on SPINT1 levels compared to placebo ($n = 63$); (**b**) SPINT1 levels were decreased in SGA pregnancies ($n = 95$), relative to AGA (birthweight $\geq$ 10th centile) controls ($n = 40$); (**c**) this difference was most marked in severe SGA (birthweight <3rd centile, $n = 77$), with no significant decrease in moderately SGA pregnancies (birthweight centile 3rd–10th, $n = 18$) relative to controls ($n = 40$); (**d**) lnSPINT1 levels were increased with higher birthweight centile ($r^2 = 0.1520$, $p < 0.0001$); (**e**) PlGF levels were significantly decreased in severe ($n = 77$) and moderately ($n = 18$) SGA pregnancies, again most markedly in severe cases, relative to AGA controls ($n = 40$); (**f**) lnPlGF levels increased with birthweight centile ($r^2 = 0.3822$, $p < 0.0001$). Each data point represents a single patient; $n = 135$ total, ** $p < 0.01$, **** $p < 0.0001$.

3.3. A Ratio of sFlt-1/SPINT1 to Identify Placental Insufficiency Manifesting as SGA Co-Exdisting with Preterm Preeclampsia

sFlt-1 is an anti-angiogenic molecule that is highly elevated in preeclampsia [13]. A ratio of sFlt-1/PlGF offers an excellent rule-out test for patients who might develop preeclampsia in the coming weeks as it has a high negative predictive value [14]. We assessed whether sFlt-1/SPINT1 might differ in preterm preeclamptic pregnancies delivered SGA. In PIE, the sFlt-1/SPINT1 ratio (Figure 3a) showed significant elevations in those patients who ultimately delivered SGA, at both <3rd ($n = 59$, median = 1.4, IQR 0.44–2.54, $p < 0.0001$) and 3rd–10th ($n = 16$, median = 0.82, IQR 0.28–1.39, $p = 0.01$) birthweight centiles, relative to AGA controls (*n* = 22, median = 0.09, IQR 0.05–0.60). The most significant changes were observed in the <3rd birthweight centile cohort. These results were mirrored by the sFlt-1/PlGF ratio (Figure 3b; <3rd median = 655, IQR 456–1426, *p* < 0.0001; 3rd–10th median = 524, IQR 98.9–1191, *p* = 0.006; control median = 37.3, IQR 11.5–278); however, the sFlt-1/PlGF ratio demonstrated greater differentiation in the median values between 3rd–10th centile samples and controls (*p* = 0.006) than the sFlt-1/SPINT1 ratio (*p* = 0.01).

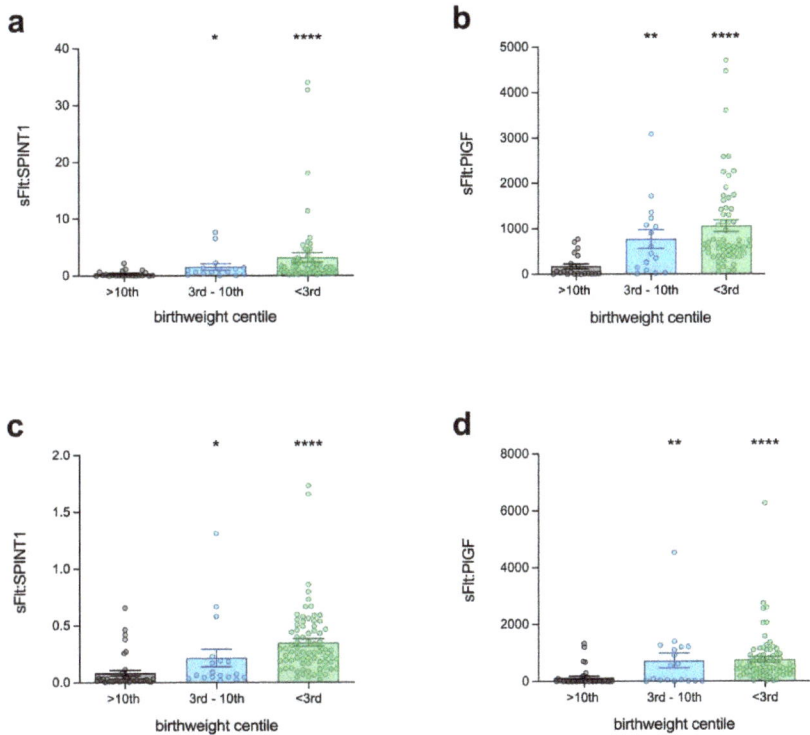

Figure 3. Association between sFlt-1 ratio and birthweight centile when substituting SPINT1 for PlGF. (**a**) The ratio of sFlt-1 to SPINT1 in PIE samples increased stepwise with decreasing birthweight centiles (<3rd *n* = 59; 3rd–10th *n* = 16; >10th *n* = 22); (**b**) the existing ratio of sFlt-1 to PlGF was also elevated with decreasing birthweight centile; (**c**) the sFlt-1 and SPINT1 ratio was again increased stepwise with SGA severity in the PI-2 samples (<3rd *n* = 77; 3rd–10th *n* = 18; >10th *n* = 40); (**d**) the sFlt-1 and PlGF ratio was again also elevated in SGA. Each data point represents a single patient; * *p* < 0.05, ** *p* < 0.01, **** *p* < 0.0001.

The analyses of the PI-2 study confirmed these changes, with the sFlt-1/SPINT1 ratio (Figure 3c) being elevated in both <3rd (*n* = 77, median = 0.27, IQR 0.17–0.48, *p* < 0.0001) and 3rd–10th (*n* = 18, median = 0.06, IQR 0.04–0.20, *p* = 0.04) birthweight centile groups, compared to AGA controls (*n* = 40, median = 0.02, IQR 0.01–0.05). The sFlt-1/PlGF ratio (Figure 3d) was similarly increased, relative to AGA controls (median = 7.45, IQR 3.58–40.43), in 3rd–10th (median = 316.3, IQR 9.59–1208, *p* = 0.001) and <3rd (median = 503.1, IQR 302.8–910.4, *p* < 0.0001) groups. Again, there was greater differentiation between 3rd–10th centile samples and controls using the sFlt-1/PlGF ratio (*p* = 0.001), compared to the sFlt-1/SPINT1 ratio *p* = 0.04); although both ratios demonstrated significant elevations in both severe and moderate SGA (indicated by a birthweight centile <3rd and 3rd–10th, respectively).

4. Discussion

Preterm FGR, though less common than term FGR, is associated with a poorer prognosis [15] and often co-exists with preeclampsia. In the search for biomarkers for placental insufficiency, we identified SPINT1 as a promising candidate. This study explored the potential that SPINT1 might be associated with preterm FGR in the presence of coexisting preeclampsia (around 30 weeks' gestation). Indeed, we found in two separate cohorts that SPINT1 was markedly reduced in the plasma of patients with preeclampsia delivering SGA infants and preeclampsia, relative to those women with preeclampsia carrying appropriately grown infants. As expected, PlGF was particularly reduced in the pregnancies complicated by both preeclampsia and FGR, while a ratio of sFlt-1/SPINT1 was significantly elevated in a similar manner to that observed for sFlt-1/PlGF.

We previously reported significantly reduced SPINT1 concentrations in the circulation of normotensive pregnancies complicated by preterm FGR [3], however this is the first time SPINT1 has been examined in association with preterm preeclampsia. Decreased circulating SPINT1 was found to be strongly associated with severe growth restriction (birthweight <3rd centile) within preeclamptic pregnancies. While PlGF performs very strongly in this cohort with established disease, further analyses in an unselected cohort collected before disease onset are needed to compare the true predictive capacity of both proteins in preterm disease. Certainly, our data in an unselected cohort at 36 weeks' gestation suggests that SPINT may perform better than PlGF in SGA prediction at term [3].

In both cohorts, it was found that the gestation at delivery and the interval between sampling and delivery was reduced in preeclamptic pregnancies delivering an SGA infant compared to AGA controls (Tables S1 and S2). This earlier delivery may relate to clinical actions that were taken in respect to suspected SGA or due to physiological factors in the pregnancy itself. Future work is required to specifically investigate whether there are changes in the predictive capability of each biomarker in cases where clinical action was taken due to suspected SGA or due to underlying maternal co-morbidities.

Our finding that SPINT1 is differentially expressed in pregnancies complicated by both preeclampsia and FGR provides further understanding of the pathogenesis of these disorders. SPINT1 is a protein highly expressed in the placenta, and our prior work demonstrates an association of decreased circulating levels with reduced placental weight [3]. Though both preeclampsia and FGR are considered to be disorders of placental insufficiency, our data herein suggest some differences in placental mechanisms underlying the manifestation of preeclampsia in the presence or absence of FGR. Animal [7,8,16] and human [3,17] placental studies provide strong evidence that SPINT1 is involved in placental development. Whether there are alterations in placental development in preeclampsia complicated by FGR, relative to preeclamptic placentas that facilitate normal growth, has not been carefully studied and should be the focus of ongoing work.

In this study, there were more cases of coexisting preeclampsia and SGA (FGR) than those with preeclampsia uncomplicated by SGA (Tables S1 and S2). This is because preeclampsia and FGR tend to concurrently arise at preterm gestations due to early placental insufficiency. FGR is less common as a comorbidity of preeclampsia diagnosed at term, which highlights the importance of carefully selecting biomarkers that could stratify those at risk during preterm gestations.

There remains a dearth of biomarkers that can accurately predict preterm or term SGA or FGR, which is an ongoing challenge within the field. Current clinical tools, such as maternal and fetal risk factors, or ultrasound measures, perform modestly [1,18]. SPINT1 is a novel biomarker that we recently reported as being differentially expressed in pregnancies destined to deliver small for gestational age at term gestations, performing better than PlGF in that setting. To date, universal ultrasound in the third trimester in nulliparouns women provides the highest sensitivity for prediction of term SGA, sitting at 57% compared to 20% for selective, or clinically indicated ultrasound [19]. Thirty-six-week SPINT1 performs similarly to selective ultrasound for predicting SGA, however its utility if combined with other biomarkers or clinical measures remains the focus of ongoing work. This new study provides the first insights into SPINT1 possibly being deranged in preterm growth restriction, irrespective of co-existing preeclampsia. Validation of this finding, however, would require a very large prospective collection, which might also include ultrasound measures so that a direct comparison between these clinical tools could be accurately assessed.

5. Conclusions

This study demonstrates that SPINT1 levels are decreased in preterm pregnancies with placental insufficiency manifesting as FGR, even in the presence of concurrent preeclampsia. It further validates the association between low SPINT1 and poor fetal growth we have previously reported [3]. In addition, this work highlights the potential of SPINT1 as a novel biomarker that could be added to the toolbox for preterm disease, but further studies are required to confirm its predictive performance.

Supplementary Materials: The following are available online at https://www.mdpi.com/article/10.3390/jcm11040901/s1, Table S1: PIE trial patient characteristics, Table S2: PI-2 trial patient characteristics.

Author Contributions: Conceptualization, T.J.K.-L., S.P.W., S.T. and T.M.M.; methodology, C.A.C., S.P.W., S.T., T.J.K.-L., E.K. and C.N.M.; formal analysis, E.K., R.H. and C.N.M.; investigation, P.C. and C.N.M.; resources, F.C.B., T.J.K.-L., N.J.H., S.T. and S.P.W.; data curation, C.A.C., R.H., T.M.M. and E.K.; writing—original draft preparation, C.N.M. and T.J.K.-L.; writing—review and editing, all co-authors; funding acquisition, T.J.K.-L., S.P.W. and S.T. All authors have read and agreed to the published version of the manuscript.

Funding: Funding for this work was provided by the National Health and Medical Research Council (#1065854, #116071, #20000732) as well as National Health and Medical Research Council Fellowships to T.K.L. (#1159261), N.J.H. (#1146128), S.T. (#1136418), and R.H. (#1176922). The funders played no role in study design or analysis.

Institutional Review Board Statement: This study was conducted in accordance with the Declaration of Helsinki and approved by the Stellenbosch University Health Research Ethics Committee FWAN00001372, IRB0005239 (M14/09/038 & M16/09/037).

Informed Consent Statement: Informed consent was obtained from all subjects involved in the study.

Data Availability Statement: Raw data are available upon request to corresponding author.

Conflicts of Interest: T.J.K., T.M.M., S.P.W. and S.T. hold a provisional patent (PCT/AU2019/050516) relating to the use of SPINT1 and syndecan as diagnostic markers in pregnancy. The remaining authors have no conflicts of interests to declare.

References

1. Gardosi, J.; Madurasinghe, V.; Williams, M.; Malik, A.; Francis, A. Maternal and fetal risk factors for stillbirth: Population based study. *BMJ* **2013**, *346*, f108. [CrossRef] [PubMed]
2. Peter, J.R.; Ho, J.J.; Valliapan, J.; Sivasangari, S. Symphysial fundal height (SFH) measurement in pregnancy for detecting abnormal fetal growth. *Cochrane Database Syst. Rev.* **2015**, *2015*, Cd008136.
3. Kaitu'u-Lino, T.U.; MacDonald, T.M.; Cannon, P.; Nguyen, T.V.; Hiscock, R.J.; Haan, N.; Myers, J.E.; Hastie, R.; Dane, K.M.; Middleton, A.L.; et al. Circulating SPINT1 is a biomarker of pregnancies with poor placental function and fetal growth restriction. *Nat. Commun.* **2020**, *11*, 2411. [CrossRef] [PubMed]
4. Tu'uhevaha, J.; Tong, S.; Walker, S.P.; MacDonald, T.M.; Cannon, P.; Nguyen, T.V.; Sadananthan, S.A.; Tint, M.T.; Ong, Y.Y.; Ling, L.S.; et al. Maternal circulating SPINT1 is reduced in small-for-gestational age pregnancies at 26 weeks: Growing up in Singapore towards health outcomes (GUSTO) cohort study. *Placenta* **2021**, *110*, 24–28.
5. Kataoka, H.; Meng, J.Y.; Itoh, H.; Hamasuna, R.; Shimomura, T.; Suganuma, T.; Koono, M. Localization of hepatocyte growth factor activator inhibitor type 1 in Langhans' cells of human placenta. *Histochem. Cell Biol.* **2000**, *114*, 469–475. [CrossRef]
6. Szabo, R.; Lantsman, T.; Peters, D.E.; Bugge, T.H. Delineation of proteolytic and non-proteolytic functions of the membrane-anchored serine protease prostasin. *Development* **2016**, *143*, 2818–2828. [CrossRef]
7. Szabo, R.; Molinolo, A.; List, K.; Bugge, T.H. Matriptase inhibition by hepatocyte growth factor activator inhibitor-1 is essential for placental development. *Oncogene* **2007**, *26*, 1546–1556. [CrossRef] [PubMed]
8. Hong, L.; He, Y.; Tan, C.; Wu, Z.; Yu, M. HAI-1 regulates placental folds development by influencing trophoblast cell proliferation and invasion in pigs. *Gene* **2020**, *749*, 144721. [CrossRef] [PubMed]

9. Cluver, C.A.; Walker, S.P.; Mol, B.W.; Theron, G.B.; Hall, D.R.; Hiscock, R.; Hannan, N.; Tong, S. Double blind, randomised, placebo-controlled trial to evaluate the efficacy of esomeprazole to treat early onset pre-eclampsia (PIE Trial): A study protocol. *BMJ Open* **2015**, *5*, e008211. [CrossRef] [PubMed]
10. Cluver, C.A.; Hannan, N.J.; van Papendorp, E.; Hiscock, R.; Beard, S.; Mol, B.W.; Theron, G.B.; Hall, D.R.; Decloedt, E.H.; Stander, M.; et al. Esomeprazole to treat women with preterm preeclampsia: A randomized placebo controlled trial. *Am. J. Obs. Gynecol.* **2018**, *219*, 388.e1–388.e17. [CrossRef] [PubMed]
11. Cluver, C.; Walker, S.P.; Mol, B.W.; Hall, D.; Hiscock, R.; Brownfoot, F.C.; Tu'uhevaha, J.; Tong, S. A double blind, randomised, placebo-controlled trial to evaluate the efficacy of metformin to treat preterm pre-eclampsia (PI2 Trial): Study protocol. *BMJ Open* **2019**, *9*, e025809. [CrossRef] [PubMed]
12. Cluver, C.A.; Hiscock, R.; Decloedt, E.H.; Hall, D.R.; Schell, S.; Mol, B.; Brownfoot, F.; Kaitu'u-Lino, T.U.; Walker, S.; Tong, S. Metformin to treat Preterm Pre-eclampsia (PI-2): A randomised, double blind, placebo-controlled trial. *Am. J. Obstet. Gynecol.* **2021**, *224*, S20. [CrossRef]
13. Levine, R.J.; Maynard, S.E.; Qian, C.; Lim, K.H.; England, L.J.; Yu, K.F.; Schisterman, E.F.; Thadhani, R.; Sachs, B.P.; Epstein, F.H.; et al. Circulating Angiogenic Factors and the Risk of Preeclampsia. *N. Engl. J. Med.* **2004**, *350*, 672–683. [CrossRef] [PubMed]
14. Zeisler, H.; Llurba, E.; Chantraine, F.; Vatish, M.; Staff, A.C.; Sennström, M.; Olovsson, M.; Brennecke, S.P.; Stepan, H.; Allegranza, D.; et al. Predictive Value of the sFlt-1:PlGF Ratio in Women with Suspected Preeclampsia. *N. Engl. J. Med.* **2016**, *374*, 13–22. [CrossRef] [PubMed]
15. Hannan, N.J.; Stock, O.; Spencer, R.; Whitehead, C.; David, A.L.; Groom, K.; Petersen, S.; Henry, A.; Said, J.M.; Seeho, S.; et al. Circulating mRNAs are differentially expressed in pregnancies with severe placental insufficiency and at high risk of stillbirth. *BMC Med.* **2020**, *18*, 145. [CrossRef] [PubMed]
16. Tanaka, H.; Nagaike, K.; Takeda, N.; Itoh, H.; Kohama, K.; Fukushima, T.; Miyata, S.; Uchiyama, S.; Uchinokura, S.; Shimomura, T.; et al. Hepatocyte growth factor activator inhibitor type 1 (HAI-1) is required for branching morphogenesis in the chorioallantoic placenta. *Mol. Cell Biol.* **2005**, *25*, 5687–5698. [CrossRef] [PubMed]
17. Kohama, K.; Kawaguchi, M.; Fukushima, T.; Lin, C.Y.; Kataoka, H. Regulation of pericellular proteolysis by hepatocyte growth factor activator inhibitor type 1 (HAI-1) in trophoblast cells. *Hum. Cell* **2012**, *25*, 100–110. [CrossRef] [PubMed]
18. Fadigas, C.; Saiid, Y.; Gonzalez, R.; Poon, L.C.; Nicolaides, K.H. Prediction of small-for-gestational-age neonates: Screening by fetal biometry at 35-37 weeks. *Ultrasound Obs. Gynecol.* **2015**, *45*, 559–565. [CrossRef] [PubMed]
19. Sovio, U.; White, I.R.; Dacey, A.; Pasupathy, D.; Smith, G.C. Screening for fetal growth restriction with universal third trimester ultrasonography in nulliparous women in the Pregnancy Outcome Prediction (POP) study: A prospective cohort study. *Lancet* **2015**, *386*, 2089–2097. [CrossRef]

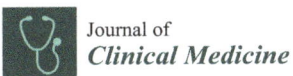

Article

Impact of Co-Existing Placental Pathologies in Pregnancies Complicated by Placental Abruption and Acute Neonatal Outcomes

Dorsa Mavedatnia [1], Jason Tran [1], Irina Oltean [2,3], Vid Bijelić [2], Felipe Moretti [1], Sarah Lawrence [1,*] and Dina El Demellawy [1,3,*]

1. Department of Medicine, University of Ottawa, Ottawa, ON K1H 8M5, Canada; dmave060@uottawa.ca (D.M.); trn.jason@gmail.com (J.T.); fmoretti@toh.ca (F.M.)
2. Children's Hospital of Eastern Ontario Research Institute, Ottawa, ON K1H 8L1, Canada; IOltean@cheo.on.ca (I.O.); VBijelic@cheo.on.ca (V.B.)
3. Department of Pathology, Children's Hospital of Eastern Ontario, Ottawa, ON K1H 8L1, Canada
* Correspondence: sllawrence@cheo.on.ca (S.L.); deldemellawy@cheo.on.ca (D.E.D.); Tel.: +1-613-737-7600 (ext. 3846) (D.E.D.)

Abstract: Placental abruption (PA) is a concern for maternal and neonatal morbidity. Adverse neonatal outcomes in the setting of PA include higher risk of prematurity. Placental pathologies include maternal vascular malperfusion (MVM), fetal vascular malperfusion (FVM), acute chorioamnionitis, and villitis of unknown etiology (VUE). We aimed to investigate how placental pathology contributes to acute neonatal outcome in PA. A retrospective cohort study of all placentas with PA were identified. Exposures were MVM, FVM, acute chorioamnionitis and VUE. The primary outcome was NICU admission and the secondary outcomes included adverse base deficit and Apgar scores, need for resuscitation, and small-for-gestational age. A total of 287 placentas were identified. There were 160 (59.9%) of placentas with PA alone vs 107 (40.1%) with PA and additional placental pathologies. Odds of NICU admission were more than two times higher in pregnancies with placental pathologies (OR = 2.37, 95% CI 1.28–4.52). These estimates were in large part mediated by prematurity and birthweight, indirect effect acting through prematurity was OR 1.79 (95% CI 1.12–2.75) and through birthweight OR 2.12 (95% CI 1.40–3.18). Odds of Apgar score ≤ 5 was more than four times higher among pregnancies with placental pathologies (OR = 4.56, 95% CI 1.28–21.26). Coexisting placental pathology may impact Apgar scores in pregnancies complicated by PA. This knowledge could be used by neonatal teams to mobilize resources in anticipation of the need for neonatal resuscitation.

Keywords: infant; newborn; female; pregnancy; abruptio placentae; Apgar score; pregnant women; gestational age; placenta

Citation: Mavedatnia, D.; Tran, J.; Oltean, I.; Bijelić, V.; Moretti, F.; Lawrence, S.; El Demellawy, D. Impact of Co-Existing Placental Pathologies in Pregnancies Complicated by Placental Abruption and Acute Neonatal Outcomes. *J. Clin. Med.* **2021**, *10*, 5693. https://doi.org/10.3390/jcm10235693

Academic Editor: Johannes Ott

Received: 11 November 2021
Accepted: 1 December 2021
Published: 3 December 2021

Publisher's Note: MDPI stays neutral with regard to jurisdictional claims in published maps and institutional affiliations.

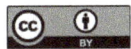

Copyright: © 2021 by the authors. Licensee MDPI, Basel, Switzerland. This article is an open access article distributed under the terms and conditions of the Creative Commons Attribution (CC BY) license (https://creativecommons.org/licenses/by/4.0/).

1. Introduction

Placental abruption remains a critical concern for maternal, fetal, and neonatal morbidity and mortality [1,2]. In fact, it is a rare but serious complication affecting 3 to 10 per 1000 pregnancies worldwide [3], accounting for around 10–20% of all neonatal deaths in developed countries [4]. Maternal complications associated with placental abruption include hemorrhagic shock, disseminated intravascular coagulation (DIC), kidney failure, organ ischemia and necrosis, and death, related to coronary heart disease and stroke [5,6]. Adverse neonatal outcomes in cases of severe placental abruption, include higher risk of fetal-growth restriction, stillbirth, prematurity, and birth asphyxia [7–11]. However, not all cases of abruption result in poor neonatal outcomes [12]. In the context of placental abruption, obstetricians may face difficulties in deciding when to intervene and deliver. Typically, in severe placental abruption cases, emergent cesarean section with shorter onset-to-delivery time is recommended, to prevent intrauterine fetal death, neonatal morbidity and mortality [13]. In addition to onset-to-delivery time, obstetricians must weigh the severity and chronicity of placental abruption and the mother's clinical status with the gestational age of the fetus [13–15] in deciding the best timing for delivery to optimize obstetric and neonatal outcomes. The potential impact of maternal underlying placental pathologies in cases of PA may help contribute to the decision making.

Underlying placental pathologies include maternal vascular malperfusion (MVM), fetal vascular malperfusion (FVM), acute chorioamnionitis, and villitis of unknown etiology (VUE) [16]. These pathologies are independently associated with the presence of neonatal complications [17–20]. In particular, MVM is prevalent in cases of hypertensive disorders of pregnancy [21], fetal-growth restriction [22], preeclampsia [23], and is highly associated with preterm labour and premature rupture of membranes [24–27]. Recent literature also suggests that pregnancy complications can recur in subsequent pregnancies, regardless of the presence of MVM lesions [28]. Moreover, severe onset of FVM can increase the chance of fetal growth restriction, fetal central nervous system (CNS) damage and neurodevelopmental delays, and stillbirth [29,30]. Chorioamnionitis can result in postpartum uterine infections [31,32], fetal death and neonatal sepsis [33,34], intraventricular hemorrhage (IVH), asphyxia, and cerebral white matter damage [35–37]. VUE can impede fetal growth and contribute to recurrent reproductive loss [38].

The aim of this present study is to investigate if placental pathologies can adversely affect acute neonatal outcome in pregnancies complicated with PA. Our hypothesis is that additional placental pathologies will deplete placenta reserve, impair placental function prior to any abruption event, and thus contribute adversely to neonatal outcome. This is knowledge needed to inform best clinical practice for obstetricians in Canada.

2. Material and Methods

2.1. Data Collection

A retrospective cohort study was conducted at The Ottawa Hospital (TOH) and the Children's Hospital of Eastern Ontario (CHEO). All placentas with the pathologic or clinical diagnosis of placental abruption and/or retroplacental hematoma from 1 October 2013 to 30 April 2020 were identified from the pathology archives using the Laboratory Information Service Program (EPIC-Hyperspace) [39]. Data on maternal demographics, neonatal outcomes, and the gross and histopathological findings of the placenta were collected using EPIC-Hyperspace and recorded on RedCap [40]. The clinical diagnosis of abruption was defined as either Obstetric ultrasound with direct visualization of subchorionic or retroplacental hematoma or clinical presentation of vaginal bleeding, abdominal pain, uterine contractions and/or uterine tenderness, as defined on the TOH electronic medical records (EMRs). The pathological diagnosis was then confirmed post-delivery, through the CHEO EPIC report, using the reports on placental examination for the presence of retroplacental clot(s). A total of 287 placentas were identified. Placentas were excluded if maternal-neonatal linked charts could not be located ($n = 26$) or there were missing data on study outcomes (percent missing ranged from 18 % to 28%). Institutional approval was obtained prior to study initiation (CHEOREB# 20/22X).

We divided the dataset into clinically diagnosed placental abruption only (presence of adherent retroplacental clot and typical findings defined above) versus placental abruption with any placental pathologies of MVM, FVM, acute chorioamnionitis, and VUE. The criteria for diagnosing placental lesions followed the 2016 Amsterdam consensus statement [16]. Of note, we considered the presence of any independent lesion external from the section taken in the area of placental abruption. For there to be a definitive MVM diagnosis, accelerated villous maturation had to be present in all cases. More importantly, infarction in the section of abruption alone is not taken as a sign of MVM. Further details regarding the definitions for each lesion are found in the Supplementary Materials (S1). Our primary outcome was NICU admission, while the secondary outcomes included BD 10–15.9 or BD $\geq$ 16, cord pH $\leq$ 7 or 7.1–7.15, Apgar score $\leq$ 5 at 10min, need for resuscitation, and small-for-gestational age (SGA).

2.2. Statistical Analysis

Demographic and anthropometric characteristics were summarised descriptively with median and interquartile range (IQR) for continuous variables, and frequencies and percentages for categorical variables and compared between the group with co-occurring placental lesions) versus the group of placental abruption only, using the Wilcoxon rank sum for continuous variables and Fischer's exact test for discrete variables. The effect of placental pathology on NICU admission was investigated using unadjusted and adjusted logistic regression. Directed acyclic graph (DAG) [41] was constructed to guide the selection of confounding and mediating variables and to inform the final multivariable analysis of the primary outcome, NICU admission. The extent to which placental lesions contribute to NICU admission was assessed using the causal mediation analysis with prematurity and birthweight as mediators. The effect of each mediator was analyzed separately. We considered the exposure-mediator interaction between placental pathology and prematurity (GA < 37 weeks) and interaction between placental pathology and birthweight. Interactions were not significant and were removed from the final mediation analysis. Both mediation analyses were adjusted for maternal smoking, maternal hypertension/preeclampsia, and maternal diabetes. The effect of placental pathology on secondary outcomes were investigated using unadjusted logistic regression. Two-sided p values less than 0.05 and odds ratios (ORs) with 95% confidence intervals (CI) excluding one, were considered statistically significant. All analysis were performed in R statistical software version 4.0.2 (R Core Team, Vienna, Austria) [42]. Mediation analyses were performed using an R package medflex [43]. DAGitty, an online-based platform, was used to formally evaluate causal associations [44].

3. Results

Table 1 demonstrates the maternal and neonatal characteristics of our sample population. There were 160 (59.9%) of placentas with PA alone vs 107 (40.1%) with PA and additional placental pathologies. Examining the full cohort with delivery mode data available, 37% of all placental abruption cases were performed via C-section (97/261) vs 63% (164/261) vaginally. Of data available for placental localization, 62% (68/110) of all placental abruption cases from the full cohort presented with marginal localization vs 38% (42/110) with central localization. Briefly, women in both groups were around 30 years of age and had similar lifestyle behaviours, though a higher percentage of hypertensive diseases of pregnancy were reported in placentas with additional pathologies vs PA alone (20.6% vs 8.6%, respectively). Babies were born in their third trimester (Table 1). Out of the full cohort, 58% (156/267) of babies were born prematurely (gestational age < 37 weeks).

After listwise deletion (n = 37, 13.9%), 142 (61.7%) placentas with PA alone and 88 (38.3%) placentas with additional pathologies remained for the analysis of primary outcome, NICU admission. NICU admission was more frequent among placentas with additional pathologies (n = 68, 77.3%) than placentas with PA alone (n = 83, 58.5%). Table 2 depicts the effect of additional pathologies (i.e., placental lesions) on primary outcome, NICU admission. The total effect of placental lesions represents the sum of the direct effect of placental lesions to NICU admission and indirect effects (e.g., acting through prematurity). Figure 1 represents the conceptual model of mediation analysis with direct and indirect pathways from the placental lesions to the primary outcome, NICU admission. Results from the adjusted and unadjusted models indicate higher odds of NICU admission in pregnancies complicated by placental lesions. In the adjusted model OR was 2.37 (1.28–4.52; p = 0.01). Indirect effect acting through prematurity was OR 1.79 (95% CI 1.12–2.75; p = 0.01) and through birthweight OR 2.12 (95% CI 1.40–3.18; p < 0.001). There was no evidence for a significant direct effect in either prematurity (p = 0.29) or birthweight (p = 0.69) mediated analysis. No evidence was found for exposure-mediator interaction between placental lesions and prematurity (p = 0.36) or between placental lesions and birthweight (p = 0.56).

Table 1. Characteristics of the Cohorts (n = 287).

Maternal Demographics	Placentas with Placental Abruption Only (n = 160, 59.9%)	Placentas with Additional Pathologies (n = 107, 40.1%)	p Value
Maternal age (mean, SD)	31.1 (6.1)	30.4 (5.3)	0.20
Parity (mean, SD)	0.5 (3.0)	0.3 (0.6)	0.68
Pre-pregnancy BMI value (mean, SD)	25.1 (6.0)	25.6 (6.5)	0.94
Diabetes (n, %)	24 (15.0)	7 (6.5)	0.05
Previous smoker (n, %)	25 (16.6)	11 (11.0)	0.27
Previous history of abruption (n, %)	10 (7.7)	4 (4.7)	0.42
Chronic hypertension, Gestational Hypertension or preeclampsia (n, %)	13 (8.6)	20 (20.6)	0.01
Other medical conditions (Pregestational diabetes, gestational diabetes, thrombophilia) (n, %)	111 (71.2))	67 (66.3)	0.49
Neonatal Demographics			
Gestational age in weeks (mean, SD)	35.7 (4.2)	33.1 (5.6)	<0.001
Birthweight (g) (mean, SD)	2638.1 (793.9)	2015.7 (967.9)	<0.001
Sex (Female, %)	68 (43.6)	53 (51.5)	0.25

BMI, body mass index; SD, standard deviation.

Table 2. Placental lesions and neonatal intensive care unit (NICU) admission.

Term	OR (95% CI)	p Value
Unadjusted logistic regression		
Placental lesions	2.42 (1.34, 4.48)	0.004
Adjusted logistic regression		
Placental lesions	2.37 (1.28, 4.52)	0.01
Maternal Smoking	3.45 (1.33, 10.77)	0.02
Maternal Hypertension/Preeclampsia	1.58 (0.65, 4.29)	0.33
Maternal Diabetes	0.31 (0.13, 0.73)	0.01
Mediation analysis; mediator = Prematurity [a]		
Natural Direct Effect	1.32 (0.78, 2.19)	0.29
Natural Indirect Effect	1.79 (1.12, 2.75)	0.01
Total Effect	2.37 (1.17, 4.51)	0.01
Mediation analysis; mediator = Birthweight		
Natural Direct Effect	1.12 (0.62, 1.99)	0.69
Natural Indirect Effect	2.12 (1.40, 3.18)	<0.001
Total Effect	2.38 (1.19, 4.63)	0.01

[a] Gestational age < 37 weeks.

Table 3 shows the effect of placental lesions on the diagnosis of small-for-gestational age (<10th percentile), base deficit, and cord pH. Of the records available for analysis, 38.1% of women with pregnancies complicated by placental abruption and lesions gave birth to SGA babies. However, this proportion was very similar to the percentage (37.8%) of women giving birth to babies of appropriate gestational age. More women with pregnancies complicated by placental abruption and placental lesions (80%) gave birth to babies requiring chest compressions and resuscitation than babies who did not require chest compressions and resuscitation (38%). Similarly, more women with such pregnancies gave birth to babies with low Apgar scores (72.7%) vs Apgar > 5 at 10-min (36.9%) (Table 3).

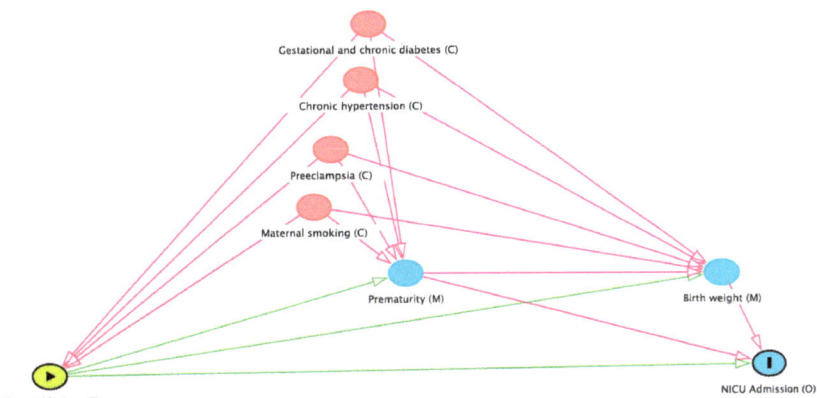

Figure 1. Directed Acyclic Graph (DAG) showing the assumed confounding effects of maternal smoking, preeclampsia, chronic hypertension, and gestational or chronic diabetes with the mediators of prematurity and birthweight between placental lesions and NICU admission. E—exposure; O—outcome; C—confounder; M—mediator.

Table 3. The effect of placental abruption and underlying lesions on perinatal outcomes.

Perinatal Outcome	Placental Lesions (n, %)	OR (95% CI)	p Value
SGA [a] (n = 42)	16 (38.1)	1.01 (0.50–2.00)	0.97
Appropriate weight [b] (n = 188)	71 (37.8)		
BD 10–15.9 or BD 16 (n = 42)	14 (33.3)	0.88 (0.42–1.77)	0.72
Normal BD (n = 171) [c]	62 (36.3)		
Cord pH 7 or 7.1–7.15 (n = 42)	15 (35.7)	1.02 (0.49–2.04)	0.97
Normal cord pH (n = 164) [d]	58 (35.4)		
Apgar 5 at 10-min (n = 11)	8 (72.7)	4.56 (1.28–21.26)	0.03
Apgar > 5 at 10-min (n = 225)	83 (36.9)		
Need for resuscitation (n = 5) [e]	4 (80.0)	6.57 (0.95–129.74)	0.09
No need for resuscitation (n = 230)	87 (37.8)		

[a] Small-for-gestational age < 10th percentile; [b] 10–90th percentile; [c] Base deficit < 10; [d] Cord pH > 7.16; [e] Need for chest compressions and/or epinephrine in the delivery room. SGA, small-for-gestational age; BD, base deficit; OR, odds ratio; CI, confidence interval.

There was no statistically significant difference in the odds of SGA or having an adverse neonatal BD value among women with pregnancies complicated by placental abruption and additional lesions, versus pregnancies complicated with abruption only (OR 1.01, 95% CI 0.50–2.00, p = 0.97; OR 0.88, 95% CI 0.42–1.77, p = 0.72). Similarly, there was no difference in having an adverse cord pH value (OR 1.02, 95% CI 0.49–2.04, p = 0.97; Table 3).

Interestingly, women with pregnancies complicated by placental abruption and lesions were more likely to have a baby with Apgar score $\leq$ 5 at 10-min than pregnancies complicated with abruption only, alone (OR 4.56, 95% CI 1.28–21.26, p = 0.03). Lastly, there was no difference in the need for newborn resuscitation between the two groups (OR 6.6, 95% CI 0.95–129.74, p = 0.09; Table 3).

4. Discussion

This study sought to compare the odds of adverse, neonatal outcomes in women with isolated placental abruption vs placental abruption with underlying placental pathologies. There is an added concern when placentas of pregnant women with placental abruption show MVM, FVM, and VUE, as evidence suggests compromised fetal outcome [17–20]. Based on our study findings, we conclude that women with pregnancies complicated by placental abruption and co-occurring lesions are more likely to have a baby admitted to the

NICU and a low Apgar score at 10-min than pregnancies with placental abruption alone. Moreover, these differences were mostly mediated through prematurity and birthweight.

In the adjusted and unadjusted analysis, we found a significant association between pregnancies complicated by placental abruption and pathologies to NICU admission. Our mediation analyses suggest that these effects act through prematurity and birthweight; however, future studies are needed to validate our finding. Neonatologists follow strict criteria for NICU admission, including evaluating the full clinical picture of the neonate. Specifically, gestational age and weight are factors they consider during admission. Studies demonstrate that maternal health history (i.e., smoking and prior placental abruption diagnosis) can impact subsequent risk of placental abruption [4,45,46]. Therefore, if the neonatologist knows the clinical history of the mother in addition to gestational age and weight, these factors together could potentially influence their decision to admit.

The presence of underlying placental lesions, as well as placental abruption, are suggested to be associated with a diverse range of neonatal problems, including lower Apgar scores and neonatal asphyxia. Specifically, lower Apgar scores at 1 and 5 min are associated with the placental lesions of maternal vascular malperfusion and intrauterine infection [47,48]. Beebe et al. determined a relationship between a high rate of chorioamnionitis in term and premature infants and low Apgar scores at 1-min [47]. Lower Apgar scores might loosely indicate other respiratory outcomes, such as neonatal RDS or neonatal asphyxia [49]. Prevalent lesions associated with neonatal asphyxia are typically vascular in nature, referring to chorioamnionitis with fetal vasculitis and fetal thrombotic vasculopathy [50,51].

Interestingly, reports in the literature show that placental lesions are associated with decreased incidence of respiratory distress syndrome (RDS) [45,49]. Specifically, the incidence of RDS is lower in infants exposed to chorioamnionitis (ORs 0.1–0.6 95% CI 0.02–0.8) [52–54]. The biological mechanism behind placental inflammation in RDS stems from increased amounts of interleukin-1 beta (IL-1β) in chorioamnionitis. IL-1β stimulates corticotrophin-releasing factor and corticotrophin [55–57]. Production of these hormones elevates cortisol production, which accelerates lung maturation and decreases RDS incidence [57]. Moreover, the lung mesenchymal tissue decreases, while the epithelial surface area and airspace lung volume increase. This leads to mature lung development and supports gas exchange [54,58,59]. In contrast, very preterm infants exposed to chorioamnionitis were at higher risk for bronchopulmonary dysplasia (BPD), due to elevated levels of IL-8, granulocyte colony-stimulating factor, and anti-inflammatory IL-10 after adjusting for duration of gestation and severity of respiratory distress during the first day after birth [60].

There is less focus in the literature on exclusively Apgar scores. In fact, only few publications have linked placental abruption to relatable outcomes, such as increased acidosis risk (a marker of hypoxia) and elevated need for resuscitation [61–63]. The increased risk in these outcomes is affected by the interaction between placental abruption status, preterm birth, hypoxia, and blood loss (i.e., fetomaternal hemorrhage) [64].

A low Apgar score at later intervals could be used as a proxy for neurological impairment, including cerebral palsy [65]. Recent studies suggest a strong correlation between low Apgar score and cerebral palsy in children born to term or with normal birth weight [66,67]. In particular, among children with a birth weight of 2500 g or more, those with an Apgar score of less than 4 at 5-min were more likely to have cerebral palsy than children who had an Apgar score of more than 8 (OR 125, 95% CI 91 to 170) [65]. In placental abruption cases, evidence supports the impact of immaturity, birthweight, gestational age, and malformations of the central nervous system decreasing Apgar scores, potentially contributing to respiratory difficulties, and possibly increasing the risk for cerebral palsy [68–70]. Furthermore, there is increasing evidence showing maternal infection causing fetal inflammation, leading to neonatal brain injury [48]. In particular, inflammatory cytokines are neurotoxic in vitro [71] and in vivo [72] and are shown to inhibit oligodendryocytes in the developing white matter [73]. Histological chorioamnionitis and neonatal blood inflammatory cytokines are likely significantly higher in infants with cerebral palsy [74,75]. Hence, the inflammatory environment at birth plays a role in neonatal brain injury.

4.1. Strengths & Limitations

There are numerous strengths of this study. Unlike previous placental pathology literature, we adjusted for known confounders (maternal smoking, maternal hypertension/preeclampsia, maternal diabetes) during our NICU admission analysis. Moreover, we followed thorough statistical approaches to test if birthweight and prematurity were mediators. We separated our neonatal outcomes, rather than combining them in order to tailor specific recommendations to pathologists and neonatologists. Fortunately, our robust sample size permitted us to examine outcomes in this manner. Data entry was performed by two extractors and consequently validated. However, there remains a possibility of misclassification bias when organizing the placental pathologies, as well as missing data or incompleteness on EMRs for SGA. Further analysis of outcomes of interest such as IVH could not be performed due to insufficient numbers.

4.2. Future Directions

A future study is underway to examine identical outcomes in connection with the specific pathologies of interest. Chorioamnionitis with respiratory outcomes and Apgar scores will be explored in detail. Another notable endeavor is to develop a national registry of prospectively collected data, to pool rare neonatal outcomes such as IVH across institutions and thus increase sample size. Assessment of coexisting placental pathology(ies) in pregnancies complicated with abruption and its potential impact on infant developmental outcome (i.e., cerebral palsy) might be warranted.

5. Conclusions

Coexisting placental pathology(ies) could potentially impact acute neonatal outcomes, such as NICU admission and Apgar scores in pregnancies complicated by PA. However, future multi-institutional studies of robust sample sizes are needed to ascertain these findings to greater certainty. This pilot study can be replicated by other institutions to determine if obstetrical and neonatal teams should mobilize resources in anticipation of the need for neonatal resuscitation. Since placental pathologies such as VUE may recur in certain cases of subsequent pregnancies [38], our next step is to examine neonatal risks by placental pathology type to inform future neonatal delivery interventions.

Supplementary Materials: The following are available online at https://www.mdpi.com/article/10.3390/jcm10235693/s1, Placental lesion definitions.

Author Contributions: Conceptualization, D.E.D., S.L. and F.M.; Methodology, D.E.D., S.L., F.M. and I.O.; Software, V.B.; Validation, D.M., J.T., I.O. and V.B.; Formal analysis, V.B.; Investigation, D.E.D., S.L., F.M., D.M., J.T., I.O. and V.B.; Resources, D.E.D., S.L., F.M. and I.O.; Data curation, D.M., J.T. and V.B.; Writing—Original Draft Preparation, D.M., J.T. and I.O.; Writing—Review & Editing, D.M., J.T., I.O., D.E.D., S.L., F.M. and V.B.; Visualization, V.B.; Supervision, D.E.D., S.L., F.M. and I.O.; Project Administration, D.M., J.T. and I.O. All authors have read and agreed to the published version of the manuscript.

Funding: This research received no external funding.

Institutional Review Board Statement: The study was approved by the Institutional Review Board of Children's Hospital of Eastern Ontario (CHEO) Research Institute (CHEOREB# 20/22X, 21 February 2020).

Informed Consent Statement: Patient consent was waived due to minimal risk to confidentiality.

Data Availability Statement: The data presented in this study are available on request from the corresponding authors.

Conflicts of Interest: The sponsors had no role in the design, execution, interpretation, or writing of the study.

References

1. Ananth, C.V. Ischemic Placental Disease: A Unifying Concept for Preeclampsia, Intrauterine Growth Restriction, and Placental Abruption. *Semin. Perinatol.* **2014**, *38*, 131–132. [CrossRef] [PubMed]
2. Elsasser, D.A.; Ananth, C.V.; Prasad, V.; Vintzileos, A.M. Diagnosis of Placental Abruption: Relationship between Clinical and Histopathological Findings. *Eur. J. Obstet. Gynecol. Reprod. Biol.* **2010**, *148*, 125–130. [CrossRef] [PubMed]
3. Ananth, C.V.; Keyes, K.M.; Hamilton, A.; Gissler, M.; Wu, C.; Liu, S.; Luque-Fernandez, M.A.; Skjærven, R.; Williams, M.A.; Tikkanen, M.; et al. An International Contrast of Rates of Placental Abruption: An Age-Period-Cohort Analysis. *PLoS ONE* **2015**, *10*, e0125246. [CrossRef]
4. Tikkanen, M. Placental Abruption: Epidemiology, Risk Factors and Consequences. *Acta Obstet. Gynecol. Scand.* **2011**, *90*, 140–149. [CrossRef]
5. Ananth, C.V.; Berkowitz, G.S.; Savitz, D.A.; Lapinski, R.H. Placental Abruption and Adverse Perinatal Outcomes. *J. Am. Med. Assoc.* **1999**, *282*, 1646–1651. [CrossRef] [PubMed]
6. Ananth, C.; Haylea, P.; Ananth, S.; Zhang, Y.; Kostis, W.; Schuster, M. Maternal Cardiovascular and Cerebrovascular Health after Placental Abruption: A Systematic Review and Meta-Analysis. *Am. J. Epidemiol.* **2021**, *143*, 1–36. [CrossRef] [PubMed]
7. Dandapat, A.; Pande, B.; Dora, S.; Mohapatra, K.; Nayak, L. A Retrospective Study on Adherent Placenta—Its Management, Maternal and Perinatal Outcome. *J. Evol. Med. Dent. Sci.* **2017**, *6*, 2278–4802.
8. Sengodan, S.S.; Dhanapal, M. Abruptio Placenta: A Retrospective Study on Maternal and Perinatal Outcome. *Int. J. Reprod. Contracept. Obstet. Gynecol.* **2017**, *6*, 4389. [CrossRef]
9. Soomro, P.; Pirzada, S.; Maheshwari, M.; Bhatti, N. Frequency, Predictors and Outcomes of Placental Abruption in Rural Sindh. *Pak. J. Med. Res.* **2021**, *60*, 57–61.
10. Satti, I.; Hassan, F.; Salim, N.A.; Mansor, A.; Ali, H. Immediate Maternal and Fetal Outcome of Placental Abruption/ Omdurman/ SUDAN (Multicentric Study). *Multi-Knowl. Electron. Compr. J. Educ. Sci. Publ.* **2021**, *41*, 1–9.
11. Qiu, Y.; Wu, L.; Xiao, Y.; Zhang, X. Clinical Analysis and Classification of Placental Abruption. *J. Matern. Neonatal Med.* **2021**, *34*, 2952–2956. [CrossRef]
12. Kramer, M.; Usher, R.; Pollack, R.; Boyd, M.; Usher, S. Etiologic Determinants of Abruptio Placenta. *Obstet. Gynecol.* **1997**, *89*, 221–226. [CrossRef]
13. Onishi, K.; Tsuda, H.; Fuma, K.; Kuribayashi, M.; Tezuka, A.; Ando, T.; Mizuno, K. The Impact of the Abruption Severity and the Onset-to-Delivery Time on the Maternal and Neonatal Outcomes of Placental Abruption. *J. Matern. Neonatal Med.* **2020**, *33*, 3775–3783. [CrossRef] [PubMed]
14. Iitani, Y.; Tsuda, H.; Ito, Y.; Moriyama, Y.; Nakano, T.; Imai, K.; Kotani, T.; Kikkawa, F. Simulation Training Is Useful for Shortening the Decision-To-Delivery Interval in Cases of Emergent Cesarean Section. *Obstet. Gynecol. Surv.* **2019**, *74*, 3–5. [CrossRef]
15. Soltanifar, S.; Russell, R. The National Institute for Health and Clinical Excellence (NICE) Guidelines for Caesarean Section, 2011 Update: Implications for the Anaesthetist. *Int. J. Obstet. Anesth.* **2012**, *21*, 264–272. [CrossRef]
16. Khong, T.Y.; Mooney, E.E.; Ariel, I.; Balmus, N.C.M.; Boyd, T.K.; Brundler, M.A.; Derricott, H.; Evans, M.J.; Faye-Petersen, O.M.; Gillan, J.E.; et al. Sampling and Definitions of Placental Lesions Amsterdam Placental Workshop Group Consensus Statement. *Arch. Pathol. Lab. Med.* **2016**, *140*, 698–713. [CrossRef]
17. Wright, E.; Audette, M.C.; Ye, X.Y.; Keating, S.; Hoffman, B.; Lye, S.J.; Shah, P.S.; Kingdom, J.C. Maternal Vascular Malperfusion and Adverse Perinatal Outcomes in Low-Risk Nulliparous Women. *Obstet. Gynecol.* **2017**, *130*, 1112–1120. [CrossRef] [PubMed]
18. Awuah, S.P.; Okai, I.; Ntim, E.A.; Bedu-Addo, K. Prevalence, Placenta Development, and Perinatal Outcomes of Women with Hypertensive Disorders of Pregnancy at Komfo Anokye Teaching Hospital. *PLoS ONE* **2020**, *15*, e0233817. [CrossRef]
19. Scifres, C.M.; Parks, W.T.; Feghali, M.; Caritis, S.N.; Catov, J.M. Placental Maternal Vascular Malperfusion and Adverse Pregnancy Outcomes in Gestational Diabetes Mellitus. *Placenta* **2017**, *49*, 10–15. [CrossRef] [PubMed]
20. Heider, A. Fetal Vascular Malperfusion. *Arch. Pathol. Lab. Med.* **2017**, *141*, 1484–1489. [CrossRef] [PubMed]
21. Bustamante Helfrich, B.; Chilukuri, N.; He, H.; Cerda, S.R.; Hong, X.; Wang, G.; Pearson, C.; Burd, I.; Wang, X. Maternal Vascular Malperfusion of the Placental Bed Associated with Hypertensive Disorders in the Boston Birth Cohort. *Placenta* **2017**, *52*, 106–113. [CrossRef] [PubMed]
22. Hendrix, M.L.E.; Bons, J.A.P.; Alers, N.O.; Severens-Rijvers, C.A.H.; Spaanderman, M.E.A.; Al-Nasiry, S. Maternal Vascular Malformation in the Placenta Is an Indicator for Fetal Growth Restriction Irrespective of Neonatal Birthweight. *Placenta* **2019**, *87*, 8–15. [CrossRef] [PubMed]
23. Redline, R.W.; Boyd, T.; Campbell, V.; Hyde, S.; Kaplan, C.; Khong, T.Y.; Prashner, H.R.; Waters, B.L. Maternal Vascular Underperfusion: Nosology and Reproducibility of Placental Reaction Patterns. *Pediatr. Dev. Pathol.* **2004**, *7*, 237–249. [CrossRef] [PubMed]
24. Visser, L.; van Buggenum, H.; van der Voorn, J.P.; Heestermans, L.A.P.H.; Hollander, K.W.P.; Wouters, M.G.A.J.; de Groot, C.J.M.; de Boer, M.A. Maternal Vascular Malperfusion in Spontaneous Preterm Birth Placentas Related to Clinical Outcome of Subsequent Pregnancy. *J. Matern. Neonatal Med.* **2021**, *34*, 2759–2764. [CrossRef] [PubMed]
25. Arias, F.; Rodriquez, L.; Rayne, S.C.; Kraus, F.T. Maternal Placental Vasculopathy and Infection: Two Distinct Subgroups among Patients with Preterm Labor and Preterm Ruptured Membranes. *Am. J. Obstet. Gynecol.* **1993**, *168*, 585–591. [CrossRef]
26. Holzman, C.; Kelly, R.; Senagore, P.; Wang, J.; Tian, Y.; Rahbar, M.H.; Chung, H. Placental Vascular Pathology Findings and Pathways to Preterm Delivery. *Am. J. Epidemiol.* **2009**, *170*, 148–158. [CrossRef]

27. Kim, Y.M.; Chaiworapongsa, T.; Gomez, R.; Bujold, E.; Yoon, B.H.; Rotmensch, S.; Thaler, H.T.; Romero, R. Failure of Physiologic Transformation of the Spiral Arteries in the Placental Bed in Preterm Premature Rupture of Membranes. *Am. J. Obstet. Gynecol.* **2002**, *187*, 1137–1142. [CrossRef] [PubMed]
28. Christians, J.K.; Huicochea Munoz, M.F. Pregnancy Complications Recur Independently of Maternal Vascular Malperfusion Lesions. *PLoS ONE* **2020**, *15*, e0228664. [CrossRef] [PubMed]
29. Redline, R.W. Severe Fetal Placental Vascular Lesions in Term Infants with Neurologic Impairment. *Am. J. Obstet. Gynecol.* **2005**, *192*, 452–457. [CrossRef] [PubMed]
30. Redline, R.W.; Ravishankar, S. Fetal Vascular Malperfusion, an Update. *Apmis* **2018**, *126*, 561–569. [CrossRef] [PubMed]
31. Mark, S.P.; Croughan-Minihane, M.S.; Kilpatrick, S.J. Chorioamnionitis and Uterine Function. *Obstet. Gynecol.* **2000**, *95*, 909–912. [CrossRef]
32. Satin, A.J.; Maberry, M.C.; Leveno, K.J.; Sherman, M.L.; Kline, D.M. Chorioamnionitis: A Harbinger of Dystocia. *Obstet. Gynecol.* **1992**, *79*, 913–915. [CrossRef]
33. Tita, A.T.N.; Andrews, W.W. Diagnosis and Management of Clinical Chorioamnionitis. *Clin. Perinatol.* **2010**, *37*, 339–354. [CrossRef]
34. Hauth, J.C.; Gilstrap, L.C.; Hankins, G.D.V.; Connor, K.D. Term Maternal and Neonatal Complications of Acute Chorioamnionitis. *Obstet. Gynecol.* **1985**, *66*, 59–62.
35. Morales, W. The Effect of Chorioamnionitis on the Developmental Outcome of Preterm Infants at One Year. *Obstet. Gynecol.* **1987**, *70*, 183–185. [PubMed]
36. Lau, J.; Magee, F.; Qiu, Z.; Houbé, J.; Von Dadelszen, P.; Lee, S.K. Chorioamnionitis with a Fetal Inflammatory Response Is Associated with Higher Neonatal Mortality, Morbidity, and Resource Use than Chorioamnionitis Displaying a Maternal Inflammatory Response Only. *Am. J. Obstet. Gynecol.* **2005**, *193*, 708–713. [CrossRef]
37. Aziz, N.; Cheng, Y.W.; Caughey, A.B. Neonatal Outcomes in the Setting of Preterm Premature Rupture of Membranes Complicated by Chorioamnionitis. *J. Matern. Neonatal Med.* **2009**, *22*, 780–784. [CrossRef] [PubMed]
38. Redline, R.W. Villitis of Unknown Etiology: Noninfectious Chronic Villitis in the Placenta. *Hum. Pathol.* **2007**, *38*, 1439–1446. [CrossRef] [PubMed]
39. Weber, D.E.; Held, J.D.; Jandarov, R.A.; Kelleher, M.; Kinnear, B.; Sall, D.; O'Toole, J.K. Development and Establishment of Initial Validity Evidence for a Novel Tool for Assessing Trainee Admission Notes. *J. Gen. Intern. Med.* **2020**, *35*, 1078–1083. [CrossRef]
40. Harris, P.A.; Taylor, R.; Minor, B.L.; Elliott, V.; Fernandez, M.; O'Neal, L.; McLeod, L.; Delacqua, G.; Delacqua, F.; Kirby, J.; et al. The REDCap Consortium: Building an International Community of Software Platform Partners. *J. Biomed. Inform.* **2019**, *95*, 103208. [CrossRef] [PubMed]
41. Greenland, S.; Pearl, J.; Robins, J.M. Causal Diagrams for Epidemiologic Research. *Epidemiology* **1999**, *10*, 37–48. [CrossRef] [PubMed]
42. R Core Team. *R: A Language and Environment for Statistical Computing*; R Foundation for Statistical Computing: Vienna, Austria, 2020. Available online: https://www.R-project.org/ (accessed on 15 March 2021).
43. Steen, J.; Loeys, T.; Moerkerke, B.; Vansteelandt, S. Medflex: An R Package for Flexible Mediation Analysis Using Natural Effect Models. *J. Stat. Softw.* **2017**, *76*. [CrossRef]
44. Textor, J.; van der Zander, B.; Gilthorpe, M.S.; Liśkiewicz, M.; Ellison, G.T. Robust Causal Inference Using Directed Acyclic Graphs: The R Package "Dagitty". *Int. J. Epidemiol.* **2016**, *45*, 1887–1894. [CrossRef] [PubMed]
45. Downes, K.L.; Shenassa, E.D.; Grantz, K.L. Neonatal Outcomes Associated with Placental Abruption. *Am. J. Epidemiol.* **2017**, *186*, 1319–1328. [CrossRef] [PubMed]
46. Sheiner, E.; Shoham-Vardi, I.; Hallak, M.; Hadar, A.; Gortzak-Uzan, L.; Katz, M.; Mazor, M. Placental Abruption in Term Pregnancies: Clinical Significance and Obstetric Risk Factors. *J. Matern. Neonatal Med.* **2003**, *13*, 45–49. [CrossRef]
47. Beebe, L.; Cowan, L.; Altshuler, G. The Epidemiology of Placental Features: Associations with Gestational Age and Neonatal Outcome. *Obstet. Gynecol.* **1996**, *5*, 771–778. [CrossRef]
48. Ogunyemi, D.; Murillo, M.; Jackson, U.; Hunter, N.; Alperson, B. The Relationship between Placental Histopathology Findings and Perinatal Outcome in Preterm Infants. *J. Matern. Neonatal Med.* **2003**, *13*, 102–109. [CrossRef]
49. Roescher, A.M.; Timmer, A.; Erwich, J.J.H.M.; Bos, A.F. Placental Pathology, Perinatal Death, Neonatal Outcome, and Neurological Development: A Systematic Review. *PLoS ONE* **2014**, *9*, e89419. [CrossRef]
50. De Laat, M.W.M.; Franx, A.; Bots, M.L.; Visser, G.H.A.; Nikkels, P.G.J. Umbilical Coiling Index in Normal and Complicated Pregnancies. *Obstet. Gynecol.* **2006**, *107*, 1049–1055. [CrossRef]
51. Wintermark, P.; Boyd, T.; Gregas, M.C.; Labrecque, M.; Hansen, A. Placental Pathology in Asphyxiated Newborns Meeting the Criteria for Therapeutic Hypothermia. *Am. J. Obstet. Gynecol.* **2010**, *203*, 579.e1–579.e9. [CrossRef]
52. Richardson, B.S.; Wakim, E.; da Silva, O.; Walton, J. Preterm Histologic Chorioamnionitis: Impact on Cord Gas and PH Values and Neonatal Outcome. *Am. J. Obstet. Gynecol.* **2006**, *195*, 1357–1365. [CrossRef]
53. Sato, M.; Nishimaki, S.; Yokota, S.; Seki, K.; Horiguchi, H.; An, H.; Ishida, F.; Fujita, S.; Ao, K.; Yatake, H. Severity of Chorioamnionitis and Neonatal Outcome. *J. Obstet. Gynaecol. Res.* **2011**, *37*, 1313–1319. [CrossRef] [PubMed]
54. Kramer, B.W.; Kallapur, S.; Newnham, J.; Jobe, A.H. Prenatal Inflammation and Lung Development. *Semin. Fetal Neonatal Med.* **2009**, *14*, 2–7. [CrossRef] [PubMed]

55. Sapolsky, R.; Rivier, C.; Yamamoto, G.; Plotsky, P.; Vale, W. Interleukin-1 Stimulates the Secretion of Hypothalamic Corticotropin-Releasing Factor. *Science* **1987**, *238*, 522–524. [CrossRef]
56. Bernton, E.W.; Beach, J.E.; Holaday, J.W.; Smallridge, R.C.; Fein, H.G. Release of Multiple Hormones by a Direct Action of Lnterleukin-1 on Pituitary Cells. *Obstet. Gynecol. Surv.* **1988**, *43*, 420–422. [CrossRef]
57. Lock, M.; Mcgillick, E.V.; Orgeig, S.; Mcmillen, I.C.; Morrison, J.L. Regulation of Fetal Lung Development in Response to Maternal Overnutrition. *Clin. Exp. Pharmacol. Physiol.* **2013**, *40*, 803–816. [CrossRef]
58. Bry, K.; Lappalainen, U.; Hallman, M. Intraamniotic Interleukin-1 Accelerates Surfactant Protein Synthesis in Fetal Rabbits and Improves Lung Stability after Premature Birth. *J. Clin. Investig.* **1997**, *99*, 2992–2999. [CrossRef] [PubMed]
59. Willet, K.E.; Jobe, A.H.; Ikegami, M.; Newnham, J.; Brennan, S.; Sly, P.D. Antenatal Endotoxin and Glucocorticoid Effects on Lung Morphometry in Preterm Lambs. *Pediatr. Res.* **2000**, *48*, 782–788. [CrossRef] [PubMed]
60. Paananen, R.; Husa, A.-K.; Vuolteenaho, R.; Herva, R.; Kaukola, T.; Hallman, M. Blood Cytokines during the Perinatal Period in Very Preterm Infants. *J. Pediatr.* **2009**, *154*, 39–43.e3. [CrossRef]
61. Boisramé, T.; Sananès, N.; Fritz, G.; Boudier, E.; Aissi, G.; Favre, R.; Langer, B. Placental Abruption: Risk Factors, Management and Maternal-Fetal Prognosis. Cohort Study over 10 Years. *Eur. J. Obstet. Gynecol. Reprod. Biol.* **2014**, *179*, 100–104. [CrossRef]
62. Furukawa, S.; Doi, K.; Furuta, K.; Sameshima, H. The Effect of Placental Abruption on the Outcome of Extremely Premature Infants. *J. Matern. Neonatal Med.* **2015**, *28*, 705–708. [CrossRef] [PubMed]
63. Andreani, M.; Locatelli, A.; Assi, F.; Consonni, S.; Malguzzi, S.; Paterlini, G.; Ghidini, A. Predictors of Umbilical Artery Acidosis in Preterm Delivery. *Am. J. Obstet. Gynecol.* **2007**, *197*, 303.e1–303.e5. [CrossRef] [PubMed]
64. Downes, K.L.; Grantz, K.L.; Shenassa, E.D. Maternal, Labor, Delivery, and Perinatal Outcomes Associated with Placental Abruption: A Systematic Review. *Am. J. Perinatol.* **2017**, *34*, 935–957. [CrossRef] [PubMed]
65. Lie, K.K.; Grøholt, E.K.; Eskild, A. Association of Cerebral Palsy with Apgar Score in Low and Normal Birthweight Infants: Population Based Cohort Study. *BMJ* **2010**, *341*, 817. [CrossRef] [PubMed]
66. Moster, D.; Lie, R.T.; Irgens, L.M.; Bjerkedal, T.; Markestad, T. The Association of Apgar Score with Subsequent Death and Cerebral Palsy: A Population-Based Study in Term Infants. *J. Pediatr.* **2001**, *138*, 798–803. [CrossRef]
67. Thorngren-Jerneck, K.; Herbst, A. Perinatal Factors Associated with Cerebral Palsy in Children Born in Sweden. *Obstet. Gynecol.* **2006**, *108*, 1499–1505. [CrossRef] [PubMed]
68. Grether, J.K.; Nelson, K.B.; Emery, E.S.; Cummins, S.K. Prenatal and Perinatal Factors and Cerebral Palsy in Very Low Birth Weight Infants. *J. Pediatr.* **1996**, *128*, 407–414. [CrossRef]
69. Hegyi, T.; Carbone, T.; Anwar, M.; Ostfeld, B.; Hiatt, M.; Koons, A.; Pinto-Martin, J.; Paneth, N. The Apgar Score and Its Components in the Preterm Infant. *Pediatrics* **1998**, *101*, 77–81. [CrossRef]
70. Pinheiro, J.M.B. The Apgar Cycle: A New View of a Familiar Scoring System. *Arch. Dis. Child. Fetal Neonatal Ed.* **2009**, *94*, 70–72. [CrossRef] [PubMed]
71. Yoon, C.Y.; Shim, Y.J.; Kim, E.H.; Lee, J.H.; Won, N.H.; Kim, J.H.; Park, I.S.; Yoon, D.K.; Min, B.H. Renal Cell Carcinoma Does Not Express Argininosuccinate Synthetase and Is Highly Sensitive to Arginine Deprivation via Arginine Deiminase. *Int. J. Cancer* **2007**, *120*, 897–905. [CrossRef]
72. Dommergues, M.A.; Patkai, J.; Renauld, J.C.; Evrard, P.; Gressens, P. Proinflammatory Cytokines and Interleukin-9 Exacerbate Excitotoxic Lesions of the Newborn Murine Neopallium. *Ann. Neurol.* **2000**, *47*, 54–63. [CrossRef]
73. Yoon, B.; Kim, C.; Park, J.; Gomez, R. Experimentally-Induced Intrauterine Infection Causes Fetal Brain White Matter Lesions in Rabbits. *Am. J. Obstet. Gynecol.* **2000**, *176*, S40. [CrossRef]
74. Wu, Y.W.; Colford, J.M. Chorioamnionitis as a Risk Factor for Cerebral Palsy A Meta-Analysis. *J. Am. Med. Assoc.* **2000**, *284*, 1417–1424. [CrossRef] [PubMed]
75. Yoon, B.H.; Romero, R.; Park, J.S.; Kim, C.J.; Kim, S.H.; Choi, J.H.; Han, T.R. Fetal Exposure to an Intra-Amniotic Inflammation and the Development of Cerebral Palsy at the Age of Three Years. *Am. J. Obstet. Gynecol.* **2000**, *182*, 675–681. [CrossRef] [PubMed]

Article

Clinical Validation of a Proteomic Biomarker Threshold for Increased Risk of Spontaneous Preterm Birth and Associated Clinical Outcomes: A Replication Study

Julja Burchard [1], Ashoka D. Polpitiya [1], Angela C. Fox [1], Todd L. Randolph [1], Tracey C. Fleischer [1,*], Max T. Dufford [1], Thomas J. Garite [1], Gregory C. Critchfield [1], J. Jay Boniface [1], George R. Saade [2] and Paul E. Kearney [1]

1 Sera Prognostics, Incorporated, Salt Lake City, UT 84109, USA; jburchard@seraprognostics.com (J.B.); ashoka@seraprognostics.com (A.D.P.); afox@seraprognostics.com (A.C.F.); trandolph@seraprognostics.com (T.L.R.); mdufford@seraprognostics.com (M.T.D.); tgarite@seraprognostics.com (T.J.G.); gcritchfield@seraprognostics.com (G.C.C.); jboniface@seraprognostics.com (J.J.B.); pkearney@data-incites.com (P.E.K.)
2 Department of Obstetrics & Gynecology, University of Texas Medical Branch, Galveston, TX 77555, USA; gsaade@utmb.edu
* Correspondence: tfleischer@seraprognostics.com; Tel.: +1-801-990-0597

Abstract: Preterm births are the leading cause of neonatal death in the United States. Previously, a spontaneous preterm birth (sPTB) predictor based on the ratio of two proteins, IBP4/SHBG, was validated as a predictor of sPTB in the Proteomic Assessment of Preterm Risk (PAPR) study. In particular, a proteomic biomarker threshold of −1.37, corresponding to a ~two-fold increase or ~15% risk of sPTB, significantly stratified earlier deliveries. Guidelines for molecular tests advise replication in a second independent study. Here we tested whether the significant association between proteomic biomarker scores above the threshold and sPTB, and associated adverse outcomes, was replicated in a second independent study, the Multicenter Assessment of a Spontaneous Preterm Birth Risk Predictor (TREETOP). The threshold significantly stratified subjects in PAPR and TREETOP for sPTB ($p = 0.041$, $p = 0.041$, respectively). Application of the threshold in a Kaplan–Meier analysis demonstrated significant stratification in each study, respectively, for gestational age at birth ($p < 0.001$, $p = 0.0016$) and rate of hospital discharge for both neonate ($p < 0.001$, $p = 0.005$) and mother ($p < 0.001$, $p < 0.001$). Above the threshold, severe neonatal morbidity/mortality and mortality alone were 2.2 ($p = 0.0083$), and 7.4-fold higher ($p = 0.018$), respectively, in both studies combined. Thus, higher predictor scores were associated with multiple adverse pregnancy outcomes.

Keywords: preterm birth; IBP4; SHBG; biomarkers

1. Introduction

Preterm birth (PTB), including both spontaneous (sPTB) and medically indicated (miPTB) birth before 37 weeks gestation, occurs in approximately 10% of all births in the US and is a leading cause of neonatal morbidities, mortality and long-term health consequences worldwide [1,2]. PTB and associated morbidities, such as respiratory distress, can require extended stays and care in neonatal intensive care nurseries, along with increased costs [3]. The application of existing interventions such as progestogens and systems of care coordination, and the effective development of new interventions depend on screening tools to identify pregnancies at risk. Clinical markers associated with an increased risk of sPTB are present in only a minority of pregnancies, limiting their overall utility. A history of previous sPTB is a traditional predictor of recurrent sPTB but applies to only approximately 4% of all pregnancies and 11% of all sPTBs [4,5]. Similarly, a short cervical length measured by transvaginal ultrasound is a predictor of sPTB, but accounts for only an additional 2% of all pregnancies and 6% of all sPTBs [6,7].

In accordance with the National Academy of Medicine's guidelines [8] for the rigorous development of multi-biomarker tests, clinical validity is ideally replicated in a second study, independent from the one in which the test was originally developed. Additionally, it is desirable for a test to have a prespecified threshold to risk-stratify subjects so that clinicians can easily interpret and act upon test results. In the Proteomic Assessment of Preterm Risk (PAPR) study, Saade et al. reported the development and clinical validation of a serum test for sPTB prediction that utilizes the proteomic biomarker of insulin-like growth factor binding protein-4 (IBP4) and sex hormone binding globulin (SHBG) [9]. These two proteins, used in combination, were found to be the most predictive pair of biomarkers amongst hundreds of proteins screened during a systems biology approach in the PAPR study. IBP4 is expressed in syncytiotrophoblasts and negatively regulates insulin-like growth factors [10], key regulators of placental development [11]. SHBG, primarily secreted by the liver, is also placentally expressed [12], and circulating SHBG levels increase ~5-fold during pregnancy [13]. SHBG regulates the bioavailability of sex hormones, is associated with diabetes and insulin resistance [14] and is negatively regulated by proinflammatory cytokines [15] implicated in etiologies of PTB.

In the subsequent validation of IBP4/SHBG, in addition to demonstrating a statistically significant area under the receiver operating characteristic (AUC) curve for predicting preterm birth, the study reported that subjects with a proteomic biomarker score at or above -1.37 delivered earlier than those with lower proteomic biomarker scores [9]. The study showed that subjects at or above a proteomic biomarker threshold of -1.37, corresponding to a risk probability of ~15%, are at approximately 2-fold or greater increased risk of sPTB as compared to the average risk of singleton pregnancies in the United States.

The primary objective of the current analysis was to demonstrate that significance of proteomic biomarker thresholds is replicated across independent studies. Of particular importance was extending the work of Saade and colleagues [9] by demonstrating that the risk of sPTB is significantly elevated at the proteomic biomarker threshold of -1.37 in two additional cohorts. First, an expanded, but partially overlapping, cohort of subjects from the PAPR study was utilized to verify that sPTB remains significantly elevated in patients with a score above the threshold. Second, we conducted a validation of the threshold in a large and completely independent cohort, the Multicenter Assessment of a Spontaneous Preterm Birth Risk Predictor (TREETOP) study (NCT02787213) [16]. In clinical practice, risk probabilities are utilized rather than proteomic biomarker thresholds. We present performance results for the proteomic biomarker threshold of -1.37 which has been shown to correspond to the risk probability of 15% [9].

The second objective was to assess whether the threshold can identify elevated risk of all PTB (sPTB and medically indicated PTB) and pregnancy complications associated with prematurity: increased lengths of maternal and neonatal hospital stay and severe neonatal morbidity and mortality. Such results are particularly important as not all premature pregnancies result in adverse outcomes, and so, demonstrating that the proteomic biomarker threshold also stratifies pregnancies by adverse neonatal and maternal outcomes adds direct evidence to the potential clinical utility of the proteomic biomarker predictor. We note that a previous exploration of the proteomic biomarker on the TREETOP cohort did not address threshold validity [16]; that is, the work did not validate a pre-specified threshold, nor did it assess the ability of the proteomic biomarker to stratify patients at any specific predictor score threshold for any outcome.

2. Materials and Methods

2.1. PAPR and TREETOP Subpopulation Selection

Subpopulations of the PAPR (NCT01371019) and TREETOP (NCT02787213) studies were selected to conduct this prospective-retrospective cohort analysis as described below. We refer to these two subpopulations as the verification and validation cohorts, respectively, in accordance with the National Academy of Medicine's Guidelines for test development [8].

The proteomic biomarker and a specific threshold were developed and fully defined in the original study [9]. The verification cohort for the current analysis was the subpopulation of PAPR consisting of all subjects (n = 549) meeting the following criteria: did not receive progesterone on or after 14 weeks gestation, underwent sample collection in the validated gestational age window ($19^{1/7}$–$20^{6/7}$ weeks) [9] and gave consent for future research use of their deidentified samples and data. Of the 549 subjects in this verification phase, only 32 were previously used for discovery of the classifier in the original study [9].

The validation cohort for the current analysis was the subpopulation of TREETOP consisting of a randomly selected subset (n = 847), or 34% of all subjects who underwent sample collection in the validated gestational age window ($19^{1/7}$–$20^{6/7}$ weeks) [16]. TREE-TOP is an observational study of pregnant women who did not receive progesterone on or after 14 weeks gestation and included iatrogenic and spontaneous PTBs, term births and co-morbid conditions. The TREETOP subjects that were not selected for the current analysis remain blinded for future studies. Importantly, the validation cohort is fully independent of the original training and verification cohorts with no subjects in common.

As a measure of neonatal outcome and accounting for major morbidity in the prematurely delivered newborns, we adapted a previously reported Neonatal Morbidity and Mortality Index (NMI, range 0 to 4) [6]. For a surviving neonate, the reported index can be 0, 1, 2 or 3 based on newborn intensive care unit length of stay or associated diagnoses, whichever is higher. For the NICU length of stay, 1–4 days stay gives a score of 1, 5–20 days a score of 2 and >20 days a score of 3. For the associated diagnoses, a unit is added for each diagnosis of respiratory distress syndrome, bronchopulmonary dysplasia, intraventricular hemorrhage grade III or IV, necrotizing enterocolitis, periventricular leukomalacia or proven severe sepsis, up to a maximum of 3. A score of 4 is assigned to perinatal mortality. Since we did not record whether the neonate was admitted to the NICU in PAPR, total length of newborn hospital stay was used in place of NICU length of stay to calculate NMI. Because all neonates had at least one day of hospital stay, our modified scale does not start at 0 as in the PREGNANT trial [6], but with an NMI of 1. Data collection through 28 days of life allowed for confirmation of all conditions contributing to NMI.

2.2. Sample Analysis

All subject samples from PAPR and TREETOP were analyzed in a certified lab according to standard operating protocol using a methodology previously validated and documented [17]. Briefly, serum samples were depleted of the top fourteen most abundant proteins (MARS14, Agilent Technologies, Inc., Santa Clara, CA, USA), reduced, alkylated, and digested with trypsin [9,17]. Following digest, the samples were spiked with stable isotope standard (SIS) peptides for proteins of interest, desalted and analyzed by reversed-phase liquid chromatography multiple reaction monitoring mass spectrometry [9,17]. The extended PAPR cohort samples were analyzed retrospectively for this study. Importantly, the TREETOP samples were analyzed prospectively, as they were collected, as would be the case in actual clinical use. Relative levels of IBP4 and SHBG were expressed as response ratios (RR) of the peak area for the endogenous peptide divided by the peak area of the SIS peptide [9,17]. The IBP4/SHBG proteomic biomarker was calculated as: $\ln(RR_{IBP4}/RR_{SHBG})$.

2.3. Data Analysis Methodology

Clinical and demographic variables were compared between the two study cohorts, with significance ($p < 0.05$) determined by Fisher's exact test for categorical variables and Welch's T-test for continuous variables. Variables including pre-pregnancy weight, race, ethnicity, and maternal education were self-reported, whereas obstetric history, delivery, and neonatal outcomes were collected from medical records review. Gestational age was based on best obstetrical estimate with LMP confirmed by ultrasound, with first trimester ultrasound confirmation required in TREETOP [18].

All analyses were pre-specified in a study protocol, including the fixed sequence of proteomic biomarker thresholds per outcome and the hypothesis test. Outcomes included sPTB and overall PTB, gestational age at birth (GAB), neonatal and maternal lengths of hospital stay and NMI. The hypothesis test was prespecified as a regression test with covariates and was utilized for both categorical and continuous outcomes. A binary variable for threshold (1 for proteomic biomarker scores greater than or equal to the threshold and 0 for values below the threshold) was tested as a predictor of adverse outcomes in regression with body mass index (BMI) as a covariate, indicated by the reported influence of BMI stratification reported by Saade and colleagues [9]. The significance of contribution of the binary predictor to the regression test was used as the measure of significance of prediction. Missing BMI values were found in 12/847 TREETOP subjects and 10/549 PAPR subjects; these subjects were dropped from the regression analyses. The protocol prespecified a hypothesis of increased PTB risk above the proteomic biomarker threshold. The regression analysis tested for one-sided significance of the binary threshold variable in prediction of an adverse outcome at alpha of 0.05. The same test of significance was used in the verification (PAPR) and validation (TREETOP) cohorts to avoid bias. To correct for multiple testing, outcomes were tested in a prespecified order in a fixed sequence approach, with alpha of 0.05. An independent statistician (see Acknowledgements) conducted pre-specified fixed sequence hypotheses testing. In exploratory analyses, statistical significance for Kaplan–Meier analysis was assessed by the log-rank statistic. To obtain even more robust estimates of threshold performance, the verification (PAPR) and validation (TREETOP) subjects were also combined for post-hoc analyses. The sensitivity and specificity of the threshold to be validated were compared to the sensitivity and specificity of the proteomic biomarker at the threshold of maximum accuracy [9] using McNemar's test. As a descriptive statistic, the fold change in the occurrence of outcomes above and below the threshold was calculated as the ratio of the rate of the outcome amongst subjects with proteomic biomarker scores at or above the threshold to the rate amongst those with proteomic biomarker scores below the threshold. All analyses were performed in R version 3.5.1 [19] using packages data.table [20], demoGraphic [21], and survival [22,23].

3. Results

The characteristics of the verification (PAPR) and validation (TREETOP) subpopulations included in this analysis are summarized in Table 1. Compared to subjects in TREETOP, women in PAPR were younger, with a higher BMI, less educated, less likely to identify as non-white, and more likely to have had a prior sPTB. They also were more likely to have delivered preterm in the index pregnancy (Table 1). Other clinical variables were not significantly different between the two cohorts.

Table 1. A comparison of the PAPR and TREETOP cohorts.

Variable	PAPR (n = 549)	TREETOP (n = 847)	p-Value
Maternal age (years) Mean (SD)	27.47 (5.88)	29.23 (5.36)	<0.001
Body mass index (kg/m^2) Mean (SD)	28.57 (7.77)	27.49 (6.96)	0.010
Maternal education n (%)			
Unknown	2 (0.36)	3 (0.35)	<0.001
No high school graduation	144 (26.23)	128 (15.11)	
High school graduation or GED	278 (50.64)	381 (44.98)	
College graduation with 4-year degree or higher	125 (22.77)	335 (39.55)	
Race n (%)			
Black or African American	89 (16.21)	173 (20.43)	<0.001
Other	52 (9.47)	165 (19.48)	
White	408 (74.32)	509 (60.09)	

Table 1. Cont.

Variable	PAPR (n = 549)	TREETOP (n = 847)	p-Value
Ethnicity n (%)			
Hispanic or Latino	192 (34.97)	335 (39.55)	0.095
Non-Hispanic or Latino	357 (65.03)	510 (60.21)	
Unknown	0 (0.00)	2 (0.24)	
Gravida n (%)			
Multigravida	389 (70.86)	570 (67.30)	0.174
Primigravida	160 (29.14)	277 (32.70)	
Prior Full-term Birth n (%)			
First Pregnancy	160 (29.14)	277 (32.70)	0.289
None	76 (13.84)	101 (11.92)	
One or more	313 (57.01)	469 (55.37)	
Prior sPTB n (%)			
First Pregnancy	160 (29.14)	277 (32.70)	<0.001
None	324 (59.02)	546 (64.46)	
One or more	65 (11.84)	24 (2.83)	
Delivery n (%)			
miPTB	29 (5.28)	32 (3.78)	0.027
sPTB	37 (6.74)	34 (4.01)	
Term	483 (87.98)	781 (92.21)	
Fetal Gender n (%)			
Ambiguous	0 (0.00)	1 (0.12)	0.771
Female	282 (51.37)	422 (49.82)	
Male	267 (48.63)	424 (50.06)	
Neonatal morbidity and mortality index n (%)			
1	482 (87.80)	767 (90.55)	0.083
2	50 (9.11)	55 (6.49)	
3	10 (1.82)	21 (2.48)	
4	7 (1.28)	4 (0.47)	

p-value (Fisher's exact test or Welch's t-test) is provided for statistical comparisons.

All outcomes were significantly predicted in TREETOP by at least the first threshold specified in the fixed sequence. Of particular interest, the proteomic biomarker threshold of -1.37 highlighted by Saade et al. [9] was statistically significant for increased sPTB in PAPR and in TREETOP (each, coincidentally, at p-value 0.041). Similarly, subjects at or above the threshold delivered earlier than those below the threshold in both studies by log-rank test (PAPR: p-value < 0.001; TREETOP: p-value 0.0016). In the combined cohort, preterm birth was significantly elevated in frequency at and above the threshold (sPTB, $p = 0.0067$, $1.8\times$; miPTB, $p = 0.0052$, $2.1\times$; PTB < 37 weeks gestation, $p < 0.001$, $1.9\times$; PTB < 35, $p = 0.011$, $2.1\times$; PTB < 32, $p = 0.0064$, $4.3\times$). The previously reported sensitivity and specificity measures for sPTB were 75% and 74%, respectively, at the proteomic biomarker threshold of maximum accuracy [9]. Sensitivity and specificity at the clinically used risk probability threshold of 15% (corresponding to a proteomic biomarker threshold of -1.37) specified in this study, were not statistically different (McNemar's test, $p = 0.48$), with significant prediction and elevation of sPTB for scores at and above the threshold ($p = 0.019$, $3.2\times$).

Neonates delivered to subjects with proteomic biomarker scores at or above the threshold had longer hospital stay than those below in both PAPR (p-value <0.001) and TREETOP (p-value 0.0053) studies (Figure 1).

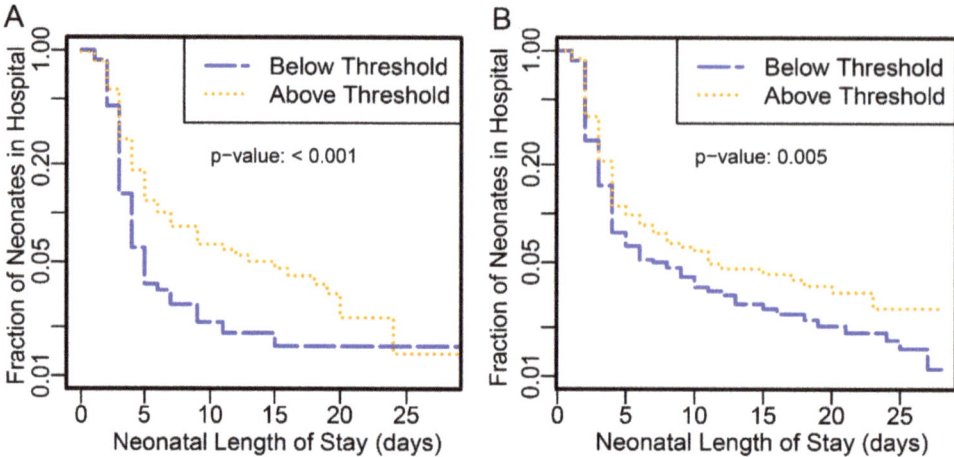

Figure 1. Kaplan–Meier curve of neonatal length of stay in days for all neonates. The fraction of neonates remaining in the hospital is plotted as a function of the length of hospital stay in days. Neonates without recorded hospital stays were omitted (A:9, B:3). Verification phase subjects from the PAPR study (**A**) and validation phase subjects from the TREETOP study (**B**) were stratified into higher- (gold) and lower-risk (blue) groups defined by the proteomic biomarker threshold −1.37.

Those preterm neonates with stays >10 days or perinatal mortality were increased by close to 3-fold at or above the threshold (Table 2, p-value < 0.001).

Table 2. Comparisons of maternal and neonatal outcomes in the combined PAPR and TREETOP populations at or above versus below the threshold of −1.37.

Threshold	NMI = 3 n (%)	NMI = 4 n (%)	Maternal Length of Hospital Stay ≥7 Days n (%)	Neonatal Length of Hospital stay >10 Days or Mortality, PTB < 37, n (%)	Neonatal Length of Hospital stay >10 Days or Mortality, PTB < 35, n (%)
Below (negative test)	18 (2.1%)	2 (0.2%)	9 (1.0%)	21 (2.4%)	17 (2.0%)
At or above (positive test)	24 (4.5%)	9 (1.7%)	23 (4.4%)	34 (6.4%)	29 (5.5%)
p-value	0.0083	0.0018	<0.001	<0.001	<0.001
Fold change	2.2	7.4	4.2	2.7	2.8

NMI = neonatal morbidity and mortality index. Counts included all infants (term or preterm) with NMI = 3 (severe morbidity) or 4 (neonatal mortality). Likewise, any mother with record of hospital stay ≥7 days was included, regardless of timing of delivery. Lastly, infants with hospital stays >10 days or perinatal mortality that delivered preterm (<37 and <35, respectively), either spontaneous or iatrogenic, were tallied.

Likewise, maternal length of stay was significantly longer amongst those subjects with scores above the proteomic biomarker threshold than below for PAPR (p-value < 0.001) and TREETOP (p-value < 0.001) (Figure 2).

Maternal length of stay ≥7 days was increased more than 4-fold at this threshold (Table 2, p < 0.001). While PAPR reported total maternal stay only, TREETOP reported antenatal and postnatal stays separately. In TREETOP, subjects at or above the threshold were hospitalized longer, both before and after delivery, than those below the threshold (antepartum p-value 0.0013; postpartum p-value 0.0027). Antepartum stay ≥5 days was increased 5.3-fold while postpartum stay ≥5 days was increased 2.5-fold. Finally, proteomic biomarker score was associated with levels of severity of NMI (Figure 3, Kendall's rank correlation p-value < 0.001).

Severe NMI (≥3) and mortality were 2.2- and 7.4-fold higher, respectively, in those at or above the proteomic biomarker threshold compared with those below (Table 2, p-values 0.0083 and 0.0018, respectively).

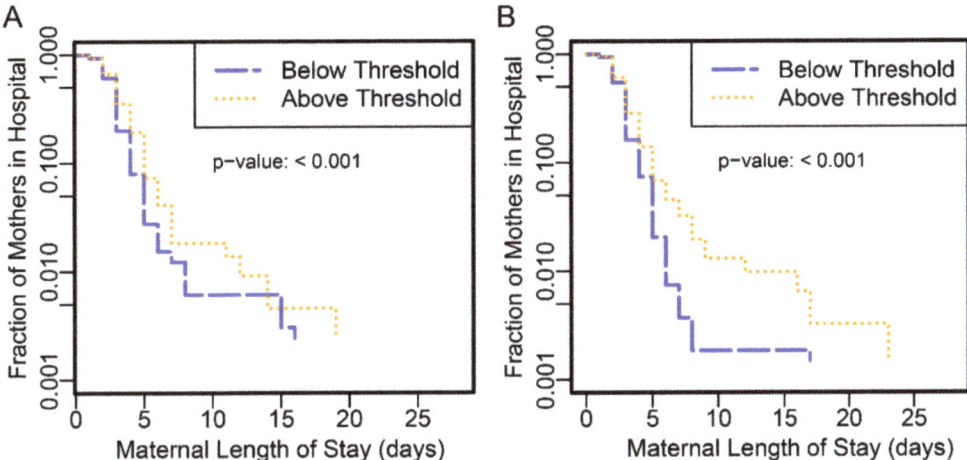

Figure 2. Kaplan–Meier curve of maternal length of stay in days. The fraction of mothers remaining in the hospital is plotted as a function of the length of hospital stay in days. Women without recorded hospital stays were omitted (**A**:3, **B**:0). Verification phase subjects from the PAPR study (**A**) and validation phase subjects from the TREETOP study (**B**) were stratified into higher- (gold) and lower-risk (blue) groups defined by the proteomic biomarker threshold of −1.37.

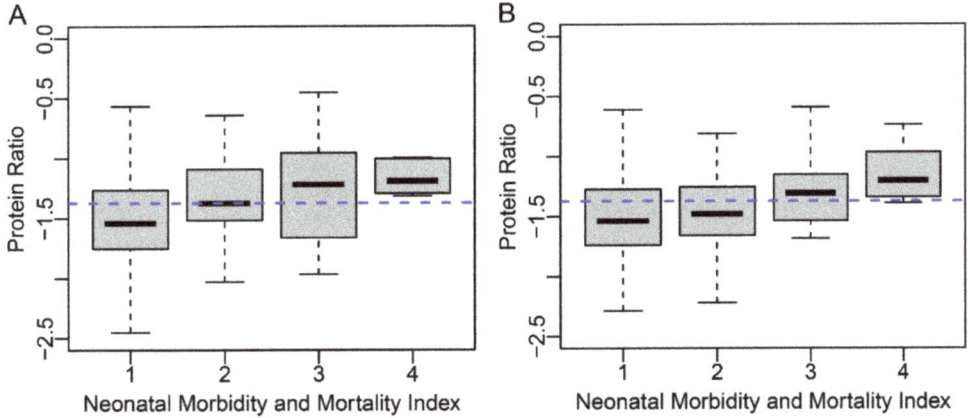

Figure 3. Distribution of all subjects by test score and NMI index. NMI distribution by proteomic biomarker in verification phase subjects from the PAPR study (**A**) and in validation phase subjects from the TREETOP study (**B**) are represented by box plots (box, interquartile range; line, mean; whiskers, remaining range of scores to a maximum of 1.5 box widths). The blue dashed line indicates the proteomic biomarker threshold of −1.37.

4. Discussion

Two large studies have been published validating the ability of the ratio of IBP4 to SHBG to risk stratify preterm delivery and associated adverse outcomes [9,16]. The National Academy of Medicine has developed and published guidelines for newly developed molecular tests which advise that such tests be replicated in a second independent study at a specific actionable threshold. Following these guidelines, we assessed an actionable threshold learned in one study and applied to the second in a critical and rigorous manner to show that not only the likelihood of spontaneous preterm delivery is similarly significantly predicted, but also the associated and clinically adverse end points are well predicted and similarly elevated at or above the threshold. A test to predict premature delivery is far more important if it can be shown that it predicts not only premature delivery, but also early premature delivery and the adverse outcomes associated with prematurity, so that interventions can be utilized, developed and tested to decrease the likelihood and/or lessen the severity of the potentially devastating complications of prematurity. Currently, for example, progesterone therapy has been shown to decrease preterm birth [24,25] and, in some studies, improve outcomes [6], but the indications for its use, women with previous spontaneous preterm delivery or short cervix, apply to a small proportion of the pregnancies that ultimately deliver prior to term. In contrast, the two studies of the IBP4/SHBG proteomic biomarker show the ratio's potential to predict the majority of preterm birth based on tested populations in excess of 1000 subjects, and for predicting associated newborn complications of prematurity as well [9,16].

The primary objective of this research was to demonstrate that statistically significant thresholds of prediction of adverse pregnancy outcomes in PAPR are also significant in the independent TREETOP population. It was of particular interest to test the proteomic biomarker threshold corresponding to a two-fold increased risk of sPTB published in Saade et al. Indeed, in this study the proteomic biomarker threshold of -1.37, corresponding to a risk probability threshold of ~15%, has been clinically validated for predicting elevated sPTB, longer neonatal and maternal length of hospital stays, and more severe neonatal outcomes.

An additional strength of this comparison of the PAPR and TREETOP studies is that while the subpopulations analyzed are both in the same intended use population for the proteomic biomarker, they are notably different on several demographic and baseline characteristics (maternal age, BMI, education, race, prior sPTB, etc.). As well, the eligible PAPR and TREETOP subjects for this study were enrolled at 10 and 14 clinical sites, respectively. All of these factors would provide further confidence that despite these demographic differences and diversity in site enrollment, the same proteomic biomarker threshold identifies pregnancies of increased risk of sPTB and associated adverse outcomes. This is strong evidence of the robust reproducibility and generalizability of the test and the validated risk threshold.

One limitation is that despite the large number of total subjects in the combined studies, the most severe and rare phenotypes analyzed had small numbers of subjects (e.g., eleven delivering with infant mortality and eighteen delivering earlier than 32 weeks).

In conclusion, we have demonstrated consistency and accordance of the proteomic biomarker in two large studies for predicting preterm delivery in a large diverse segment of low-risk pregnant women tested at a time in the second trimester when most women are seen for their anatomic ultrasound. This provides confidence that pregnancies can be robustly risk-stratified by the proteomic biomarker.

Author Contributions: Conceptualization, J.B., G.C.C., J.J.B., G.R.S. and P.E.K.; Data Curation, A.C.F. and M.T.D.; Formal Analysis, J.B., A.D.P. and P.E.K.; Investigation, J.B., T.L.R. and T.C.F.; Methodology, J.B., J.J.B. and P.E.K.; Project Administration, P.E.K.; Supervision, J.J.B. and P.E.K.; Visualization, M.T.D.; Writing—Original Draft, J.B., T.C.F., T.J.G., J.J.B. and P.E.K.; Writing—Review and Editing, J.B., A.D.P., A.C.F., T.L.R., T.C.F., M.T.D., T.J.G., G.C.C., J.J.B., G.R.S. and P.E.K. All authors have read and agreed to the published version of the manuscript.

Funding: This study was funded by Sera Prognostics. Sera Prognostics employees and consultants played a role in study design, data collection and analysis, manuscript preparation and decision to submit.

Institutional Review Board Statement: The following is a listing of all TREETOP (NCT02787213) IRBs: IRB for Human Research Medical University of South Carolina (Pro00057002, 23-May-2016), Office of Human Research Ethics The University of North Carolina at Chapel Hill (18-1544, 11-July-2018), Maricopa Integrated Health System IRB (2016-038, 7-October-2016), Oregon Health & Science University IRB (STUDY00018309, 9-May-2018), University of Texas Medical Branch IRB (17-0154, 06-July-2017), Boston Medical Center IRB (H-35437, 31-August-2016), Ochsner Clinic Foundation IRB (2016.165.B, 16-July-2016), University of California, San Diego Human Research Protections Program (161184, 29-August-2016), Northwestern University IRB (STU00203521,15-August-2016), Indiana University IRB (1606246056, 2-November-2016), Duke Medicine IRB for Clinical Investigations (Pro00080957, 31-March-2017), Greenville Health System IRB (Pro00080513, 2-August-2018),

Western IRB [used by Denver Health & Hospital Authority (20161196, 05-August-2016), University of Colorado-Denver (20161196, 21-June-18), UC-Irvine (20161196, 20-August-2016), Thomas Jefferson University (20161196, 13-October-2016), Regional Obstetrical Consultants (20161196, 23-July-2016), and Baystate Medical Center (20161196, 26-March-2017)]. The following is a listing of all PAPR (NCT01371019) IRBs: Institutional Review Board for Human Research, Office of Research Integrity, Medical University of South Carolina (Pro00012552, 11-October-2011), Office of Human Research Ethics, University of North Carolina (11-1641, 13-September-2011), Maricopa Integrated Health System Institutional Review Board (2011-078, 18-October-2011), Baystate Medical Center Institutional Review Board (BH-12-020, 23-December-2011), Research Integrity Office, Oregon Health Sciences University (IRB00008131, 7-February-2012), University of Texas Medical Branch Institutional Review Board (12-046, 29-March-2012), Christiana Care Institutional Review Board (32234, 28-December-2012), Western IRB [used by Ohio State University (20112063, 13-December-2011), San Diego Perinatal Center (20112063, 10-February-2012), Regional Obstetrical Consultants (20112063, 20-November-2012)]. All IRBs gave approval. All necessary patient/participant consent has been obtained and the appropriate institutional forms have been archived.

Informed Consent Statement: Informed consent was obtained from all subjects involved in the study.

Data Availability Statement: Data supporting the results presented here can be requested at data-sharing@seraprognostics.com. Data will not be made publicly available, or in any format, that may violate a subject's right to privacy. For example, dating information or identifiers that would allow data to be integrated, thereby enabling the potential identification of study subjects, are protected.

Acknowledgments: We thank the Principal Investigators of the PAPR clinical trial (NCT01371019): Kim A. Boggess, Scott A. Sullivan, Glenn R. Markenson, Jay D. Iams, Dean V. Coonrod, Leonardo M. Pereira, M. Sean Esplin, Larry M. Cousins, Garrett K. Lam, Matthew K. Hoffman, and TREE-TOP(NCT02787213): Glenn R. Markenson, Louise C. Laurent, Kent D. Heyborne, Dean V. Coonrod, Corina N. Schoen, Jason K. Baxter, David M. Haas, Sherri Longo, William A. Grobman, Scott A. Sullivan, Carol A. Major, Sarahn M. Wheeler, Leonardo M. Pereira, Emily J. Su, Kim A. Boggess, Angela F. Hawk, and Amy H. Crockett for contributing samples and clinical data. We also thank Glenn R. Markenson for critical review of the manuscript. Finally, we thank Babak Shahbaba, who conducted fixed sequence hypotheses testing.

Conflicts of Interest: The authors of this manuscript have the following competing interests: J.B., A.C.F., T.C.F., M.T.D., T.J.G., G.C.C. and J.J.B. are employees and stockholders of Sera Prognostics. A.D.P., T.L.R. and P.E.K. are consultants and stockholders for Sera Prognostics. G.R.S. does not have competing interests.

References

1. Blencowe, H.; Vos, T.; Lee, A.C.; Philips, R.; Lozano, R.; Alvarado, M.R.; Cousens, S.; Lawn, J.E. Estimates of neonatal morbidities and disabilities at regional and global levels for 2010: Introduction, methods overview, and relevant findings from the Global Burden of Disease study. *Pediatr. Res.* **2013**, *74* (Suppl. 1), 4–16. [CrossRef]
2. Martin, J.A.; Hamilton, B.E.; Osterman, M.J.K.; Driscoll, A.K.; Drake, P. Births: Final Data for 2017. *Natl. Vital Stat. Rep.* **2018**, *67*, 1–50. [PubMed]
3. Waitzman, N.J.; Jalali, A.; Grosse, S.D. Preterm birth lifetime costs in the United States in 2016: An update. *Semin. Perinatol.* **2021**, *45*, 151390. [CrossRef] [PubMed]
4. Laughon, S.K.; Albert, P.S.; Leishear, K.; Mendola, P. The NICHD Consecutive Pregnancies Study: Recurrent preterm delivery by subtype. *Am. J. Obs. Gynecol.* **2014**, *210*, 131.e1–131.e8. [CrossRef] [PubMed]
5. Petrini, J.R.; Callaghan, W.M.; Klebanoff, M.; Green, N.S.; Lackritz, E.M.; Howse, J.L.; Schwarz, R.H.; Damus, K. Estimated effect of 17 alpha-hydroxyprogesterone caproate on preterm birth in the United States. *Obs. Gynecol.* **2005**, *105*, 267–272. [CrossRef] [PubMed]
6. Hassan, S.S.; Romero, R.; Vidyadhari, D.; Fusey, S.; Baxter, J.K.; Khandelwal, M.; Vijayaraghavan, J.; Trivedi, Y.; Soma-Pillay, P.; Sambarey, P.; et al. Vaginal progesterone reduces the rate of preterm birth in women with a sonographic short cervix: A multicenter, randomized, double-blind, placebo-controlled trial. *Ultrasound Obs. Gynecol.* **2011**, *38*, 18–31. [CrossRef] [PubMed]
7. McIntosh, J.; Feltovich, H.; Berghella, V.; Manuck, T. The role of routine cervical length screening in selected high- and low-risk women for preterm birth prevention. *Am. J. Obs. Gynecol.* **2016**, *215*, B2–B7. [CrossRef]
8. Micheel, C.M.; Nass, S.J.; Omenn, G.S. (Eds.) *Evolution of Translational Omics: Lessons Learned and the Path Forward*; National Academies Press: Cambridge, MA, USA, 2012.

9. Saade, G.R.; Boggess, K.A.; Sullivan, S.A.; Markenson, G.R.; Iams, J.D.; Coonrod, D.V.; Pereira, L.M.; Esplin, M.S.; Cousins, L.M.; Lam, G.K.; et al. Development and validation of a spontaneous preterm delivery predictor in asymptomatic women. *Am. J. Obs. Gynecol.* **2016**, *214*, 633.e1–633.e24. [CrossRef] [PubMed]
10. Crosley, E.J.; Dunk, C.E.; Beristain, A.G.; Christians, J.K. IGFBP-4 and -5 are expressed in first-trimester villi and differentially regulate the migration of HTR-8/SVneo cells. *Reprod. Biol. Endocrinol.* **2014**, *12*, 123. [CrossRef] [PubMed]
11. Forbes, K.; Westwood, M. Maternal growth factor regulation of human placental development and fetal growth. *J. Endocrinol.* **2010**, *207*, 1–16. [CrossRef] [PubMed]
12. Larrea, F.; Diaz, L.; Carino, C.; Larriva-Sahd, J.; Carrillo, L.; Orozco, H.; Ulloa-Aguirre, A. Evidence that human placenta is a site of sex hormone-binding globulin gene expression. *J. Steroid. Biochem. Mol. Biol.* **1993**, *46*, 497–505. [CrossRef]
13. O'Leary, P.; Boyne, P.; Flett, P.; Beilby, J.; James, I. Longitudinal assessment of changes in reproductive hormones during normal pregnancy. *Clin. Chem.* **1991**, *37*, 667–672. [CrossRef] [PubMed]
14. Wallace, I.R.; McKinley, M.C.; Bell, P.M.; Hunter, S.J. Sex hormone binding globulin and insulin resistance. *Clin. Endocrinol. (Oxf.)* **2013**, *78*, 321–329. [CrossRef] [PubMed]
15. Simo, R.; Saez-Lopez, C.; Barbosa-Desongles, A.; Hernandez, C.; Selva, D.M. Novel insights in SHBG regulation and clinical implications. *Trends Endocrinol. Metab.* **2015**, *26*, 376–383. [CrossRef] [PubMed]
16. Markenson, G.R.; Saade, G.R.; Laurent, L.C.; Heyborne, K.D.; Coonrod, D.V.; Schoen, C.N.; Baxter, J.K.; Haas, D.M.; Longo, S.; Grobman, W.A.; et al. Performance of a proteomic preterm delivery predictor in a large independent prospective cohort. *Am. J. Obstet. Gynecol. MFM* **2020**, *2*, 100140. [CrossRef]
17. Bradford, C.; Severinsen, R.; Pugmire, T.; Rasmussen, M.; Stoddard, K.; Uemura, Y.; Wheelwright, S.; Mentinova, M.; Chelsky, D.; Hunsucker, S.W.; et al. Analytical validation of protein biomarkers for risk of spontaneous preterm birth. *Clin. Mass Spectrom.* **2017**, *3*, 25–38. [CrossRef]
18. ACOG. Committee opinion no 611: Method for estimating due date. *Obs. Gynecol* **2014**, *124*, 863–866. [CrossRef] [PubMed]
19. R Core Team. *R: A Language and Environment for Statistical Computing*; R Foundation for Statistical Computing: Vienna, Austria, 2014.
20. Dowle, M.; Srinivasan, A. data.table: Extension of 'data.frame', R Package Version 1.11.4. Available online: https://CRAN.R-project.org/package=data.table (accessed on 1 July 2018).
21. Robinson, L. *demoGraphic: Providing Demographic Table with the p-Value, Standardized Mean Difference Value*; R package version 0.1.0; R Foundation for Statistical Computing: Vienna, Austria, 2019.
22. Therneau, T.M. A Package for Survival Analysis in R. Available online: https://CRAN.R-project.org/package=survival (accessed on 1 February 2021).
23. Therneau, T.M.; Grambsch, P.M. *Modeling Survival Data: Extending the {C}ox Model*; Springer: Berlin/Heidelberg, Germany, 2000.
24. da Fonseca, E.B.; Bittar, R.E.; Carvalho, M.H.; Zugaib, M. Prophylactic administration of progesterone by vaginal suppository to reduce the incidence of spontaneous preterm birth in women at increased risk: A randomized placebo-controlled double-blind study. *Am. J. Obs. Gynecol.* **2003**, *188*, 419–424. [CrossRef]
25. Meis, P.J.; Klebanoff, M.; Thom, E.; Dombrowski, M.P.; Sibai, B.; Moawad, A.H.; Spong, C.Y.; Hauth, J.C.; Miodovnik, M.; Varner, M.W.; et al. Prevention of Recurrent Preterm Delivery by 17 Alpha-Hydroxyprogesterone Caproate. *N. Engl. J. Med.* **2003**, *348*, 2379–2385. [CrossRef] [PubMed]

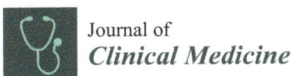

Journal of
Clinical Medicine

Article

Sildenafil Citrate Downregulates PDE5A mRNA Expression in Women with Recurrent Pregnancy Loss without Altering Angiogenic Factors—A Preliminary Study

Monika Kniotek [1], Aleksander Roszczyk [1], Michał Zych [1], Małgorzata Wrzosek [2,3,*], Monika Szafarowska [4], Radosław Zagożdżon [1,5] and Małgorzata Jerzak [2,3,6]

1. Department of Clinical Immunology, Medical University of Warsaw, 59 Nowogrodzka St., 02-006 Warsaw, Poland; monika.kniotek@wum.edu.pl (M.K.); aleksander.roszczyk@wum.edu.pl (A.R.); michal.zych@wum.edu.pl (M.Z.); radoslaw.zagozdzon@wum.edu.pl (R.Z.)
2. Department of Biochemistry and Pharmacogenomics, Faculty of Pharmacy, Medical University of Warsaw, 1 Banacha St., 02-097 Warsaw, Poland; mmjerzak@wp.pl
3. Laboratory of Biochemistry and Clinical Chemistry, Preclinical Research Center, Medical University of Warsaw, 1 Banacha St., 02-097 Warsaw, Poland
4. Department of Gynecology and Oncological Gynecology, Military Institute of Medicine, 128 Szaserów St., 04-141 Warsaw, Poland; monika.szafarowska@wp.pl
5. Department of Immunology, Transplantology and Internal Diseases, Medical University of Warsaw, 59 Nowogrodzka St., 02-006 Warsaw, Poland
6. m-CLINIC 77/U9 Puławska St., 02-595 Warsawa, Poland
* Correspondence: malgorzata.wrzosek@wum.edu.pl

Citation: Kniotek, M.; Roszczyk, A.; Zych, M.; Wrzosek, M.; Szafarowska, M.; Zagożdżon, R.; Jerzak, M. Sildenafil Citrate Downregulates PDE5A mRNA Expression in Women with Recurrent Pregnancy Loss without Altering Angiogenic Factors—A Preliminary Study. *J. Clin. Med.* **2021**, *10*, 5086. https://doi.org/10.3390/jcm10215086

Academic Editors: Alex Heazell and Sylvie Girard

Received: 27 July 2021
Accepted: 25 October 2021
Published: 29 October 2021

Publisher's Note: MDPI stays neutral with regard to jurisdictional claims in published maps and institutional affiliations.

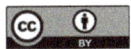

Copyright: © 2021 by the authors. Licensee MDPI, Basel, Switzerland. This article is an open access article distributed under the terms and conditions of the Creative Commons Attribution (CC BY) license (https://creativecommons.org/licenses/by/4.0/).

Abstract: In our previous study, we showed that sildenafil citrate (SC), a selective PDE5A blocker, modulated NK cell activity in patients with recurrent pregnancy loss, which correlated with positive pregnancy outcomes. It was found that NK cells had a pivotal role in decidualization, angiogenesis, spiral artery remodeling, and the regulation of trophoblast invasion. Thus, in the current study, we determined the effects of SC on angiogenic factor expression and production, as well as idNK cell activity in the presence of nitric synthase blocker L-NMMA. Methods: NK cells (CD56$^+$) were isolated from the peripheral blood of 15 patients and 15 fertile women on MACS columns and cultured in transformation media containing IL-15, TGF-β, and AZA—a methylation agent—for 7 days in hypoxia (94% N_2, 1% O_2, 5% CO_2). Cultures were set up in four variants: (1) with SC, (2) without SC, (3) with NO, a synthase blocker, and (4) with SC and NO synthase blocker. NK cell activity was determined after 7 days of culturing as CD107a expression after an additional 4h of stimulation with K562 erythroleukemia cells. The expression of the *PDE5A*, *VEGF-A*, *PlGF*, *IL-8*, and *RENBP* genes was determined with quantitative real-time PCR (qRT-PCR) using TaqMan probes and ELISA was used to measure the concentrations of VEGF-A, PLGF, IL-8, Ang-I, Ang-II, IFN-γ proteins in culture supernatants after SC supplementation. Results: SC downregulated *PDE5A* expression and had no effect on other studied angiogenic factors. *VEGF-A* expression was increased in RPL patients compared with fertile women. Similarly, VEGF production was enhanced in RPL patients' supernatants and SC increased the concentration of PlGF in culture supernatants. SC did not affect the expression or concentration of other studied factors, nor idNK cell activity, regardless of NO synthase blockade.

Keywords: RPL; NK cells; sildenafil; PDE5A; VEGF-A; angiotensin

1. Introduction

Unexplained recurrent pregnancy loss [1] is a growing health problem worldwide. It is estimated that RPL affects over 1% of the general population and only half of the cases can be explained after a medical investigation. Each miscarriage increases the risk of another miscarriage to 15% [2,3]. Recurrent pregnancy loss [2] was defined according to the WHO definition as three or more consecutive spontaneous miscarriages before the 20th week of gestation [4,5]. ESHRE guidelines indicated immunological diagnostics in case of two idiopathic pregnancy losses [1]. Despite well-described causes of RPL, such as chromosomal abnormalities, uterine anatomical malformations, endocrine dysfunctions, thrombophilic factors, and immune disorders, the reasons remain unknown in approximately 50% of RPL cases [6].

It was reported that sildenafil citrate (SC) could be applied for the treatment of such complications during pregnancy as intrauterine fetal growth restriction (FGR) [7–10], low birth weight [11], preeclampsia, or idiopathic recurrent pregnancy losses [10–15]. However, recent findings have emphasized the lack of action of sildenafil on FGR and suggested further studies to assess the safety and efficacy of SC in utero, in addition to the implications on long-term health [16]. Clinical research showed that SC might increase the risk of neonatal pulmonary hypertension [17]. Nonetheless, our previous clinical research showed decreased NK activity in in vivo and in vitro research in 40 RPL patients treated with SC suppositories BEFORE conception, which correlated with positive pregnancy outcomes: live births and the lack of complications during pregnancy [12]. Therefore, SC may modulate the immune response to the trophoblast antigens and endometrial environment by the modification of NK cell function [12,13,18–20].

SC increases cellular cGMP levels through competition for the phosphodiesterase binding site with cGMP, thus inhibiting the degradation of cGMP to GMP [21]. A high level of cGMP results in increased NO production and subsequently causes the relaxation of vascular smooth muscles and increases vasodilation [7,21,22]. Vaginal sildenafil acting through NO improves uterine artery blood flow and sonographic endometrial thickness in patients with previous failed assisted reproductive cycles due to poor endometrial response. While improving uterine blood flow in the proliferative phase, NO may exert a detrimental effect on the development of the endometrium during the implantation window [11,12]. NO mediates the release of cytokines such as tumor necrosis factor-α [6,23] secreted from activated natural killer cells [24] which was implicated as a cause of implantation failure [12]. Normally, NK cells, which account for approx. A total of 70% of the decidual immune cells as so-called 'decidual NK cells (dNK)' [25] have a high capacity of producing cytokines such as IFN-γ, TNF-α, GM-CSF, TGF-β, and IL-10. Previous reports implied that this special population of dNK cells was involved in decidualization, angiogenesis [24], the regulation of trophoblast invasion [18], and spiral artery remodeling [26] by promoting the production of certain cytokines and factors, e.g., interferon gamma-induced protein 10 (IP-10), vascular endothelial growth factor A (VEGF-A), and IFN-γ [27]. The expression of placental growth factor (PlGF), angiogenin, endostatin, and sIL-2R increased by dNK cells may contribute to pregnancy disorders associated with poor spiral artery remodeling [25]. It was shown that angiotensin II induced vascular dysfunction dependent on IFN-γ production by NK cells [28]. Jurewicz et al. demonstrated that NK cells were fully equipped with renin–angiotensin system elements: renin, the renin receptor, angiotensinogen, and angiotensin-converting enzymes, which were capable of producing and delivering Ang II to the sites of inflammation [29]. The local renin–angiotensin system in the placenta plays an extremely important role in placental development. It was established that most of the circulating and local RAS components were over-expressed during normal pregnancy and the disruption of the balance might cause pregnancy complications [30].

dNK cells are characterized by limited cytotoxicity and they control embryo implantation and spiral artery formation [18,29]. However, several studies showed that women with recurrent pregnancy loss had a higher cytotoxic activity of NK cells both in the periphery and in the endometrium compared with healthy fertile women [31–33]. Our previous research showed that SC decreased peripheral blood NK activity in women with RPL treated with SC suppositories, which was correlated with positive pregnancy outcomes [12].

In 2013, Cadeira et al. proposed an in vitro model of the conversion of peripheral blood NK cells (pbNK) into induced decidual NK cells (idNK cells), which resembled dNK cells phenotypically and functionally [34].

In the current study we attempted to establish whether SC influenced the activity of idNK cells, obtained via the above-mentioned method, through blocking phosphodiesterase 5A (PDE5A) and increasing the level of cGMP or NO synthase activation. To determine if SC can influence idNK cell angiogenic activity, we used a real-time polymerase chain reaction to measure the mRNA levels of VEGF-A, PlGF, CXCL8 (IL-8), and PDE5A in idNK cells cultured with or without SC. Additionally, we measured VEGF-A, PLGF, IL-8, IFN-γ, angiotensin I (Ang I), and angiotensin II (Ang II) concentrations in the supernatants obtained from the cultures.

2. Material and Methods

The study was approved by the Bioethics Committee of the Medical University of Warsaw (No. KB/192/2015). All measurements, interventions, and blood collections were performed after informed consent had been obtained.

2.1. Control Group

The control group consisted of 15 fertile women without a history of obstetric-gynecological and internal disorders. None of the subjects included in the control group reported any problems regarding conception; all subjects declared a normal course of pregnancy and delivery. Moreover, none of the control subjects were treated for any internal disorders. Women on oral hormonal contraception and other forms of hormonal treatment, or women with hormonal intrauterine devices, were excluded from the study. Transvaginal ultrasound scans were performed in all the patients between day 3 and day 5 of the menstrual cycle to reveal the normal morphology of the uterus, endometrium, and appendages.

2.2. Study Group

One hundred and fifty patients with RPL were evaluated. However, only fifteen patients with RPL were finally included in the study group because of very strict exclusion criteria. Recurrent pregnancy loss was defined according to the WHO definition as three or more consecutive spontaneous miscarriages before the 20th week of gestation [35]. All studied patients had experienced the last miscarriage at least 6 months before the research. Therefore, the immunological status of patients had normalized before the study. A complete medical, surgical, and social history was obtained in all cases. All the women with a history of RPL were investigated in terms of any identifiable causes of abortion. Hysterosalpingography or hysteroscopy revealed no abnormalities in the patients' uteri. The study group underwent peripheral blood chromosome assessment which revealed normal karyotypes. Patients with anatomic, genetic, microbiological, immunological, and hormonal causes of abortions were excluded from the research. The women with RPL were tested for thrombophilia and immunological markers such as aPL and none of them exhibited any defects. The characteristics of the study group, including age and the number of spontaneous pregnancy losses, are listed in Table S1.

3. Methods

3.1. The Isolation of Peripheral Blood Mononuclear Cells and CD56$^+$ Cells

Peripheral blood mononuclear cells (PBMC) were isolated from the peripheral blood of 15 women with recurrent miscarriages and 15 healthy volunteers via Ficoll gradient centrifugation. After being washed twice in phosphate-buffered saline (PBS, Biomed, Lublin, Poland), the cells were suspended in 1 mL of cold MACS buffer (MiltenyiBiotec, Auburn, CA, USA) The cells were counted and stained according to the manufacturer's instructions with the appropriate amount of CD56$^+$ microbeads. After washing, the stained cells were separated with MidiMACS manual separator (MiltenyiBiotec, Auburn, CA, USA) according to the manufacturer's instructions (MiltenyiBiotec, Auburn, CA, USA). After isolation, we obtained approximately 2×10^6 CD56-positive cells with 96% purity.

3.2. Cell Culture

Isolated CD56-positive cells were cultured in 24-well plates (SPL Life Sciences Co., Ltd., Naechon-Myeon, Gyeonggi-do, South Korea), in Opti-MEM Reduced Serum Media (Gibco, Thermo Fisher Scientific, Waltham, MA, USA) containing 10% FCS (MERK, KGaA, Darmstadt, Germany), 1 U/ML penicillin/streptomycin/100 µg/mL [11], 2 mM glutamine (Sigma Aldrich), 1 mM sodium pyruvate (Fluka), nonessential amino acids ((MERK, KGaA, Darmstadt, Germany), 55 mM 2-mercaptoethanol, 10 ng/mL recombinant human IL-15 (MERK, KGaA, Darmstadt, Germany), 2 ng/mL recombinant human TGF-β-1 (R&D), and 1 µM 5-aza-2′deoxycytidine (AZA, (MERK, KGaA, Darmstadt, Germany), in a hypoxic (94% N_2, 5% CO_2, 1% O_2) environment [24].

The cells were cultured at a concentration of 1×10^6/mL in 4 variants: NK cells in the medium, NK cells with 400 ng/mL of sildenafil citrate (MERK, KGaA, Darmstadt, Germany), NK cells with 500 µM of NOS inhibitor—NG-Monomethyl-L-arginine, monoacetate salt (L-NMMA, (MERK, KGaA, Darmstadt, Germany), NK cells with 500 µM of L-NMMA and SC (both from MERK, KGaA, Darmstadt, Germany), [36,37]. The concentration of SC used in the experiments was consistent with the physiological concentration of 200 mg of orally administered Viagra in the blood of a healthy man [38]. Hypoxic conditions were obtained by culturing cells in a sealed anaerobic workstation incubator (Modular Incubator Chamber, MIC-101, Billups-Rothenberg, Inc., Del Mar, CA, USA), incorporated with a gas flow measurement system (DFM 3002, Biogenet, Józefów, Poland) and flushed with a mixture of 1% O_2, 5% CO_2, and 94% N_2. The entry and exit ports of the chambers were subsequently clamped, and the chambers were placed in a 37 °C incubator. After 5 days of culturing, the cells were harvested for the determination of idNK cell degranulation and activity or gene expression pattern.

3.3. Degranulation of idNK Cells—CD107a Expression Determination

After 5 days of culturing, idNK cells were seeded with the E:T ratio of 2:1 and 1:1 in falcon tubes in RPMI full medium and incubated for 4 h at 37 °C and 5% CO_2. For functional assays, anti-CD107a APC was added together with monensin (GolgiStop TM, Becton Dickinson, Franklin Lakes, NJ, USA) and brefeldin A (GolgiPlug TM, Becton Dickinson, Franklin Lakes, NJ, USA) at the beginning of the assay. At the end of the assay, the cells were stained for CD3-FITC, CD56-PE surface markers to identify the CD3$^-$CD56$^+$ idNK-cell subsets. Gating strategy and cut-off values of positive fluorescence were based on a fluorescence minus one (FMO) experiment and are shown in supplementary data (Figure S1). Cell readouts were acquired using a Becton Dickinson FACSCanto II cytometer (BD FACS Canto II, Becton Dickinson, Franklin Lakes, NJ, USA) and analyzed with BD FACS Diva 6.1.3. software. Analyses were conducted on live cells only [39].

3.4. The Determination of the Gene Expression of Selected Angiogenic Factors

Cultures for gene expression determination were performed in 2 versions: The culture of idNK cells and idNK cells supplemented with SC. The cells were centrifuged at 800 *g* for 10 min., culture supernatants were collected and frozen at −80 °C for subsequent analysis with the enzyme-linked immunosorbent assay (ELISA) and idNK cells were suspended in a lysis buffer (RLT buffer, Qiagen, Hilden, Germany). RNA was extracted from frozen idNK cells using the guanidinium-thiocyanate-based RNA extraction (Qiagen RNeasy Mini Kit, Qiagen, Valencia, CA) followed by column-based purification. RNA concentration and the purity were evaluated with a micro-volume UV-Vis spectrophotometer (Quawell Q3000, Quawell Technology Inc., San Jose, CA, USA). Quantitative RT-PCR was carried out with the RNA-to-C_T™ 1-Step kit [(Applied Biosystems (AB), Foster City, CA, USA]. The TaqMan Gene Expression Assays (Thermo Fisher Scientific Inc., Waltham, MA, USA) were performed with the use of a ViiA™7 Real-Time PCR system (Applied Biosystems; Thermo

Fisher Scientific, Inc.) under the following thermocycling conditions: 48 °C for 15 min, 95 °C for 10 min and 40 cycles of 95 °C for 15 sec and 60 °C for 1 min. TaqMan Probes used for RT-PCR are presented in Table 1. Data were normalized to the reference genes (GAPDH and B2M, Table 1) and the relative expression level of each target gene was expressed as $2^{-(Ct;\ Target\ gene\ -Ct;\ Reference\ gene)}$. All qRT-PCR experiments were run in triplicate, and the mean value was used for the determination of mRNA levels [40,41].

Table 1. TaqMan probes used for RT-PCR in determination of the gene expression of selected angiogenic factors.

Gene Name	Gene Symbol	Assay ID
Phosphodiesterase 5A	PDE5A	Hs00153649_m1
Vascular endothelial growth factor A	VEGF-A	Hs00900055_m1
Placental growth factor	PIGF	Hs00182176_m1
Renin binding protein	RENBP	Hs00234138_m1
C-X-C motif chemokine ligand 8	CXCL8 (IL-8)	Hs00174103_m1
Glyceraldehyde-3-phosphate dehydrogenase	GAPDH	Hs99999905_m1
Beta-2-microglobulin	B2M	Hs99999907_m1

3.5. The Determination of the Concentration of Angiogenic Factors

The concentrations of selected cytokines and angiogenic factors (VEGF-A, PIGF, IL-8, IFN-γ, Ang I, Ang II) were measured in idNK culture supernatants twice via the enzyme-linked immunosorbent assay (ELISA) according to the manufacturer's instructions. The concentrations of cytokines were calculated from a standard curve of linear regression according to the manufacturer's instructions (ELISA kits, Bioassay Technology Laboratory, Shanghai, China). The sensitivity of ELISA kits were: VEGF-A—1.52 ng/L, PIGF—4.02 ng/mL, INF-γ—0.49 ng/mL, IL-8—2.51 ng/L, angiotensin I (Ang I) < 75 pg/mL, angiotensin II (Ang II)—18.75 pg/mL. The intra-assay CV was < 8% and the inter-assay CV was < 10% for all used kits [42].

3.6. Statistical Analysis

All statistical analyses were performed with Graph Pad Prism 9.00. The normal distribution of data was determined with the Shapiro–Wilk test. In order to determine the statistical significance between the control and study group samples, the unpaired t-test was used in case of the normal distribution of data, and the Mann–Whitney U test was used in case of non-normal distribution. The analyses of data inside the groups (samples after culturing with SC) were performed with the Wilcoxon signed-rank test in case of non-normal distribution and the paired t-test for the normal distribution of samples. The p values below 0.05 ($p < 0.05$) were considered statistically significant. The data were shown as the median and interquartile range (IQR) in the figures.

4. Results

No difference was observed as regards the age between RPL patients (36.70 $\pm$ 4.48) and healthy women (37.40 $\pm$ 1.90).

4.1. The Determination of the Gene Expression of PDE5A and Selected Angiogenic Factors

The PDE5A enzyme was expressed in idNK cells, and its expression was significantly higher in RPL women than in healthy women (Figures 1 and 2) The addition of 400 ng/mL SC to the culture decreased the expression of *PDE5A* in RPL patients (Figure 1). We also found a significantly higher expression of *VEGF-A* in RPL patients than in the control group (Figure 2). No significant differences occurred in the mRNA expression of *PIGF, RNEBP,* and *CXCL8 (IL-8)* between the studied groups. However, the expression of IL-8 showed a wide range in RPL and control group (Figures 1 and 2).

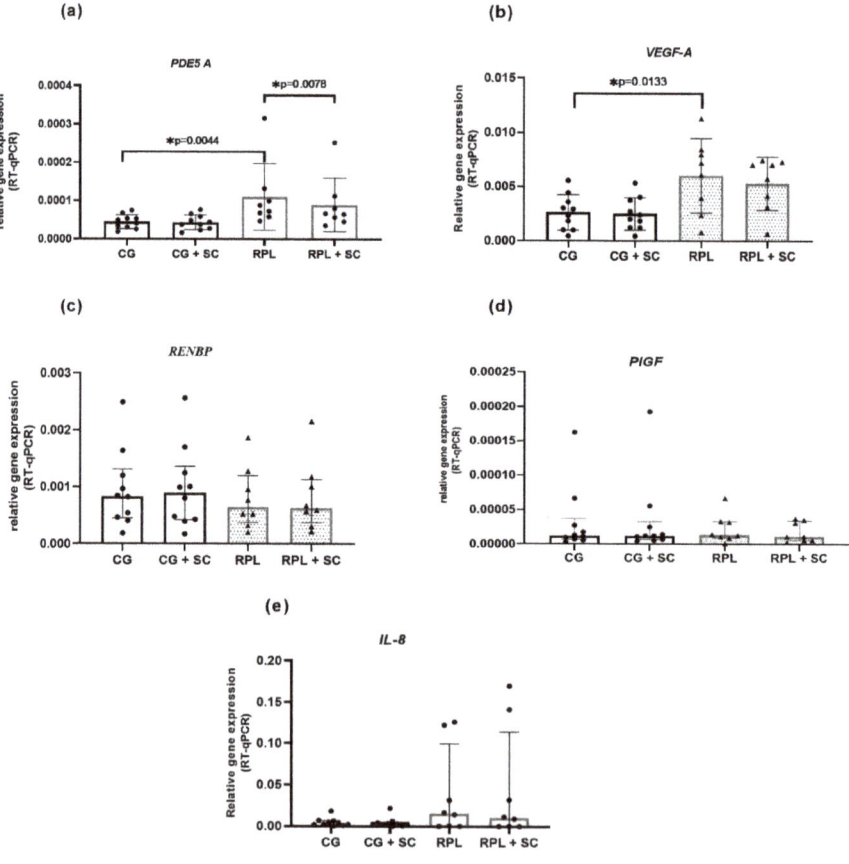

Figure 1. PDE5A, VEGF-A, ANG-I, PIGF, IL-8 expression after SC treatment in the idNK cells of healthy and RPL women, data shown as the mean ± SD compared with idNK cells maintained without SC (green points, CG—control group, $n = 10$; red points—RPL patients, $n = 8$; statistical significance * $p < 0.05$).

Figure 2. The expression of *PDE5A* and *VEGF-A* is upregulated in the idNK cells of patients with RPL. SC downregulated *PDE5A* gene expression in RPL group, (**a**) a genomic meta-analysis of PDE5A gene expression in idNK cells, (**b**) a genomic meta-analysis of *VEGF-A* gene expression in idNK cells (**c**) a genomic meta-analysis of *RNEBP* gene expression in idNK cells, (**d**) a genomic meta-analysis of *PIGF* gene expression in idNK cells, (**e**) a genomic meta-analysis of *IL-8* gene expression in idNK cells; data are shown as the median and interquartile range, CG—control group $n = 10$, RPL patients $n = 8$, circles and triangles represents single samples; SC—sildenafil citrate 400 ng/mL, statistical significance marked as star—* $p < 0.05$.

4.2. The Levels of Angiogenic Factors in the Culture Supernatants of idNK Cells

The concentrations of IL-8, IFN-γ, and angiogenic factors (VEGF-A, PlGF, angiotensin I, angiotensin II) were measured in the culture supernatants of idNK cells with the ELISA method. Surprisingly, we found no difference in protein levels between the studied groups before or after SC treatment (Figure 3). Similarly to gene expression, we found that VEGF-A concentration was upregulated in RPL patients. Moreover, PlGF level was enhanced after SC treatment.

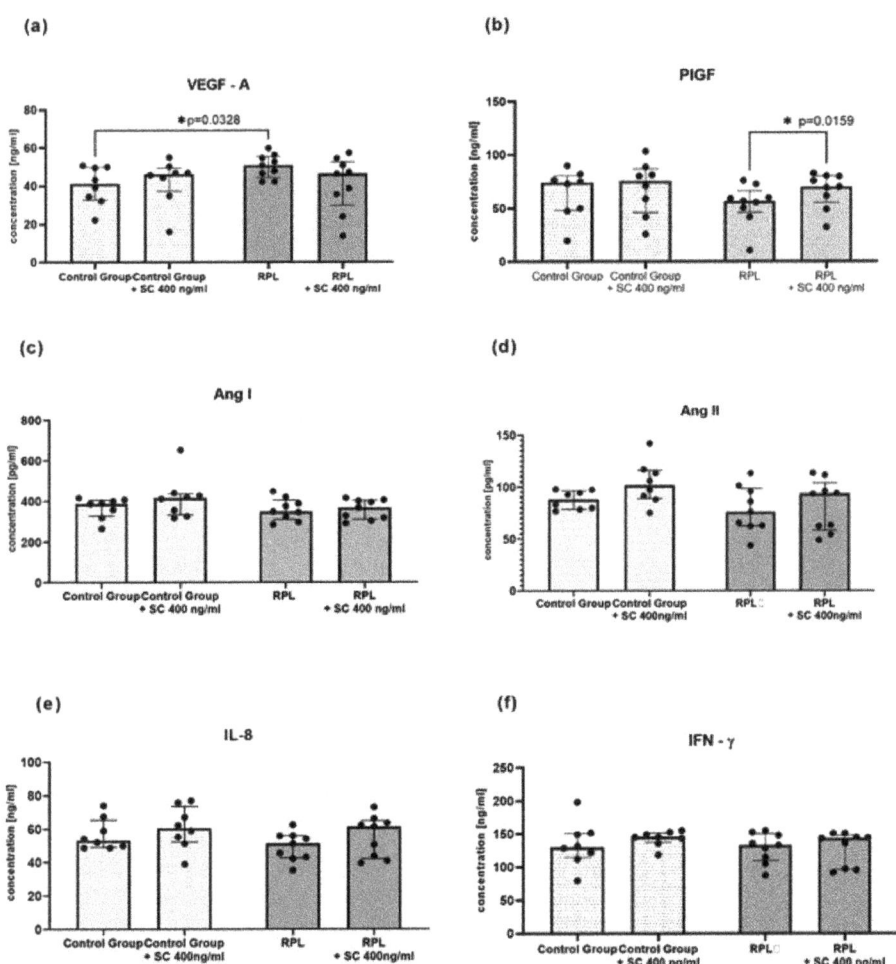

Figure 3. The concentrations of angiogenic factors and cytokines in idNK cultures with and without sildenafil citrate: (**a**) VEGF-A, (**b**) PlGF, (**c**) Ang I, (**d**) Ang II, (**e**) IL-8; (**f**) IFN-γ; Control group $n = 9$, RPL patients $n = 8$; dots on the figures reflects numbers of determined samples, SC—sildenafil citrate 400 ng/mL, statistical significance marked as star—* $p < 0.05$.

4.3. idNK Cell Activity and CD107a Expression

The flow cytometry determination of idNK cell cytotoxicity and degranulation did not reveal any differences between the groups. The blockage of NO synthase with L-NMMA did not alter idNK activity or the expression of CD107a in the studied groups. Sildenafil citrate did not influence idNK cell function in any of the studied variants (Figure S2).

5. Discussion

Decidualization, which involves a dramatic morphological and functional differentiation of human endometrial stromal and immune cells, plays an important role in promoting placental formation to support pregnancy [43]. dNK cells are the most abundant population of immune cells in the decidua. Almost a decade has passed since researchers pointed out that increased pbNk cell activity reflected the activity of decidual NK cells [29]. Further studies on dNK cells revealed their regulatory function during a physiological pregnancy, including the creation of optimal conditions for blastocyst invasion, control of the invasion process depending on gestation terms, as well as taking part in the uterus spiral artery remodeling and uterus–placenta normal blood flow establishment [25,44–46].

In our previous study, we observed that sildenafil citrate decreased pbNK cell activity, and improved uterine blood flow and the endometrial thickness of women with RPL [12]. Thus, in the present study, we verified the influence of SC on the activity and angiogenic properties of idNK cells. We found that supplementing the culture with a low dose of sildenafil citrate downregulated *PDE5* gene expression. To the best of our knowledge, it is the first study investigating the expression of *PDE5A* phosphodiesterase in human NK cells and idNK cells. Furthermore, we showed the expression of the gene was significantly higher in RPL patients, which suggests a faster conversion of cGMP to GMP in the dNK cells of RPL patients. CGMP indirectly activates NO synthases, and it is known that nitric oxide (NO) improves endometrial thickness by enhancing uterine blood flow (7, 9). It also improves NK activity [36]. The shortage of cGMP in the cells of RPL patients may disturb NO release and, subsequently, cause an inadequate cytotrophoblast invasion of the uterine spiral arteries and endometrium growth, as well as embryonic cell proliferation decrease [12,47–49]. The downregulation of *PDE5* gene expression by SC may restore the required level of cGMP and improve NO production demanded during trophoblast implantation. However, further research is needed.

We performed cultures of idNK cells with and without a blocker of NO synthase (L-NMMA) supplementation in a hypoxic (1% of oxygen) environment to determine if SC influenced iNOs synthase and modulated NK activity. Cifoni et al. showed that NO synthase inhibitors impaired NK cell-mediated target cell killing [50]. However, L-NMMA, SC, or both compounds did not affect idNK activity towards K562 tumor cells or the expression of lysosomal-associated membrane protein-1 (LAMP-1; CD107a) in our research. Sanson and Malagoni reported that even in the presence of L-NMMA, NO generation occurred following hypoxia [51]. Therefore, it was probably hypoxia which abolished the effect of L-NMMA in our study. Moreover, transformation media for idNK cell cultures contained IL-15 cytokine which plays a dominant role in NK cell activation. It was shown that brief priming with IL-15 markedly enhanced the antitumor response of $CD56^{bright}$ NK cells [52]. Furthermore, we observed no changes in the CD107a expression on idNK cells after SC addition. The data are in opposition to our previous results obtained from the cultures of PBMC, where SC decreased pbNK cell activity after 48 h of culturing [12]. It may also suggest an influence of other immune cells controlling NK activity and the impact of hypoxia on idNK cells. According to some authors, hypoxia improves NO release, and subsequently improves NK cell activity [6,24,50].

It was found that hypoxia was the principal regulator of VEGF expression [53]. We noted a higher expression of VEGF mRNA in the idNK cells of RPL patients in hypoxia which was reflected in the concentration of VEGF in culture supernatants. Atalay et al. and Pan et al. reported a higher level of VEGF in the serum of RPL patients than in fertile women [54,55]. It was demonstrated that VEGF increased microvascular permeability and promoted coagulation, which is directly related to the pathogenesis of preeclampsia [23]. Others claimed that VEGF-A level in the serum of RPL patients was not correlated with NK cell function and level [56].

Several studies demonstrated that dNK cells produced angiogenic factors and cytokines such as PlGF, IL-8, IFN-γ, Ang I, Ang II, which influenced endothelial integrity, and the imbalanced expression resulted in endothelial barrier dysfunction and vascular permeability in RPL patients [18,27,57]. In 2016, Cavalli et al. showed that idNK cells obtained from pbNK cells by culturing in transformation media in hypoxia expressed similar factors [24]. After the implementation of cultures similar to those described by Cavali et al., we tested the levels of the aforementioned factors in culture supernatants. Turner et al. reported that women who required emergency operative deliveries as a result of fetal distress had low pre-labor levels of placental growth factor (PIGF), which declined as labor progressed. During a recent phase 2 randomized controlled trial (RCT), they showed that women in the placebo cohort had a greater decline in PIGF levels than those receiving SC [58]. A clinical case study of a 26-year-old woman with severe preeclampsia showed that SC increased the PLGF level measured in the serum [59]. Our RPL group of patients had lower concentrations of PIGF than the fertile group of women, which was not reflected in gene expression and SC improved the concentration of PLGF as in the mentioned studies. However, we did not test RPL women during labor or pregnancy.

It was widely reported that SC influenced angiogenic factor production. There is evidence that sildenafil decreased IL-8 level in the serum, as well as gene expression in the PBMC cultures of patients with diabetic cardiomyopathy [60]. Other researchers showed that SC decreased the production of IL-6, IL-8 and ROS in dermal fibroblast cultures isolated from patients with systemic sclerosis [60]. Dias et al. confirmed that sildenafil attenuated the morphofunctional deleterious effects of Ang II on resistance vessels [61]. Chiu et al. found that SC improved renin secretion in the serum of men [62]. However, the present research revealed no such effect of SC in our in vitro model of idNK cells. It was also reported that sildenafil reduced ionized calcium-binding adapter molecule 1 (Iba-1), IFN-γ, and IL-1β levels in an inflammatory demyelination model in INOS knockout mice [61,63]. We did not notice such a phenomenon concerning idNK cell cultures in the current research as well as in our previous research, SC did not influence the percentage of T lymphocytes producing IFN–γ in the PBMC cultures in healthy men [64].

We are aware that the presented data are preliminary, but they may aid in further understanding of SC effect on idNK cells and the practical use of idNK cells in the studies of the pathology of idiopathic recurrent pregnancy loss.

Supplementary Materials: The following are available online at https://www.mdpi.com/article/10.3390/jcm10215086/s1, Table S1: Characteristics of RPL patients included to the study group; Figure S1: Gating strategy for CD107a expressing idNK cells (CD56+ CD3-) and NKT cells (CD56+ CD3+); Figure S2: The effect of sildenafil on the degranulation (CD107a expression) of idNK cells determined after 5 days of culturing in transformation media and hypoxia, results are showed as the median and IQR, CG—control group, RPL—study group, 500µM L-arginine iNOS inhibitor (L-NMMA), SC—sildenafil citrate 400 ng/ml).

Author Contributions: Conceptualization, M.K. and M.J.; methodology, M.K. and M.W.; software, A.R.; validation, A.R., M.Z. and M.W.; formal analysis, M.S.; investigation, M.K., A.R., M.Z. and M.W.; resources, M.J. and M.S.; data curation, M.K., A.R., M.Z. and M.W.; writing—original draft preparation, M.K. and M.W.; writing—review and editing, R.Z.; visualization, M.K.; supervision, M.J.; project administration, M.K.; funding acquisition, M.K. All authors have read and agreed to the published version of the manuscript.

Funding: The research was supported by a grant from the National Science Centre, Poland (NSC) no. 2014/15/D/NZ7/01838 and Department's statutory funds 1MG/N/2019.

Institutional Review Board Statement: The study was conducted according to the guidelines of the Declaration of Helsinki and approved by the Ethics Committee of Medical University of Warsaw, (No. KB/192/2015).

Informed Consent Statement: Informed consent was obtained from all subjects involved in the study.

Data Availability Statement: The data presented in this study are available on request from the first author.

Conflicts of Interest: The authors declare that there is no conflict of interest regarding the publication of this paper.

Abbreviations

Ang II	Angiotensin II
AZA	5-aza-2′deoxycytidine
cGMP	cyclic guanosine monophosphate
dNK	decidual NK cells
GMP	guanosine monophosphate
idNK	induced decidual NK cells
IL	interleukin
IUR	intrauterine growth restriction
L-MNNA	NG-Monomethyl-L-arginine
NO	nitric oxide
NOS	nitric oxide synthase
PBS	phosphate-buffered saline
PDE-Is	phosphodiesterase inhibitors
PDEs	phosphodiesterases
RAS	renin–angiotensin system
RPL	recurrent pregnancy loss
RSA	recurrent spontaneous abortions
SC	sildenafil citrate

References

1. Atik, R.B.; Christiansen, O.B.; Elson, J.; Kolte, A.M.; Lewis, S.; Middeldorp, S.; Nelen, W.; Peramo, B.; Quenby, S.; ESHRE Guideline Group on RPL; et al. ESHRE guideline: Recurrent pregnancy loss. *Hum. Reprod. Open* **2018**, *2018*, hoy004.
2. Cho, H.Y.; Park, H.S.; Ko, E.J.; Ryu, C.S.; Kim, J.O.; Kim, Y.R.; Ahn, E.H.; Lee, W.S.; Kim, N.K. Association of Complement Factor D and H Polymorphisms with Recurrent Pregnancy Loss. *Int. J. Mol. Sci.* **2019**, *21*, 17. [CrossRef] [PubMed]
3. Kwak-Kim, J.; Yang, K.M.; Gilman-Sachs, A. Recurrent pregnancy loss: A disease of inflammation and coagulation. *J. Obstet. Gynaecol. Res.* **2009**, *35*, 609–622. [CrossRef] [PubMed]
4. Practice Committee of the American Society for Reproductive Medicine. Definitions of infertility and recurrent pregnancy loss: A committee opinion. *Fertil. Steril.* **2013**, *99*, 63. [CrossRef] [PubMed]
5. Ford, H.B.; Schust, D.J. Recurrent Pregnancy Loss: Etiology, Diagnosis, and Therapy. *Rev. Obstet. Gynecol.* **2009**, *2*, 76–83.
6. Mekinian, A.; Cohen, J.; Alijotas-Reig, J.; Carbillon, L.; Nicaise-Roland, P.; Gilles Kayem, G.; Daraï, E.; Fain, O.; Bornes, M. Unexplained Recurrent Miscarriage and Recurrent Implantation Failure: Is There a Place for Immuno-modulation? *Am. J. Reprod. Immunol.* **2016**, *76*, 8–28. [CrossRef]
7. Chen, J.; Gong, X.; Chen, P.; Luo, K.; Zhang, X. Effect of L-arginine and sildenafil citrate on intrauterine growth restriction fetuses: A meta-analysis. *BMC Pregnancy Childbirth* **2016**, *16*, 225. [CrossRef]
8. El-Sayed, M.A.; Saleh, S.A.-A.; Maher, M.A.; Khidre, A.M. Utero-placental perfusion Doppler indices in growth restricted fetuses: Effect of sildenafil citrate. *J. Matern. Neonatal Med.* **2017**, *31*, 1045–1050. [CrossRef]
9. Figueras, F. Sildenafil therapy in early-onset fetal growth restriction: Waiting for the individual patient data meta-analysis. *BJOG Int. J. Obstet. Gynaecol.* **2019**, *126*, 1007. [CrossRef]
10. Maged, M.; Wageh, A.; Shams, M.; Elmetwally, A. Use of sildenafil citrate in cases of intrauterine growth restriction (IUGR); a prospective trial. *Taiwan. J. Obstet. Gynecol.* **2018**, *57*, 483–486. [CrossRef]
11. Paauw, N.D.; Paauw, N.D.; Terstappen, F.; Ganzevoort, W.; Joles, J.A.; Gremmels, H.; Lely, A.T. Sildenafil during Pregnancy: A Preclinical Meta-Analysis on Fetal Growth and Maternal Blood Pressure. *Hypertension* **2017**, *70*, 998–1006. [CrossRef]
12. Jerzak, M.; Kniotek, M.; Mrozek, J.; Górski, A.; Baranowski, W. Sildenafil citrate decreased natural killer cell activity and enhanced chance of successful pregnancy in women with a history of recurrent miscarriage. *Fertil. Steril.* **2008**, *90*, 1848–1853. [CrossRef]
13. Jerzak, M.; Szafarowska, M.; Kniotek, M.; Gorski, A. Successful pregnancy after Intralipid addition to sildenafil and enoxaparin in woman with history of re-current pregnancy loss (RPL). *Neuro Endocrinol. Lett.* **2016**, *37*, 473–477. [PubMed]
14. Luna, R.L.; Vasconcelos, A.G.; Nunes, A.K.S.; De Oliveira, W.H.; Barbosa, K.P.D.S.; Peixoto, C.A. Effects of Sildenafil Citrate and Heparin Treatments on Placental Cell Morphology in a Murine Model of Pregnancy Loss. *Cells Tissues Organs* **2016**, *201*, 193–202. [CrossRef]
15. El-Far, M.; El-Motwally, A.E.-G.; Hashem, I.A.; Bakry, N. Biochemical role of intravaginal sildenafil citrate as a novel antiabortive agent in unexplained recurrent spontaneous miscarriage: First clinical study of four case reports from Egypt. *Clin. Chem. Lab. Med.* **2009**, *47*, 1433–1438. [CrossRef]
16. Renshall, L.J.; Cottrell, E.; Cowley, E.; Sibley, C.P.; Baker, P.N.; Thorstensen, E.B.; Greenwood, S.L.; Wareing, M.; Dilworth, M.R. Antenatal sildenafil citrate treatment increases offspring blood pressure in the placental-specific Igf2 knockout mouse model of FGR. *Am. J. Physiol. Circ. Physiol.* **2020**, *318*, H252–H263. [CrossRef]

17. Pels, A.; Derks, J.; Elvan-Taspinar, A.; van Drongelen, J.; de Boer, M.; Duvekot, H.; van Laar, J.; van Eyck, J.; Al-Nasiry, S.; Sueters, M.; et al. Maternal Sildenafil vs Placebo in Pregnant Women with Severe Early-Onset Fetal Growth Restriction: A Randomized Clinical Trial. *JAMA Netw. Open* **2020**, *3*, e205323. [CrossRef]
18. Hanna, J.H.; Goldman-Wohl, D.; Hamani, Y.; Avraham, I.; Greenfield, C.; Natanson-Yaron, S.; Prus, D.; Cohen-Daniel, L.; Arnon, T.I.; Manaster, I.; et al. Decidual NK cells regulate key developmental processes at the human fetal-maternal interface. *Nat. Med.* **2006**, *12*, 1065–1074. [CrossRef]
19. Kniotek, M.; Boguska, A. Sildenafil Can Affect Innate and Adaptive Immune System in Both Experimental Animals and Patients. *J. Immunol. Res.* **2017**, *2017*, 1–8. [CrossRef]
20. Ohams, M.; Jerzak, M.; Górski, A. Effects of sildenafil citrate and etanercept treatment on TNF-α levels in peripheral blood of women with recurrent miscarriage. *Ginekol. Pol.* **2015**, *86*, 520–524. [CrossRef] [PubMed]
21. Mehrotra, N.; Gupta, M.; Kovar, A.; Meibohm, B. The role of pharmacokinetics and pharmacodynamics in phosphodiesterase-5 inhibitor therapy. *Int. J. Impot. Res.* **2006**, *19*, 253–264. [CrossRef] [PubMed]
22. Oyston, C.; Stanley, J.L.; Oliver, M.H.; Bloomfield, F.H.; Baker, P.N. Maternal Administration of Sildenafil Citrate Alters Fetal and Placental Growth and Fetal-Placental Vas-cular Resistance in the Growth-Restricted Ovine Fetus. *Hypertension* **2016**, *68*, 760–767. [CrossRef]
23. Lee, E.S.; Oh, M.-J.; Jung, J.W.; Lim, J.-E.; Seol, H.-J.; Lee, K.J.; Kim, H.-J. The Levels of Circulating Vascular Endothelial Growth Factor and Soluble Flt-1 in Pregnancies Complicated by Preeclampsia. *J. Korean Med Sci.* **2007**, *22*, 94–98. [CrossRef]
24. Cavalli, R.C.; Cerdeira, A.S.; Pernicone, E.; Korkes, H.A.; Burke, S.D.; Rajakumar, A.; Thadhani, R.I.; Roberts, U.J.; Bhasin, M.; Karumanchi, S.A.; et al. Induced Human Decidual NK-Like Cells Improve Utero-Placental Perfusion in Mice. *PLOS ONE* **2016**, *11*, e0164353. [CrossRef]
25. Wallace, A.E.; Fraser, R.; Gurung, S.; Goulwara, S.S.; Whitley, G.S.; Johnstone, A.P.; Cartwright, J.E. Increased angiogenic factor secretion by decidual natural killer cells from pregnancies with high uterine artery resistance alters trophoblast function. *Hum. Reprod.* **2014**, *29*, 652–660. [CrossRef] [PubMed]
26. Fraser, R.; Whitley, G.S.; Johnstone, A.P.; Host, A.J.; Sebire, N.J.; Thilaganathan, B.; Cartwright, J.E. Impaired decidual natural killer cell regulation of vascular remodelling in early human pregnancies with high uterine artery resistance. *J. Pathol.* **2012**, *228*, 322–332. [CrossRef]
27. Jia, N.; Li, J. Human Uterine Decidual NK Cells in Women with a History of Early Pregnancy Enhance Angiogenesis and Trophoblast Invasion. *BioMed Res. Int.* **2020**, *2020*, 1–7. [CrossRef]
28. Kossmann, S.; Schwenk, M.; Hausding, M.; Karbach, S.H.; Schmidgen, M.I.; Brandt, M.; Knorr, M.; Hu, H.; Kröller-Schön, S.; Schönfelder, T.; et al. Angiotensin II–Induced Vascular Dysfunction Depends on Interferon-γ–Driven Immune Cell Recruitment and Mutual Activation of Monocytes and NK-Cells. *Arter. Thromb. Vasc. Biol.* **2013**, *33*, 1313–1319. [CrossRef]
29. Jurewicz, M.; McDermott, D.; Sechler, J.M.; Tinckam, K.; Takakura, A.; Carpenter, C.B.; Milford, E.; Abdi, R. Human T and Natural Killer Cells Possess a Functional Renin-Angiotensin System: Further Mechanisms of Angiotensin II–Induced Inflammation. *J. Am. Soc. Nephrol.* **2007**, *18*, 1093–1102. [CrossRef]
30. Stettner, D.; Bujak-Gizycka, B.; Olszanecki, R.; Rytlewski, K.; Huras, H.; Korbut, R. Assessment of angiotensin I metabolism in the human placenta using an LC/MS method. *Folia medica Cracoviensia* **2013**, *53*, 31–39.
31. Ramos-Medina, R.; García-Segovia, Á.; De León-Luis, J.; Alonso, B.; Tejera-Alhambra, M.; Gil, J.; Caputo, J.D.; Seyfferth, A.; Aguarón, Á.; Vicente, A.; et al. New Decision-Tree Model for Defining the Risk of Reproductive Failure. *Am. J. Reprod. Immunol.* **2013**, *70*, 59–68. [CrossRef] [PubMed]
32. Fukui, A.; Funamizu, A.; Yokota, M.; Yamada, K.; Nakamua, R.; Fukuhara, R.; Kimura, H.; Mizunuma, H. Uterine and circulating natural killer cells and their roles in women with recurrent pregnancy loss, implantation failure and preeclampsia. *J. Reprod. Immunol.* **2011**, *90*, 105–110. [CrossRef] [PubMed]
33. Yamada, H.; Morikawa, M.; Kato, E.H.; Shimada, S.; Kobashi, G.; Minakami, H. Pre-conceptional Natural Killer Cell Activity and Percentage as Predictors of Biochemical Pregnancy and Spontaneous Abortion with Normal Chromosome Karyotype. *Am. J. Reprod. Immunol.* **2003**, *50*, 351–354. [CrossRef]
34. Cerdeira, A.S.; Rajakumar, A.; Royle, C.M.; Lo, A.; Husain, Z.; Thadhani, R.I.; Sukhatme, V.P.; Karumanchi, S.A.; Kopcow, H.D. Conversion of Peripheral Blood NK Cells to a Decidual NK-like Phenotype by a Cocktail of Defined Factors. *J. Immunol.* **2013**, *190*, 3939–3948. [CrossRef] [PubMed]
35. Practice Committee of the American Society for Reproductive Medicine. Definitions of infertility and recurrent pregnancy loss. *Fertil. Steril.* **2008**, *89*, 1603. [CrossRef]
36. Padron, J.; Glaria, L.; Martínez, O.; Torres, M.; López, E.; Delgado, R.; Caveda, L.; Rojas, A. Nitric oxide modulates interleukin-2-induced proliferation in CTLL-2 cells. *Mediat. Inflamm.* **1996**, *5*, 324–327. [CrossRef] [PubMed]
37. Levesque, M.C.; Misukonis, M.A.; O'Loughlin, C.W.; Chen, Y.; Beasley, B.E.; Wilson, D.L.; Adams, D.J.; Silber, R.; Weinberg, J.B. IL-4 and interferon gamma regulate expression of inducible nitric oxide synthase in chronic lympho-cytic leukemia cells. *Leukemia* **2003**, *17*, 442–450. [CrossRef]
38. Glossmann, H.; Petrischor, G.; Bartsch, G. Molecular mechanisms of the effects of sildenafil (VIAGRA®). *Exp. Gerontol.* **1999**, *34*, 305–318. [CrossRef]

39. Oei, V.Y.S.; Siernicka, M.; Graczyk-Jarzynka, A.; Hoel, H.J.; Yang, W.; Palacios, D.; Almåsbak, H.; Bajor, M.; Clement, D.; Brandt, L.; et al. Intrinsic Functional Potential of NK-Cell Subsets Constrains Retargeting Driven by Chimeric Antigen Receptors. *Cancer Immunol. Res.* **2018**, *6*, 467–480. [CrossRef]
40. Livak, K.J.; Schmittgen, T.D. Analysis of relative gene expression data using real-time quantitative PCR and the 2(-Delta Delta C(T)) Method. *Methods* **2001**, *25*, 402–408. [CrossRef]
41. Klutzny, S.; Anurin, A.; Nicke, B.; Regan, J.; Lange, M.; Schulze, L.; Parczyk, K.; Steigemann, P. PDE5 inhibition eliminates cancer stem cells via induction of PKA signaling. *Cell Death Dis.* **2018**, *9*, 1–15. [CrossRef]
42. Jelińska, M.; Skrajnowska, D.; Wrzosek, M.; Domanska, K.; Bielecki, W.; Zawistowska, M.; Korczak, B.B. Inflammation factors and element supplementation in cancer. *J. Trace Elements Med. Biol.* **2020**, *59*, 126450. [CrossRef] [PubMed]
43. Zhang, J.; Dunk, C.E.; Shynlova, O.; Caniggia, I.; Lye, S.J. TGFb1 suppresses the activation of distinct dNK subpopulations in preeclampsia. *EBioMedicine* **2019**, *39*, 531–539. [CrossRef] [PubMed]
44. Zhang, J.; Dunk, C.; Croy, A.B.; Lye, S.J. To serve and to protect: The role of decidual innate immune cells on human pregnancy. *Cell and Tissue Research* **2015**, *363*, 249–265. [CrossRef] [PubMed]
45. Sokolov, D.I.; Mikhailova, V.A.; Agnayeva, A.O.; Bazhenov, D.; Khokhlova, E.V.; Bespalova, O.N.; Gzgzyan, A.M.; Selkov, S.A. NK and trophoblast cells interaction: Cytotoxic activity on recurrent pregnancy loss. *Gynecol. Endocrinol.* **2019**, *35*, 5–10. [CrossRef] [PubMed]
46. Wallace, A.E.; Fraser, R.; Cartwright, J.E. Extravillous trophoblast and decidual natural killer cells: A remodelling partner-ship. *Hum. Reprod Update* **2012**, *18*, 458–471. [CrossRef]
47. Zhang, Y.; Yan, L.; Liu, J.; Cui, S.; Qiu, J. cGMP-dependent protein kinase II determines β-catenin accumulation that is essential for uterine decidual-ization in mice. *Am. J. Physiol. Cell Physiol.* **2019**, *317*, C1115–C1127. [CrossRef] [PubMed]
48. Celik, O.; Celik, N.; Ugur, K.; Hatirnaz, S.; Celik, S.; Muderris, I.I.; Yavuzkir, S.; Sahin, I.; Yardim, M.; Aydin, S. Nppc/Npr2/cGMP signaling cascade maintains oocyte developmental capacity. *Cell. Mol. Biol.* **2019**, *65*, 83–89. [CrossRef]
49. Durán-Reyes, G.; Gómez-Meléndez, M.D.R.; la Brena, G.M.-D.; Mercado-Pichardo, E.; Medina-Navarro, R.; Hicks-Gómez, J.J. Nitric oxide synthesis inhibition suppresses implantation and decreases cGMP concentration and protein peroxidation. *Life Sci.* **1999**, *65*, 2259–2268. [CrossRef]
50. Cifone, M.; Ulisse, S.; Santoni, A. Natural killer cells and nitric oxide. *Int. Immunopharmacol.* **2001**, *1*, 1513–1524. [CrossRef]
51. Sanson, A.J.; Malangoni, M.A. Hypoxia increases nitric oxide concentrations that are not completely inhibited by l-NMMA. *J. Surg. Res.* **2003**, *110*, 202–206. [CrossRef]
52. Wagner, J.A.; Rosario, M.; Romee, R.; Berrien-Elliott, M.; Schneider, S.E.; Leong, J.W.; Sullivan, R.P.; Jewell, B.A.; Becker-Hapak, M.; Schappe, T.; et al. CD56bright NK cells exhibit potent antitumor responses following IL-15 priming. *J. Clin. Investig.* **2017**, *127*, 4042–4058. [CrossRef]
53. Krock, B.L.; Skuli, N.; Simon, M.C. Hypoxia-Induced Angiogenesis: Good and Evil. *Genes Cancer* **2011**, *2*, 1117–1133. [CrossRef] [PubMed]
54. Pang, L.; Wei, Z.; Li, O.; Huang, R.; Qin, J.; Chen, H.; Fan, X.; Chen, Z.-J. An Increase in Vascular Endothelial Growth Factor (VEGF) and VEGF Soluble Receptor-1 (sFlt-1) Are Associated with Early Recurrent Spontaneous Abortion. *PLOS ONE* **2013**, *8*, e75759. [CrossRef]
55. Atalay, M.A.; Ugurlu, N.; Zulfikaroglu, E.; Danisman, N. Clinical significance of maternal serum vascular endothelial growth factor (VEGF) level in idiopathic recurrent pregnancy loss. *Eur. Rev. Med. Pharm. Sci* **2016**, *20*, 2974–2982.
56. Bansal, R.; Ford, B.; Bhaskaran, S.; Thum, M.; Bansal, A. Elevated Levels of Serum Vascular Endothelial Growth Factor-A Are Not Related to NK Cell Parameters in Recurrent IVF Failure. *J. Reprod. Infertil.* **2017**, *18*, 280–287. [PubMed]
57. Lash, G.E.; Robson, S.C.; Bulmer, J.N. Review: Functional role of uterine natural killer (uNK) cells in human early pregnancy decidua. *Placenta* **2010**, *31*, S87–S92. [CrossRef] [PubMed]
58. Turner, J.; Dunn, L.; Kumar, S. Oral sildenafil citrate during labor mitigates the intrapartum decline in placental growth factor in term pregnancies. *Am. J. Obstet. Gynecol.* **2020**, *223*, 588–590. [CrossRef]
59. Brownfoot, F.C.; Tong, S.; Hannan, N.J.; Cannon, P.; Nguyen, V.; Kaitu'U-Lino, T. Effect of sildenafil citrate on circulating levels of sFlt-1 in preeclampsia. *Pregnancy Hypertens.* **2018**, *13*, 1–6. [CrossRef]
60. Giannattasio, S.; Corinaldesi, C.; Colletti, M.; Luigi, L.D.; Antinozzi, C.; Filardi, T.; Scolletta, S.; Basili, S.; Lenzi, A.; Morano, S.; et al. The phosphodiesterase 5 inhibitor sildenafil decreases the proinflammatory chemokine IL-8 in dia-betic cardiomyopathy: In Vivo and in vitro evidence. *J. Endocrinol. Invest.* **2019**, *42*, 715–725.
61. Dias, A.T.; Leal, M.A.S.; Zanardo, T.C.; Alves, G.M.; Porto, M.L.; Nogueira, B.V.; Gava, A.L.; Campagnaro, B.P.; Pereira, T.M.C.; Meyrelles, S.S.; et al. Beneficial Morphofunctional Changes Promoted by Sildenafil in Resistance Vessels in the Angiotensin II-Induced Hypertension Model. *Curr. Pharm. Biotechnol.* **2018**, *19*, 483–494. [CrossRef]
62. Chiu, Y.J.; Reid, I.A. Effect of sildenafil on renin secretion in human subjects. *Exp. Biol. Med.* **2002**, *227*, 620–625. [CrossRef]
63. Raposo, C.; de Santana Nunes, A.K.; de Almeida Luna, R.L.; da Rocha Araújo, S.M.; da Cruz-Höfling, M.A.; Peixoto, C.A. Sildenafil (Viagra) protective effects on neuroinflammation: The role of iNOS/NO system in an inflam-matory demyelination model. *Mediat. Inflamm.* **2013**, *2013*, 321460. [CrossRef]
64. Zych, M.; Roszczyk, A.; Kniotek, M.; Kaleta, B.; Zagozdzon, R. Sildenafil Citrate Influences Production of TNF-αin Healthy Men Lymphocytes. *J. Immunol. Res.* **2019**, *2019*, 8478750. [CrossRef] [PubMed]

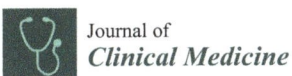

Journal of Clinical Medicine

Article

Proteomic Analysis of Maternal Urine for the Early Detection of Preeclampsia and Fetal Growth Restriction

Emmanuel Bujold [1,2,*], Alexandre Fillion [1], Florence Roux-Dalvai [1], Marie Pier Scott-Boyer [1], Yves Giguère [1,3], Jean-Claude Forest [1,3], Clarisse Gotti [1], Geneviève Laforest [1], Paul Guerby [1,4] and Arnaud Droit [1]

[1] CHU de Québec—Université Laval Research Center, Université Laval, Quebec City, QC G1V 4G2, Canada; alexandre.fillion.3@ulaval.ca (A.F.); florence.roux-dalvai@crchudequebec.ulaval.ca (F.R.-D.); marie-pier.scott-boyer.1@ulaval.ca (M.P.S.-B.); Yves.Giguere@crchudequebec.ulaval.ca (Y.G.); jean-claude.forest.med@ssss.gouv.qc.ca (J.-C.F.); clarisse.gotti@crchudequebec.ulaval.ca (C.G.); genevieve.laforest@crchudequebec.ulaval.ca (G.L.); paul.guerby@gmail.com (P.G.); arnaud.droit@crchudequebec.ulaval.ca (A.D.)

[2] Department of Obstetrics and Gynecology, Faculty of Medicine, CHU de Québec—Université Laval, Quebec City, QC G1V 4G2, Canada

[3] Department of Molecular Biology, Medical Biochemistry and Pathology, Faculty of Medicine, CHU de Québec—Université Laval, Quebec City, QC G1V 4G2, Canada

[4] Department of Obstetrics and Gynecology, Paule de Viguier Hospital, CHU de Toulouse—Université de Toulouse, 31059 Toulouse, France

* Correspondence: emmanuel.bujold@crchudequebec.ulaval.ca

Abstract: Background: To explore the use of maternal urine proteome for the identification of preeclampsia biomarkers. Methods: Maternal urine samples from women with and without preeclampsia were used for protein discovery followed by a validation study. The targeted proteins of interest were then measured in urine samples collected at 20–24 and 30–34 weeks among nine women who developed preeclampsia, one woman with fetal growth restriction, and 20 women with uncomplicated pregnancies from a longitudinal study. Protein identification and quantification was obtained using liquid chromatography–tandem mass spectrometry (LC–MS/MS). Results: Among the 1108 urine proteins quantified in the discovery study, 21 were upregulated in preeclampsia and selected for validation. Nineteen (90%) proteins were confirmed as upregulated in preeclampsia cases. Among them, two proteins, ceruloplasmin and serpin A7, were upregulated at 20–24 weeks and 30–34 weeks of gestation ($p < 0.05$) in cases of preeclampsia, and could have served to identify 60% of women who subsequently developed preeclampsia and/or fetal growth restriction at 20–24 weeks of gestation, and 78% at 30–34 weeks, for a false-positive rate of 10%. Conclusions: Proteomic profiling of maternal urine can differentiate women with and without preeclampsia. Several proteins including ceruloplasmin and serpin A7 are upregulated in maternal urine before the diagnosis of preeclampsia and potentially fetal growth restriction.

Keywords: pregnancy; preeclampsia; proteomics; urine; biomarkers

1. Introduction

Preeclampsia (PE) affects about 2% to 5% of pregnant women in developed countries and up to 10% of pregnant women in developing countries [1–3]. PE is associated with short-term and long-term adverse outcomes in mothers and infants [4–8]. About 10% to 15% of maternal deaths and 25% of neonatal deaths are attributable to PE and its complications [8,9]. In the most severe cases, PE occurs before term and is typically associated with deep placentation disorders that can also lead to fetal growth restriction [10–12].

There is a growing body of evidence that the preterm PE, severe PE, and fetal growth restriction can be predicted in early pregnancy using a combination of biophysical, biochemical and ultrasound markers [13–15]. However, such screening tools require equipment and expertise that are not readily available throughout the world. There is evidence that urine biomarkers could also be used for the early diagnosis of PE [16,17].

Mass-spectrometry-based proteomics analysis has gained popularity in the past decades for its ability to cover a large proportion of cellular or biological fluid proteomes [18]. Indeed, bottom-up proteomics have allowed for the identification and quantification of hundreds of proteins. This strategy relies on the identification and quantification of peptides resulting from the trypsin digestion of protein extracts by liquid chromatography coupled with tandem mass spectrometry (LC–MS/MS). The acquired spectra are then searched against publicly available protein databases. Protein candidates can also be accurately quantified by targeted proteomics in which up to one hundred proteins can be specifically monitored by LC–MS/MS in a single analysis [19]. The urinary proteome, which can be collected non-invasively and which contains more than 1800 protein species, is an ideal source of biomarkers for both renal/urological tract and systemic diseases [20,21].

For preeclampsia, a recent review of proteomic studies reported that at least 132 urine proteins could be used for early diagnosis [22]. More importantly, Buhimschi et al. observed that a specific urine proteomic profile combining serpin A1 and albumin could have: (1) a high accuracy in the identification of women with severe PE that required immediate delivery; and (2) could identify women at high risk to develop severe PE up to 10 to 25 weeks before its diagnosis [16]. However, these observations were limited to a small number of participants; the experiments were performed using equipment developed many years ago, and should therefore be validated in larger studies.

In the current study, we aim to assess the urine proteomic profiles in PE and to identify biomarkers that could help in the early prediction of PE.

2. Materials and Methods

We performed a secondary analysis of the PEARL case-cohort study (PreEclampsia And growth Restriction: a Longitudinal study) that included both nulliparous women with PE (cases) and a cohort of nulliparous women at low risk of PE, recruited in early pregnancy and followed until delivery (controls) [23,24]. PE was defined according to the Society of Obstetricians and Gynecologists of Canada guidelines as de novo hypertension after 20 weeks of pregnancy (i.e., Systolic BP $\geq$ 140 mmHg and/or diastolic BP $\geq$ 90 mmHg) with proteinuria ($\geq$300 mg per 24 h or $\geq$2 + protein on urine dipstick) or an adverse condition (thrombocytopenia, renal failure, liver injury, headache, seizures, vision problem or pulmonary edema) [25]. Fetal growth restriction was defined as a birth weight below the 10th percentile for gestational age based on a Canadian reference chart [26]. Urine samples were collected on the day of the diagnosis of PE for all cases and at several points during pregnancy for all controls. Urine samples were aliquoted and stored at $-80\ °C$ until analysis. All participants signed an informed consent form, and the study was approved by the ethics committee of the CHU de Québec—Université Laval (B14–07-2037).

For the purpose of the current study, we divided our population as follows: for the discovery study, 12 participants with PE (including 6 with fetal growth restriction) were matched to 12 controls without PE based on gestational age at urine collection, maternal age and maternal body mass index. For the validation study, another subset of 12 participants with PE (including 2 with fetal growth restriction) were matched to 12 controls also based on gestational age, maternal age and maternal body mass index. We used all samples available (n = 24) and divided by two for the discovery and validation study. For the longitudinal study, we used an independent cohort of women who were seen at each trimester of pregnancy: we selected 9 women who developed PE; 1 woman who developed fetal growth restriction without PE; and 20 women with uncomplicated pregnancies who provided urine samples at 20–24 and 30–34 weeks.

2.1. Mass Spectrometry Analyses

Each 500 µL sample of urine was concentrated on an Amicon Ultra-0.5 Centrifugal Filter device (Millipore, Burlington, MA, USA) by 10 min centrifugation 14,000× g, followed by a wash with 500 µL ammonium bicarbonate 50 mM and centrifugation in the same conditions. The protein concentration of the concentrated urine samples (volumes between 55 and 85 µL) was measured using Bradford assay. A total of 10 µg from each sample was then used for the subsequent steps. Briefly, the sample volume was adjusted to 50 µL with ammonium bicarbonate at 50 mM, and sodium deoxycholate was added to a final concentration of 1%. Protein denaturation was performed by heating at 95 °C for 5 min. The reduction and alkylation of cystein disulfide bridges was performed by the addition of 1,4 dithiothreitol (DTT) (final concentration 0.2 mM) and incubation at 37 °C for 30 min followed by the addition of iodoacetamide (final concentration 0.8 mM) and incubation at 37 °C for 30 min in the dark. An amount of 200 ng of trypsin enzyme was then added and samples were incubated at 37 °C overnight for proteolysis. Enzymatic digestion was stopped by acidification with 50% formic acid and the resulting peptides were purified on StageTip according to Rappsilber et al., using C18 Empore reverse phase (CDS) [27]. The samples were vacuum-dried and stored at −20 °C prior to mass spectrometry analysis. Each sample was resuspended at 0.2 µg/µL with 2% acetonitrile, 0.05% TFA. For validation and longitudinal studies only, iRT internal standard peptides (Biognosys, Schlieren, Switzerland) were added in each sample at 1X final concentration. An amount of 1µg from each sample was analyzed by liquid chromatography coupled with tandem mass spectrometry (LC–MS/MS) using a U3000 RSLCnano chromatographic system (Thermo Fisher Scientific, Waltham, MA, USA) and an Orbitrap Fusion mass spectrometer (Thermo Fisher Scientific). The chromatographic separation was performed on an Acclaim PepMap 100 C18 column (75 µm internal diameter, 3 µm particles and 500 mm length) using a 5–45% solvent B 90 min gradient (A: 5% acetonitrile, 0.1% formic acid; B: 80% acetonitrile, 0.1% formic acid).The mass spectrometer was operated in Data Dependent Acquisition mode for the discovery study, and Parallel Reaction Monitoring mode for the validation and longitudinal studies, using two peptide precursor masses for each protein selected from the discovery study.

2.2. Bioinformatics and Statistical Treatment

For the discovery study, MaxQuant software was used to obtain protein identification by searching a Uniprot human database (Human Reference Proteome UP000005640), and quantification was obtained by the Label-Free Quantification (LFQ) method [28]. LFQ intensity values of MaxQuant were used to calculate a protein fold change (FC) between the two groups of patients, and the values were then centered by the calculation of a z-score ($z = (FC - FC\ average)/FC\ standard\ deviation$). Statistical analyses were then performed using R software [29]. A Limma statistical test was applied to each protein between the two groups and the corresponding p-values were adjusted for multiple testing using the Benjamini–Hochberg method and thus obtained q-values [30]. A protein was considered as significantly regulated between the two groups if it met the following criteria: $|z| > 1.96$ and $q < 0.05$. For the validation and longitudinal studies, the data analysis was performed using the Skyline software [31]. The quantification value of each targeted peptide was obtained by integration of the corresponding chromatographic peak reconstructed from the best parent/fragment transition. Two normalizations of the quantification values were then applied. The first used the median of iRT internal standard peptides intensity to correct for LC–MS/MS variability, the second used the signal of peptides from the protein biotinidase (BTD) (Uniprot accession number P43251), which displayed no variation between the two groups in our discovery analysis, to correct for Bradford protein assay. For each sample, the intensities of the two peptides of each protein were summed to obtain a protein intensity value. A modified statistical Student's test (Welch test) was performed between the two groups of patients. Statistical analyses were conducted using R software and IBM SPSS Statistics version 26.0. Interaction network analysis was performed using the STRING database [32].

3. Results

3.1. Discovery Study

The median gestational age of the 12 participants at diagnosis of PE (31.9; IQ: 28.5–34.3 weeks) was comparable to the median gestational age of the 12 participants used as controls (32.1; IQ: 29.0–35.3 weeks). Table 1 reports participant's characteristics for the discovery, the validation and the longitudinal study.

Table 1. Characteristics of our study populations.

	Discovery Study		Validation Study		Longitudinal Study	
	Cases (n = 12)	Controls (n = 12)	Cases (n = 12)	Controls (n = 12)	Cases (n = 10)	Controls (n = 20)
Maternal age (years)	29 (27–31)	29 (27–33)	29 (27–31)	30 (28–33)	31 (27–35)	30 (29–33)
BMI (kg/m^2)	33 (28–36)	28 (26–33)	30 (28–35)	30 (25–34)	31 (29–33)	24 (22–26)
Caucasian	12 (100%)	12 (100%)	11 (92%)	12 (100%)	9 (90%)	20 (100%)
Gestational age at birth	34 (29–36)	39 (38–40)	34 (30–35)	40 (40–41)	35 (33–36)	40 (39–41)
Preeclampsia	12 (100%)	0 (0%)	12 (100%)	0 (0%)	9 (90%)	0 (0%)
Fetal growth restriction	6 (50%)	1 (8%)	2 (17%)	2 (17%)	4 (40%)	0 (0%)

Median (Interquartile range) or Number (percentage).

Our proteomic analyses allowed us to quantify 1108 proteins from urine samples which were used in a Principal Component Analysis (PCA) to explore the variability of the urinary proteomic profiles of participants (Figure 1). The PCA showed two distinct groups for control and PE revealing distinct proteomic profiles.

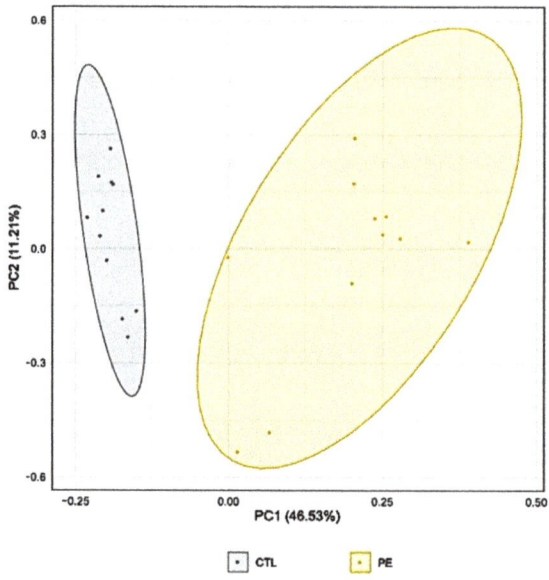

Figure 1. Principal Component Analysis (PCA) of the urinary proteomic profiles in participants with and without preeclampsia. Each point represents a participant. The axes correspond to artificial axes rebuilt by the PCA to display the maximum variability between the samples. CTL: Control; PE: Preeclampsia.

A heatmap of the intensity of the proteins quantified in this study was also generated and associated to a hierarchical clustering, which allowed us to group the most similar profiles among the urine proteomes (Figure 2).

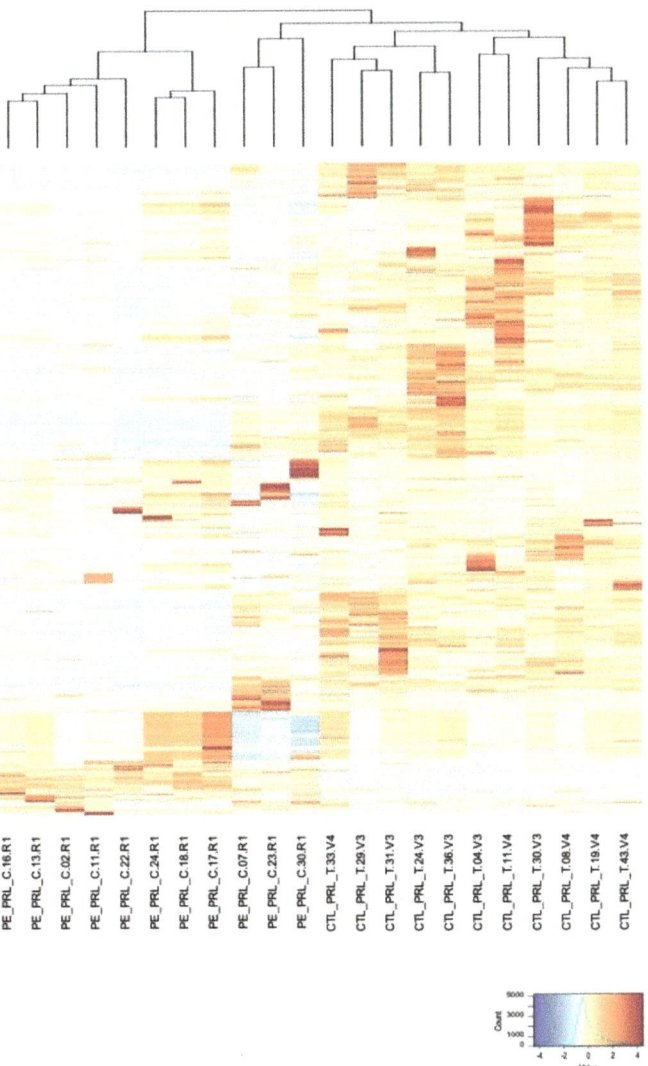

Figure 2. Heatmap of the expression of the 1108 proteins extracted from the proteomic analysis. Colors correspond to the centered intensity values of each protein in each urine sample from blue (smallest intensity) to red (highest intensity). The proteins (in lines) and the samples (in columns) are presented as clustered according to a complete linkage clustering method; the corresponding dendro-gram is shown only for samples.

Among all the quantified proteins, 62 (53 upregulated, 9 downregulated) were found statistically regulated between PE and control after filtering on z-score (obtained after centering of the protein fold change) and on the q-value associated to a Limma statistical test corrected for multiple testing (Figure 3). Twenty-one upregulated proteins were selected for further validation (A1BG; ALB; AFM; TTR; AZGP1; C3; CA1; CP; GC; HBA1; HBB; ITIH2; ORM1; ORM2; SERPINA1; SERPINA3; SERPINA6; SERPINA7; SERPINC1; SHBG; TF; see Table 2 for protein descriptions) based on their fold change, their total signal intensity and/or the sequence of their corresponding peptides (peptides carrying oxidized methionine and those containing missed trypsin cleavages were excluded). Using a STRING analysis, we found that most of them have known interactions, either direct protein interaction, gene co-expression, or are cited together in the literature (Supplementary Figure S1).

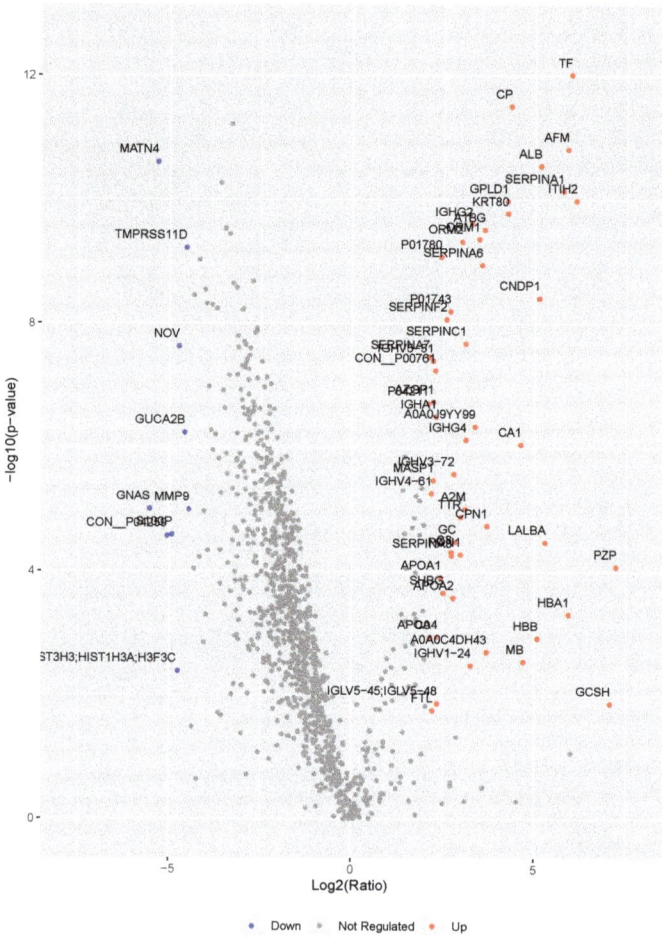

Figure 3. Volcano plot of the 1108 proteins quantified in the proteomic analysis. The x-axis corresponds to the fold change (Log2 of PE/control protein intensity ratio), the y-axis corresponds to the statistical value ($-\mathrm{Log}10$ (p-value)). Significantly regulated proteins are displayed in red (upregulated) or in blue (downregulated); non-significantly regulated proteins are displayed in grey.

3.2. Validation Study

The median gestational age at urine collection of our PE cases and term uncomplicated delivery controls was 31.5 (IQ: 29.0–34.3) weeks and 32.5 weeks (IQ: 29.6–33.9) weeks, respectively (Table 1). The 21 proteins previously selected were monitored by targeted proteomics to obtain an accurate protein quantification. Table 2 and Figure 4 report the average and distribution of intensity values for each group, PE or control, of each of the selected 21 proteins monitored by targeted proteomics. We observed that 19 (90%) of the 21 proteins were significantly upregulated in the urine of PE patients when compared to controls with a p-value < 0.05. Among them, 13 have a p-value < 0.001.

Table 2. Validation study by targeted proteomics of 21 urinary proteins in women with and without preeclampsia.

Protein Accession	Gene Name	Protein Description	Ratio	p-Value	Significance
P04217	A1BG	Alpha-1B-glycoprotein	4.85	0.00000	***
P43652	AFM	Afamin	6.89	0.00001	***
P25311	AZGP1	Zinc-alpha-2-glycoprotein	14.39	0.00005	***
P01024	C3	Complement C3	1.92	0.01029	*
P00915	CA1	Carbonic anydrase 1	6.20	0.03347	*
P00450	CP	Ceruloplasmin	6.55	0.00005	***
P02774	GC	Vitamin D-binding protein	11.31	0.00001	***
P19823	ITIH2	Inter-alpha-trypsin inhibitor heavy chain 2	6.35	0.01660	*
P02763	ORM1	Alpha-1-acid-glycoprotein 1	2.96	0.06649	
P19652	ORM2	Alpha-1-acid-glycoprotein 2	1.66	0.28634	
P01009	SERPINA1	Alpha-1-antitrypsin (serpin A1)	9.50	0.01026	*
P01011	SERPINA3	Alpha-1-antichymotrypsin (serpin A3)	3.83	0.00011	**
P08185	SERPINA6	Corticosteroid-binding globulin (serpin A6)	2.27	0.00039	**
P05543	SERPINA7	Thyroxine-binding globulin (serpin A7)	16.42	0.00013	**
P01008	SERPINC1	Antithrombin-III (serpin C1)	4.38	0.00000	***
I3L145	SHBG	Sex-hormone-binding globulin	4.35	0.00000	***
P02766	TTR	Transthyretin	4.32	0.00000	***
P02768	ALB	Albumin	2.57	0.00001	***
P69905	HBA1	Hemoglobin subunit alpha 1	3.74	0.02510	*
P68871	HBB	Hemoglobin subunit beta	24.62	0.00004	***
P02787	TF	Serotransferrin	2.82	0.02372	*

For each protein (Uniprot accession number given in the first column), average intensity ratio of PE over control groups (PE/CTL) is shown associated to its Student's test statistical p-value and the corresponding significance. * $p < 0.05$; ** $p < 0.001$; *** $p < 0.0001$.

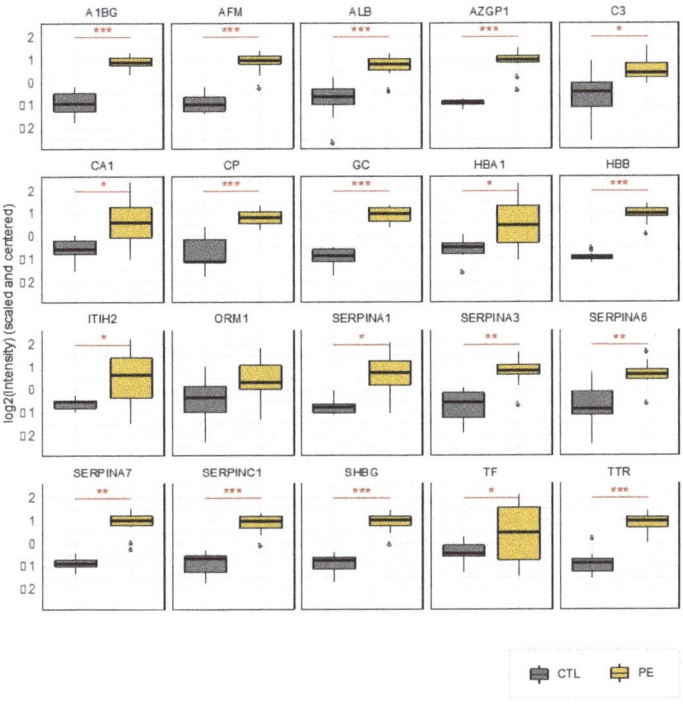

Figure 4. Validation study: Distribution of intensities measured by targeted proteomics of 21 urinary proteins in women with and without preeclampsia. The boxplots represent the distribution of intensities in each group (grey: control, yellow: PE) as well as the median (line), the interquartile (box) and the maximum and minimum values within 1.5 times the interquartile range (whisker) of 21 proteins monitored by targeted proteomics in urine samples of women with preeclampsia or women with uncomplicated pregnancies. Statistical significance is displayed above each graph: * $p < 0.05$; ** $p < 0.01$; *** $p < 0.001$.

3.3. Longitudinal Study

In the longitudinal study, we observed that 6 of the 21 proteins monitored by targeted proteomics were significantly upregulated at 30–34 weeks in women who subsequently developed PE in comparison to the control group (serpin A7; ceruloplasmin; afamin; inter-alpha-trypsin inhibitor heavy chain; transferrin; alpha-1B-glycoprotein). Two, serpin A7 and ceruloplasmin, were also found significantly upregulated at 20–24 weeks in women who subsequently developed PE in comparison to the control group (Table 3 and Figure 5).

Table 3. Longitudinal study by targeted proteomics of 21 urinary proteins in women with and without preeclampsia.

	20–24 Weeks			30–34 Weeks		
Gene Name	Ratio PE/CTL	p-Value	Significance	Ratio PE/CTL	p-Value	Significance
SERPINA7	1.42	0.04247	*	1.62	0.00966	**
CP	1.81	0.04515	*	4.87	0.01784	*
AFM	1.29	0.33745		2.48	0.01821	*
ITIH2	1.14	0.66046		3.67	0.02808	*
TF	1.86	0.27263		8.42	0.03446	*
A1BG	1.19	0.50528		2.22	0.04651	*
SERPINA3	1.39	0.22978		1.95	0.05920	
GC	1.20	0.28638		1.97	0.06296	
ALB	1.49	0.20602		5.54	0.06954	
SERPINA1	1.36	0.24731		4.11	0.07165	
C3	1.07	0.85042		1.63	0.07776	
ORM1	1.69	0.42028		2.52	0.07781	
SERPINA6	1.05	0.84649		1.97	0.08995	
ORM2	1.35	0.49657		1.52	0.19926	
TTR	1.23	0.29396		1.48	0.21370	
HBA1	5.27	0.01524	*	55.40	0.30338	
HBB	5.43	0.02956	*	30.91	0.33029	
SERPINC1	0.99	0.97216		1.28	0.34586	
AZGP1	1.44	0.59655		1.19	0.61454	
CA1	0.62	0.55159		0.70	0.63019	
SHBG	0.92	0.58530		1.07	0.72452	

For each protein (Uniprot accession number given in the first column) at two-time points (20–24 or 30–34 weeks of gestation), average intensity of PE over control groups (PE/CTL) is shown associated to its Student's test statistical p-value and the corresponding significance. * $p < 0.05$; ** $p < 0.01$.

Figure 6A,B reports the receiver operating characteristic (ROC) curves for the prediction of PE or fetal growth restriction using ceruloplasmin and serpin A7 protein concentrations in urine at 20–24 weeks and 30–34 weeks of gestation. At a false positive rate of 10%, ceruloplasmin could have predicted between 60% and 78% of the PE and/or fetal growth restriction cases at 20–24 weeks and 30–34 weeks of gestation, respectively. Interestingly, the case of fetal growth restriction without preeclampsia would have been detected with ceruloplasmin but not with serpin A7.

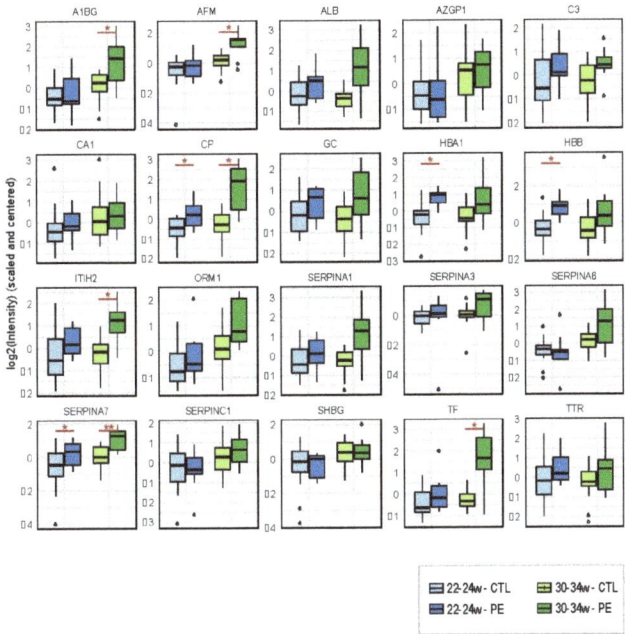

Figure 5. Longitudinal study: Distribution of intensities measured by targeted proteomics of 21 urinary proteins in women with and without preeclampsia at 20–24 or 30–34 weeks of gestation. The boxplots represent the distribution of intensities in each group as well as the median (line), the interquartile (box) and the maximum and minimum values within 1.5 times the interquartile range (whisker) of 21 proteins monitored by targeted proteomics in urine samples collected at 20–22 weeks (blue) and 30–32 weeks (green) of gestation in women with preeclampsia ($n = 9$) (dark color) or women with uncomplicated pregnancies ($n = 20$) (light color). Statistical significance is displayed above each graph: * $p < 0.05$; ** $p < 0.01$.

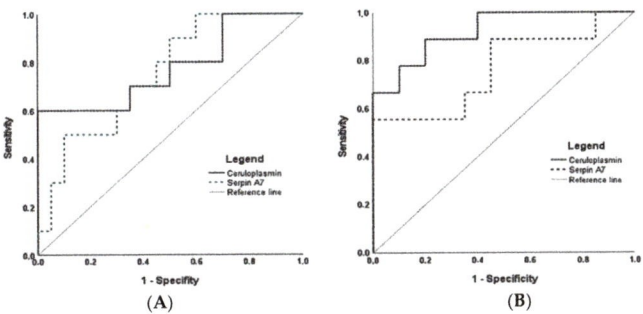

Figure 6. Receiver operating characteristic (ROC) curves for the prediction of preeclampsia and/or fetal growth restriction based on ceruloplasmin and serpin A7 proteins measured by targeted proteomics in urine of women at 20–24 and 30–34 weeks of gestation. The ROC curves present the predictive values of ceruloplasmin and serpin A7 measurements using targeted proteomic on maternal urine samples collected at 20–24 weeks of gestation (**A**) and at 30–34 weeks of gestation (**B**). The area under the ROC curves (AUC) were significant for ceruloplasmin at 20–24 weeks (AUC: 0.78; 95%CI: 0.58–0.97, $p = 0.016$); serpin A7 at 20–24 weeks (AUC: 0.75; 95%CI: 0.57–0.92, $p = 0.028$); ceruloplasmin at 30–34 weeks (AUC: 0.92; 95%CI: 0.82–1.00, $p < 0.001$); serpin A7 at 30–34 weeks (AUC: 0.77; 95%CI: 0.56–0.98, $p = 0.024$).

4. Discussion

We observed that women with preeclampsia have a different urine proteomic profile than women without preeclampsia and such differences can be present up to 12 weeks before the first signs and symptoms of preeclampsia. This observation, consistent with previous studies, suggests that women at high-risk of preeclampsia could be detected from urine biomarkers. Since fetal growth restriction shares a common mechanism of disease, it is possible that it could be detected in early pregnancy as well.

More specifically, the PCA performed on our dataset discriminates the two groups of patients (PE vs. controls). Moreover, the hierarchical clustering associated with the heatmap of protein intensities generates two main clusters containing either control or PE samples. To reveal the proteins dysregulated between PE and controls, we centered the control/PE ratios by calculating a z-score. Indeed, the proteinuria associated to PE strongly affects the protein content of the analyzed samples. Therefore, lower mass spectrometry signals obtained in PE cases, as can be observed on the heatmap of protein expressions, might result in a misinterpretation of the dysregulated proteins between the two groups. By applying a z-score correction and using a statistical test corrected for multiple testing (q-values), we could confidently identify 62 proteins with statistical differences in intensity between control and PE groups. Using targeted proteomics, known for their high accuracy in protein quantification, and another subset of patients from the same cohort, we confirmed our findings from the discovery study. The monitoring of these 21 proteins in our longitudinal study revealed that 6 of these proteins were significantly upregulated at 30–34 weeks of gestation and 2 of them (ceruloplasmin and serpin A7) were significantly upregulated at 20–24 weeks of gestation, up to 12 weeks before the clinical onset of PE. Ceruloplasmin is a copper-binding protein involved in iron transport across cellular membranes, and has antioxidant ferroxidase properties. It could be upregulated in PE as a response to placental ischemia [33,34]. As for serpin A7, also known as thyroxine-binding globulin (TBG), the major thyroid hormone transport protein in serum, studies have observed lower serum TBG in women with PE [35,36]. However, little is known about how and why serpin A7 is upregulated in the urine of PE cases.

Overall, our observations suggest that the urine proteomic profile could be used to predict preeclampsia several weeks before the first signs and symptoms manifest themselves. More specifically, we observed that at least two proteins, namely, ceruloplasmin and serpin A7, are increased in maternal urine at 20–24 and 30–34 weeks of gestation in most women who subsequently develop PE.

Our study is in agreement with the study of Buhimschi et al., who observed that serpin A1, another member of the serpin family, was significantly increased in PE cases [16]. Their study also reported misfolded proteins in the urine of women with preeclampsia bound to Congo Red dye (urine congophilia or affinity for the amyloidophilic dye Congo Red) [37]. Ultimately, their study reported promising results from a prototype point-of-care test for the detection of urine congophilia [38]. A review by Navajas et al. found nine publications from 2008 to 2020 that observed 132 proteins that were differently expressed in urine in PE cases compared to controls [22]. Nineteen of these showed high potential for PE prediction as they were consistently higher or lower in PE, including ceruloplasmin, serpin A1, serpin A5, C3, ALB, TF and HBB. Starodubtseva et al. reported that the estimation of serpin A1 peptides in urine was also related to the severity of PE [39]. Placental growth factor (PlGF), a proangiogenic protein commonly used for the prediction of PE and other placental-mediated outcomes of pregnancy is also predictive of PE and PE-related adverse outcomes when measured in urine [17,23,40]. Altogether, these studies, including ours, provide hope that rapid identification of PE and potentially early prediction of PE is possible using urine studies.

The small number of cases available at each step is a limit of our study. However, we used standardized methods for proteomic analysis and, using high-resolution LC–MS/MS, we obtained the largest urinary proteome coverage ever published on preeclampsia samples (1108 proteins quantified). One of the major strengths of the current study is the validation of our findings in an independent subset of patients and subsequent confirmation in a prospective study, which includes the collection of urine samples up to three months before the first signs and symptoms of PE.

5. Conclusions

PE is a major cause of perinatal morbidity and mortality around the world, primarily in developing countries. PE is commonly associated with fetal growth restriction, as they share a common mechanism of disease. Our study and current literature strongly suggest that PE, and potentially fetal growth restriction, are syndromes that are highly detectable in their early phases using the proteomic analysis of maternal urine. More efforts should be devoted to the development of rapid point-of-care tests on maternal urine that could help in the prevention of PE-related adverse outcomes of pregnancy.

Supplementary Materials: The following are available online at https://www.mdpi.com/article/10.3390/jcm10204679/s1, Figure S1: STRING interaction network of the 21 proteins selected for validation study.

Author Contributions: Conceptualization, E.B., A.D., F.R.-D.; methodology, E.B., P.G., F.R.-D., C.G.; software, F.R.-D., M.P.S.-B., C.G.; validation, E.B., F.R.-D., M.P.S.-B., C.G.; formal analysis, E.B., F.R.-D., C.G., G.L.; investigation, E.B., A.F., P.G.; resources, E.B.; data curation, F.R.-D.; writing—original draft preparation, E.B., F.R.-D.; writing—review and editing, E.B., A.F., G.L., P.G., Y.G., J.-C.F.; visualization, A.F.; supervision, A.D., E.B.; project administration, E.B., Y.G.; funding acquisition, E.B. All authors have read and agreed to the published version of the manuscript.

Funding: This research was funded by Jeanne et Jean-Louis Lévesque, Perinatal Research Chair—Université Laval.

Institutional Review Board Statement: The study was conducted according to the guidelines of the Declaration of Helsinki, and approved by the Institutional Review Board (or Ethics Committee) of Centre de recherché du CHU de Québec (protocol code B14-07-2037 on 7 August 2014).

Informed Consent Statement: Informed consent was obtained from all subjects involved in the study.

Data Availability Statement: The data presented in this study are available on request from the corresponding author.

Acknowledgments: We acknowledge the work of M. Michael Spanier, for the editing and review of the document.

Conflicts of Interest: The authors declare no conflict of interest. The funders had no role in the design of the study; in the collection, analyses, or interpretation of data; in the writing of the manuscript, or in the decision to publish the results.

References

1. Mol, B.W.J.; Roberts, C.T.; Thangaratinam, S.; Magee, L.A.; de Groot, C.J.M.; Hofmeyr, G.J. Pre-eclampsia. *Lancet* **2016**, *387*, 999–1011. [CrossRef]
2. Rana, S.; Lemoine, E.; Granger, J.P.; Karumanchi, S.A. Preeclampsia: Pathophysiology, Challenges, and Perspectives. *Circ. Res.* **2019**, *124*, 1094–1112. [CrossRef] [PubMed]
3. Nakimuli, A.; Chazara, O.; Byamugisha, J.; Elliott, A.M.; Kaleebu, P.; Mirembe, F.; Moffett, A. Pregnancy, parturition and preeclampsia in women of African ancestry. *Am. J. Obstet. Gynecol.* **2014**, *210*, 510–520. [CrossRef] [PubMed]
4. Murphy, M.S.; Smith, G.N. Pre-eclampsia and Cardiovascular Disease Risk Assessment in Women. *Am. J. Perinatol.* **2016**, *33*, 723–731. [CrossRef] [PubMed]
5. Wu, P.; Haththotuwa, R.; Kwok, C.S.; Babu, A.; Kotronias, R.A.; Rushton, C.; Zaman, A.; Fryer, A.A.; Kadam, U.; Chew-Graham, C.A.; et al. Preeclampsia and Future Cardiovascular Health: A Systematic Review and Meta-Analysis. *Circ. Cardiovasc. Qual. Outcomes* **2017**, *10*, e003497. [CrossRef]
6. Pinheiro, T.V.; Brunetto, S.; Ramos, J.G.; Bernardi, J.R.; Goldani, M.Z. Hypertensive disorders during pregnancy and health outcomes in the offspring: A systematic review. *J. Dev. Orig. Health Dis.* **2016**, *7*, 391–407. [CrossRef]
7. Davis, E.F.; Lazdam, M.; Lewandowski, A.J.; Worton, S.A.; Kelly, B.; Kenworthy, Y.; Adwani, S.; Wilkinson, A.R.; McCormick, K.; Sargent, I.; et al. Cardiovascular risk factors in children and young adults born to preeclamptic pregnancies: A systematic review. *Pediatrics* **2012**, *129*, e1552–e1561. [CrossRef]

8. Duley, L. The global impact of pre-eclampsia and eclampsia. *Semin. Perinatol.* **2009**, *33*, 130–137. [CrossRef]
9. Steegers, E.A.; von Dadelszen, P.; Duvekot, J.J.; Pijnenborg, R. Pre-eclampsia. *Lancet* **2010**, *376*, 631–644. [CrossRef]
10. Burton, G.J.; Redman, C.W.; Roberts, J.M.; Moffett, A. Pre-eclampsia: Pathophysiology and clinical implications. *BMJ* **2019**, *366*, l2381. [CrossRef]
11. Phipps, E.A.; Thadhani, R.; Benzing, T.; Karumanchi, S.A. Pre-eclampsia: Pathogenesis, novel diagnostics and therapies. *Nat. Rev. Nephrol.* **2019**, *15*, 275–289. [CrossRef]
12. Hod, T.; Cerdeira, A.S.; Karumanchi, S.A. Molecular Mechanisms of Preeclampsia. *Cold Spring Harb. Perspect. Med.* **2015**, *5*, a023473. [CrossRef]
13. Boutin, A.; Gasse, C.; Guerby, P.; Giguere, Y.; Tetu, A.; Bujold, E. First-Trimester Preterm Preeclampsia Screening in Nulliparous Women: The Great Obstetrical Syndrome (GOS) Study. *J. Obstet. Gynaecol. Can.* **2021**, *43*, 43–49. [CrossRef]
14. Rolnik, D.L.; Wright, D.; Poon, L.C.Y.; Syngelaki, A.; O'Gorman, N.; de Paco Matallana, C.; Akolekar, R.; Cicero, S.; Janga, D.; Singh, M.; et al. ASPRE trial: Performance of screening for preterm pre-eclampsia. *Ultrasound Obstet. Gynecol.* **2017**, *50*, 492–495. [CrossRef]
15. Mosimann, B.; Amylidi-Mohr, S.K.; Surbek, D.; Raio, L. First Trimester Screening for Preeclampsia—A Systematic Review. *Hypertens. Pregnancy* **2020**, *39*, 1–11. [CrossRef] [PubMed]
16. Buhimschi, I.A.; Zhao, G.; Funai, E.F.; Harris, N.; Sasson, I.E.; Bernstein, I.M.; Saade, G.R.; Buhimschi, C.S. Proteomic profiling of urine identifies specific fragments of SERPINA1 and albumin as biomarkers of preeclampsia. *Am. J. Obstet. Gynecol.* **2008**, *199*, 551.e1–551.e16. [CrossRef] [PubMed]
17. Lecarpentier, E.; Gris, J.C.; Cochery-Nouvellon, E.; Mercier, E.; Abbas, H.; Thadhani, R.; Karumanchi, S.A.; Haddad, B. Urinary Placental Growth Factor for Prediction of Placental Adverse Outcomes in High-Risk Pregnancies. *Obstet. Gynecol.* **2019**, *134*, 1326–1332. [CrossRef] [PubMed]
18. Parker, C.E.; Pearson, T.W.; Anderson, N.L.; Borchers, C.H. Mass-spectrometry-based clinical proteomics—A review and prospective. *Analyst* **2010**, *135*, 1830–1838. [CrossRef]
19. Uzozie, A.C.; Aebersold, R. Advancing translational research and precision medicine with targeted proteomics. *J. Proteom.* **2018**, *189*, 1–10. [CrossRef]
20. Beasley-Green, A. Urine Proteomics in the Era of Mass Spectrometry. *Int. Neurourol. J.* **2016**, *20*, S70–S75. [CrossRef]
21. Marimuthu, A.; O'Meally, R.N.; Chaerkady, R.; Subbannayya, Y.; Nanjappa, V.; Kumar, P.; Kelkar, D.S.; Pinto, S.M.; Sharma, R.; Renuse, S.; et al. A comprehensive map of the human urinary proteome. *J. Proteome Res.* **2011**, *10*, 2734–2743. [CrossRef] [PubMed]
22. Navajas, R.; Corrales, F.; Paradela, A. Quantitative proteomics-based analyses performed on pre-eclampsia samples in the 2004-2020 period: A systematic review. *Clin. Proteom.* **2021**, *18*, 6. [CrossRef] [PubMed]
23. Fillion, A.; Guerby, P.; Lachance, C.; Comeau, M.-P.; Bussières, M.-C.; Doucet-Gingras, F.-A.; Zérounian, S.; Demers, S.; Laforest, G.; Menzies, D.; et al. Placental Growth Factor and soluble Fms-like tyrosine kinase-1 in Preeclampsia: A case-cohort (PEARL) study. *J. Obstet. Gynaecol. Can.* **2020**, *42*, 1235–1242. [CrossRef] [PubMed]
24. Fillion, A.; Guerby, P.; Menzies, D.; Lachance, C.; Comeau, M.P.; Bussieres, M.C.; Doucet-Gingras, F.A.; Zerounian, S.; Bujold, E. Pathological investigation of placentas in preeclampsia (the PEARL study). *Hypertens. Pregnancy* **2021**, *40*, 56–62. [CrossRef] [PubMed]
25. Magee, L.A.; Pels, A.; Helewa, M.; Rey, E.; von Dadelszen, P. Diagnostic, evaluation et prise en charge des troubles hypertensifs de la grossesse: Resume directif. *J. Obstet. Gynaecol. Can.* **2016**, *38*, S426–S452. [CrossRef]
26. Kramer, M.S.; Platt, R.W.; Wen, S.W.; Joseph, K.S.; Allen, A.; Abrahamowicz, M.; Blondel, B.; Breart, G.; Fetal/Infant Health Study Group of the Canadian Perinatal Surveillance, S. A new and improved population-based Canadian reference for birth weight for gestational age. *Pediatrics* **2001**, *108*, E35. [CrossRef]
27. Rappsilber, J.; Mann, M.; Ishihama, Y. Protocol for micro-purification, enrichment, pre-fractionation and storage of peptides for proteomics using StageTips. *Nat. Protoc.* **2007**, *2*, 1896–1906. [CrossRef]
28. Tyanova, S.; Temu, T.; Cox, J. The MaxQuant computational platform for mass spectrometry-based shotgun proteomics. *Nat. Protoc.* **2016**, *11*, 2301–2319. [CrossRef]
29. RCoreTeam. *R: A Language and Environment for Statistical Computing*; R Foundation for Statistical Computing: Vienna, Austria, 2020.
30. Smyth, G. *Limma: Linear Models for Microarray Data*; Springer: New York, NY, USA, 2005; pp. 397–420.
31. Pino, L.K.; Searle, B.C.; Bollinger, J.G.; Nunn, B.; MacLean, B.; MacCoss, M.J. The Skyline ecosystem: Informatics for quantitative mass spectrometry proteomics. *Mass Spectrom. Rev.* **2020**, *39*, 229–244. [CrossRef]
32. Szklarczyk, D.; Gable, A.L.; Nastou, K.C.; Lyon, D.; Kirsch, R.; Pyysalo, S.; Doncheva, N.T.; Legeay, M.; Fang, T.; Bork, P.; et al. The STRING database in 2021: Customizable protein-protein networks, and functional characterization of user-uploaded gene/measurement sets. *Nucleic Acids Res.* **2021**, *49*, D605–D612. [CrossRef]
33. Serdar, Z.; Gur, E.; Develioglu, O. Serum iron and copper status and oxidative stress in severe and mild preeclampsia. *Cell Biochem. Funct.* **2006**, *24*, 209–215. [CrossRef] [PubMed]
34. Guller, S.; Buhimschi, C.S.; Ma, Y.Y.; Huang, S.T.; Yang, L.; Kuczynski, E.; Zambrano, E.; Lockwood, C.J.; Buhimschi, I.A. Placental expression of ceruloplasmin in pregnancies complicated by severe preeclampsia. *Lab. Investig.* **2008**, *88*, 1057–1067. [CrossRef] [PubMed]

35. Alemu, A.; Terefe, B.; Abebe, M.; Biadgo, B. Thyroid hormone dysfunction during pregnancy: A review. *Int. J. Reprod. Biomed.* **2016**, *14*, 677–686. [CrossRef] [PubMed]
36. Kaya, E.; Sahin, Y.; Ozkececi, Z.; Pasaoglu, H. Relation between birth weight and thyroid function in preeclampsia-eclampsia. *Gynecol. Obstet. Investig.* **1994**, *37*, 30–33. [CrossRef]
37. Buhimschi, I.A.; Nayeri, U.A.; Zhao, G.; Shook, L.L.; Pensalfini, A.; Funai, E.F.; Bernstein, I.M.; Glabe, C.G.; Buhimschi, C.S. Protein misfolding, congophilia, oligomerization, and defective amyloid processing in preeclampsia. *Sci. Transl. Med.* **2014**, *6*, 245ra292. [CrossRef]
38. Bracken, H.; Buhimschi, I.A.; Rahman, A.; Smith, P.R.S.; Pervin, J.; Rouf, S.; Bousieguez, M.; Lopez, L.G.; Buhimschi, C.S.; Easterling, T.; et al. Congo red test for identification of preeclampsia: Results of a prospective diagnostic case-control study in Bangladesh and Mexico. *EClinicalMedicine* **2021**, *31*, 100678. [CrossRef]
39. Starodubtseva, N.; Nizyaeva, N.; Baev, O.; Bugrova, A.; Gapaeva, M.; Muminova, K.; Kononikhin, A.; Frankevich, V.; Nikolaev, E.; Sukhikh, G. SERPINA1 Peptides in Urine as A Potential Marker of Preeclampsia Severity. *Int. J. Mol. Sci.* **2020**, *21*, 914. [CrossRef]
40. Levine, R.J.; Thadhani, R.; Qian, C.; Lam, C.; Lim, K.H.; Yu, K.F.; Blink, A.L.; Sachs, B.P.; Epstein, F.H.; Sibai, B.M.; et al. Urinary placental growth factor and risk of preeclampsia. *JAMA* **2005**, *293*, 77–85. [CrossRef]

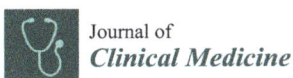

Article

Evaluating Markers of Immune Tolerance and Angiogenesis in Maternal Blood for an Association with Risk of Pregnancy Loss

Michelle A. Wyatt [1], Sarah C. Baumgarten [1], Amy L. Weaver [2], Chelsie C. Van Oort [1], Bohdana Fedyshyn [1], Rodrigo Ruano [1], Chandra C. Shenoy [1] and Elizabeth Ann L. Enninga [1,3,*]

Citation: Wyatt, M.A.; Baumgarten, S.C.; Weaver, A.L.; Van Oort, C.C.; Fedyshyn, B.; Ruano, R.; Shenoy, C.C.; Enninga, E.A.L. Evaluating Markers of Immune Tolerance and Angiogenesis in Maternal Blood for an Association with Risk of Pregnancy Loss. *J. Clin. Med.* **2021**, *10*, 3579. https://doi.org/10.3390/jcm10163579

Academic Editor: Alex Heazell

Received: 14 July 2021
Accepted: 12 August 2021
Published: 14 August 2021

Publisher's Note: MDPI stays neutral with regard to jurisdictional claims in published maps and institutional affiliations.

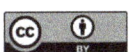

Copyright: © 2021 by the authors. Licensee MDPI, Basel, Switzerland. This article is an open access article distributed under the terms and conditions of the Creative Commons Attribution (CC BY) license (https://creativecommons.org/licenses/by/4.0/).

[1] Department of Obstetrics and Gynecology, Mayo Clinic College of Medicine, Rochester, MN 55905, USA; michelleashleywyatt@gmail.com (M.A.W.); Baumgarten.Sarah@mayo.edu (S.C.B.); Vanoort.Chelsie@mayo.edu (C.C.V.O.); Fedyshyn.Bohdana@mayo.edu (B.F.); rodrigoruano@hotmail.com (R.R.); Shenoy.Chandra@mayo.edu (C.C.S.)
[2] Department of Health Sciences Research, Mayo Clinic College of Medicine, Rochester, MN 55905, USA; weaver@mayo.edu
[3] Department of Immunology, Mayo Clinic College of Medicine, Rochester, MN 55905, USA
* Correspondence: Enninga.elizabethann@mayo.edu

Abstract: Pregnancy loss affects approximately 20% of couples. The lack of a clear cause complicates half of all miscarriages. Early evidence indicates the maternal immune system and angiogenesis regulation are both key players in implantation success or failure. Therefore, this prospective study recruited women in the first trimester with known viable intrauterine pregnancy and measured blood levels of immune tolerance proteins galectin-9 (Gal-9) and interleukin (IL)-4, and angiogenesis proteins (vascular endothelial growth factors (VEGF) A, C, and D) between 5 and 9 weeks gestation. Plasma concentrations were compared between groups defined based on (a) pregnancy outcome and (b) maternal history of miscarriage, respectively. In total, 56 women were recruited with 10 experiencing a miscarriage or pregnancy loss in the 2nd or 3rd trimester and 11 having a maternal history or miscarriage. VEGF-C was significantly lower among women with a miscarriage or pregnancy loss. Gal-9 and VEGF-A concentrations were decreased in women with a prior miscarriage. Identification of early changes in maternal immune and angiogenic factors during pregnancy may be a tool to improve patient counseling on pregnancy loss risk and future interventions to reduce miscarriage in a subset of women.

Keywords: miscarriage; pregnancy loss; immunology; vascular endothelial growth factor; galectin-9; interleukin-4

1. Introduction

A positive pregnancy test can be a momentous occasion in a person's life; however, in the United States alone, 20% of couples will experience a pregnancy loss, which can lead to long-term physical and psychological distress [1,2]. Women who have a miscarriage report feeling isolated, ashamed, and dissatisfied that their clinical care did not address their emotional well-being [3]. While approximately half of first trimester miscarriages are associated with genetic abnormalities or identifiable uterine factors, the other 50% often lack a clear cause [4,5]. Currently, we rely on clinical symptoms of vaginal bleeding and cramping as well as trending human chorionic gonadotropin (hCG) levels and early pregnancy transvaginal ultrasonography to determine an increased risk of pregnancy loss; however, these methods are often unclear in the early stages of a miscarriage and there is a need for more prognostic indicators for pregnancy viability.

Pregnancy is a unique period that requires alterations in the immune system to accept a haploidentical fetus. Despite investigation into the fetal and maternal interactions at play during gestation, there is still a limited understanding of these complex interactions [6–12].

There is increasing evidence of the importance of the immune system in the success or failure of a pregnancy. T cell immunoglobulin and mucin-containing protein 3 (Tim-3), a transmembrane protein expressed on differentiated T-helper 1 cells (Th1) and natural killer (NK) cells that functions as an immune checkpoint, has been found to be critical for suppressing allograft rejection [13–18] and, thus, it is hypothesized to play a central role in pregnancy outcomes. Studies have demonstrated that Tim-3 expression on various immune cells is increased early in the first trimester and remains elevated throughout pregnancy [19–22]. Reduced Tim-3 expression has been identified in mice prone to recurrent miscarriage and, additionally, the blockade of the Tim-3 pathway was associated with increased miscarriage rates [20,22,23].

We have previously shown that early in the first trimester plasma galectin-9 (Gal-9) levels increase in maternal blood and remain elevated throughout pregnancy [24]. Gal-9, a ligand for Tim-3, promotes Th1 cell apoptosis, resulting in the downregulation of cytotoxic activity and the promotion of immunologic tolerance [15,18,25]. Interactions between Tim-3 and Gal-9 have also been shown to suppress NK cell cytotoxicity at the maternal–fetal interface [26]. Women who have a history of miscarriage have reduced Gal-9 plasma concentrations, and the administration of Gal-9 reduced embryo loss in abortion-prone mice [22]. Interleukin-4 (IL-4), a cytokine involved in differentiation of naïve CD4+ cells into a Th2, tolerogenic phenotype, increases Tim-3 expression [21,22]. IL-4 expression increases throughout gestation [27,28]. Gal-9 also increases IL-4 concentrations, and in patients with recurrent miscarriage, IL-4 levels have been shown to be decreased [29,30]. This indicates that these interactions have an important role in pregnancy success in early gestation.

In addition to the Tim-3/Gal-9 pathway, which regulates immune tolerance at the maternal–fetal interface, angiogenic factors, such as vascular endothelial growth factor (VEGF), have been shown to have a critical role in pregnancy through ensuring vascular integrity, which supports implantation and embryo development [31–34]. Like Gal-9, VEGF concentrations increase in the decidua and serum during the first trimester and activate VEGF receptors [33,35,36]. Histological differences in VEGF expression in trophoblasts, villi endothelial cells, and decidua have been observed with reduced expression in women with a spontaneous miscarriage compared to women with a viable pregnancy [37–39].

Based on these prior studies, we hypothesized that immunologic dysregulation and alterations in angiogenesis in early pregnancy may account for some causes of unexplained miscarriage and could be measured through the profiling of maternal blood. This study aimed to determine if early plasma protein concentrations including Gal-9, IL-4, VEGF-A, VEGF-C, and VEGF-D were associated with pregnancy loss. This is critical because, despite miscarriage affecting many women, there is an incomplete understanding about the interaction between maternal immune factors, the haploidentical fetus, and angiogenesis, leaving providers with limited tools to help counsel women on risk for or cause of miscarriage or to prevent pregnancy loss.

2. Materials and Methods

2.1. Patient Selection

This study was approved by the Mayo Clinic Institutional Review Board and patients were recruited either under IRB 18-011413 ($n = 63$) or 13-008482 ($n = 3$). The latter IRB was part of an initial pilot study. A prospective, observational study recruited 66 women presenting to the obstetrical unit for prenatal care between 5 weeks and 9 weeks gestation. Patients could be presenting for either a scheduled visit or due to a pregnancy-related concern (bleeding, abdominal pain, or worsening anxiety due to prior miscarriages or ectopic pregnancy). Women, 18 years of age or older, were approached if they had a confirmed viable intrauterine pregnancy (fetal pole with cardiac activity within the uterine cavity) and were planning to deliver at our institution or health system to obtain pregnancy outcomes from their medical records. The study excluded women who were non-English speaking or less than 18 years old. Written informed consent was obtained by all participants involved in the study. Participants were asked if they had experienced any bleeding or cramping prior to enrollment and, once enrolled, they had 10 milliliters of maternal blood collected within 24 h of enrollment. Whole blood was processed with plasma separated and stored at −80 °C until use. Maternal history, pregnancy symptoms, and outcomes were obtained from a medical chart review. Study data were recorded and managed using a secure Research Electronic Data Capture system (REDCap) [40].

2.2. Enzyme Linked Immunosorbent Assays (ELISA)

The following plasma proteins were measured by ELISA to assess immune tolerance: Gal-9, IL-4, VEGF-A, VEGF-C, and VEGF-D. Sandwich ELISAs were used to quantify each protein as per the manufacturer's instructions (R&D Systems, Minneapolis, MN, USA). All samples were run in duplicate, averaged, and a seven-point standard curve was used to calculate concentrations following capture of 450 nm absorbance using a plate reader (BioTek Instruments Inc., Winooski, VT, USA).

2.3. Aims

The primary aims were to determine if Gal-9, IL-4, VEGF-A, -C, and -D concentrations differ between women who experience (a) miscarriage versus ongoing pregnancy at 12 weeks gestation or (b) pregnancy loss compared to live birth. The secondary aims were pre-specified to compare concentrations based on maternal history of miscarriage compared to no miscarriage and to determine if concentrations differed among fetal sex.

2.4. Statistical Analysis

Data are descriptively summarized using frequency counts and percentages for categorical variables, means and standard deviations (SD) for non-skewed continuous variables, and medians and interquartile ranges (IQR) for continuous variables with skewed distributions. Comparisons between groups were evaluated using the Mann–Whitney test U test. Additionally, 95% confidence intervals (95% CI) for the median difference between groups were calculated using the Hodges–Lehmann estimation of location shift, also known as Moses confidence limits. Spearman rank tests were utilized to identify correlations between plasma proteins, maternal age, and gestation age at blood draw. All calculated p-values were two sided and p-values < 0.05 were considered significant. Statistical analysis was performed using SAS version 9.4 (SAS Institute, Cary, NC, USA) and Prism 9.0 (GraphPad, San Diego, CA, USA).

The study was designed to enroll 70 patients, assuming a miscarriage rate of 15%, with the goal of obtaining data on 10 women with a miscarriage and 60 women with a viable pregnancy at 12 weeks. With this sample size, the study would have 80% power to detect a difference in groups means of 2 standard deviations and 90% power to detect a difference in groups means of 1.16 standard deviations, using a two-sided two-sample t-test with a type I error of 5%. However, given the skewed nature of the observed data, the actual data analysis utilized a non-parametric test, the Mann–Whitney U test, instead of the parametric two-sample t-test, and therefore, the statistical power of our analysis was 5–10% less than what we projected.

3. Results

In total, 74 women were approached, 66 consented to participate, and 8 declined. After enrollment, it was determined that 10 women never had a confirmed viable intrauterine pregnancy at the time of blood draw and they were excluded, leaving 56 participants. Three women recruited under IRB 13-008482 did not have VEGF-A data.

3.1. Patient Characteristics and Pregnancy Outcomes

The mean maternal age at recruitment was 30.3 (SD 4.4; range 20–38). The mean gravidity was 2.4 (SD 1.6; range 1–7) and the mean parity was 1 (SD 1.1, range 0–4). Race among participants included 52 (92.9%) self-described as Caucasian, 2 (3.5%) as Asian, 1 (1.8%) as Black, and 1 (1.8%) as other. Table 1 details maternal characteristics based on pregnancy outcomes. Among the 56 included participants, 8 women had spontaneous miscarriage diagnosed prior to 12 weeks gestation, and 2 had losses after 12 weeks gestation. In the loss group, 60% (6/10) of participants had symptoms of bleeding or abdominal pain. In the viable group, approximately a third of women (15/46) had the same concerning symptoms. Genetic testing was not performed in any patient with a pregnancy loss. Overall, 38 women had live births, and 8 women did not have known pregnancy outcomes, but had a viable pregnancy at 20 weeks gestation. (Figure 1) We did not observe strong correlations between the plasma protein concentrations and maternal age or gestational age at recruitment in our study (Supplemental Figure S1). Therefore, we did not fit multivariable models adjusting for these covariates; however, this should be explored in larger studies.

Table 1. Maternal and obstetric characteristics in women with pregnancy loss compared to women who had live birth or viable pregnancy at 20 weeks gestation.

Characteristic	Miscarriage or Pregnancy Loss (n = 10)	Viable Pregnancy or Live Birth (n = 46)
Maternal Age, mean (SD)	31.7 (3.7)	30.0 (4.6)
Body mass index pre-pregnancy, mean (SD)	30.3 (6.3)	28.2 (7.0)
Gravidity, mean (SD)	2.1 (1.8)	2.5 (1.5)
Parity, mean (SD)	0.9 (1.5)	1.0 (1.0)
Prior spontaneous miscarriage, N (%)	1 (10%)	10 (22%)
Race, N (%)		
Caucasian	9 (90%)	43 (94%)
Black	1 (10%)	0 (0%)
Asian	0 (0%)	2 (4%)
Other	0 (0%)	1 (2%)
Maternal comorbidities, N (%)		
Pregestational diabetes	0 (0%)	3 (6.5%)
Chronic hypertension	2 (20%)	0 (0%)
Thyroid disorder	0 (0%)	2 (4.3%)
Rheumatologic condition	0 (0%)	1 (2.2%)
Gestational age at recruitment, N (%)		
5 weeks	1 (10%)	3 (6.5%)
6 weeks	5 (50%)	10 (21.7%)
7 weeks	2 (20%)	6 (13.0%)
8 weeks	2 (20%)	18 (39.1%)
9 weeks	0 (0%)	9 (19.6%)
Symptoms, N (%)		
Yes	6 (60%)	15 (32.6%)
No	4 (40%)	31 (67.4%)

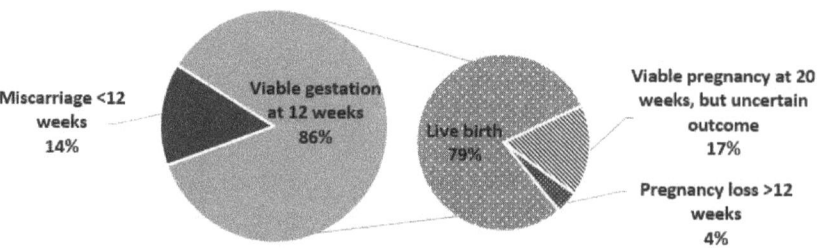

Figure 1. Pregnancy outcomes of the women enrolled on this prospective cohort.

3.2. VEGF-C Is Lower in Women with Miscarriage Prior to 12 Weeks Gestation

Plasma concentrations were compared between the 8 women who experienced a spontaneous loss prior to 12 weeks gestation versus the 48 women with viable pregnancy at 12 weeks. The median concentration of VEGF-C was significantly lower among women who experienced a miscarriage versus those who had an ongoing pregnancy at 12 weeks (1191 pg/mL vs. 2815 pg/mL, respectively, $p = 0.04$). There was no statistically significant difference in median concentrations for Gal-9, IL-4, VEGF-A, and VEGF-D between groups (Table 2).

Table 2. Plasma concentrations for immune tolerance markers and angiogenic factors based on pregnancy outcome at 12 weeks gestation.

Plasma Concentrations (pg/mL)	Miscarriage ($n = 8$) Median (IQR)	Viable Gestation ($n = 48$) Median (IQR)	95% CI for the Median Difference between Groups †	p-Value
Gal-9	513.2 (396.9, 1179.9)	662.0 (273.6, 1145.7)	−375.8 to 461.3	0.99
IL-4	36.6 (13.2, 64.1)	55.2 (30.3, 192.7)	−2.6 to 143.6	0.08
VEGF-A *	46.2 (40.2, 52.1)	52.8 (24.8, 100.9)	−19.9 to 51.8	0.65
VEGF-C	1191.0 (607.8, 2172.6)	2815.1 (1320.5, 3718.3)	80.9 to 2536.7	0.04
VEGF-D	442.2 (349.3, 1193.5)	583.2 (338.4, 1647.1)	−163.4 to 595.3	0.44

† Difference calculated as viable gestation group minus miscarriage group. * Three patients had missing VEGF-A data, two had a miscarriage prior to 12 weeks, and 1 had viable gestation.

3.3. VEGF-C Is Lower in Women with Pregnancy Loss Compared to Live Birth

We then compared plasma concentrations in 38 women who had a live birth compared to 10 with a pregnancy loss. No significant differences between groups were detected in the concentrations of Gal-9 (Figure 2A, $p = 0.64$) and IL-4 (Figure 2B, $p = 0.13$). VEGF-C levels were again found to be significantly lower among women with pregnancy loss (Figure 2D, median 932.7 vs. 3116.2 pg/mL, $p = 0.001$). Additionally, VEGF-A (Figure 2C, $p = 0.25$) and -D (Figure 2E, $p = 0.23$) concentrations were not significantly different between the two groups.

3.4. History of Miscarriage Associated with Decreased Gal-9 and VEGF-A

We then wanted to know if a history of miscarriage impacts protein levels in a subsequent pregnancy. Among our cohort, 11 women had a prior spontaneous miscarriage. We observed that their median plasma concentrations were significantly lower for Gal-9 (395.8 vs. 701.5 pg/mL, $p = 0.02$, Figure 3A) and VEGF-A (28.5 vs. 53.4 pg/mL, $p = 0.04$, Figure 3C) compared to the 45 women with no prior miscarriage. There were no significant differences in IL-4 (Figure 3B, $p = 0.52$), VEGF-C (Figure 3D, $p = 0.99$) or VEGF-D (Figure 3E, $p = 0.79$). The difference in Gal-9 levels persisted when comparing 11 women with a history of miscarriage to 24 with a prior pregnancy and no miscarriage history (median, 395.8 vs. 761.0 pg/mL, $p = 0.053$, Table 3). While the VEGF-A concentration was lower, it no longer attained statistical significance when excluding primiparous women (median, 28.5 vs. 51.5 pg/mL, $p = 0.08$). No significant differences were seen in maternal plasma concentrations of all proteins in women for which this was their first pregnancy (N = 21) compared to women with a prior positive pregnancy test (N = 35, Figure 4A–E).

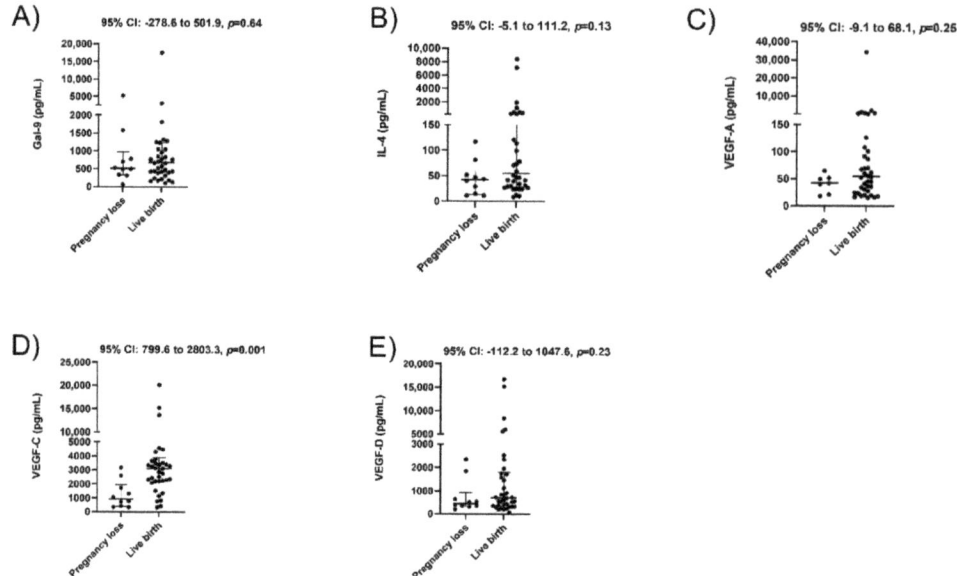

Figure 2. Plasma concentrations of immune tolerance markers and angiogenic factors among women who experience pregnancy loss versus live birth. Concentrations of Galectin-9 (**A**), IL-4 (**B**), VEGF-A (**C**), VEGF-C (**D**), and VEGF-D (**E**) as measured by ELISA. Data are displayed as median with interquartile range along with 95% CI for the median difference between groups above each panel.

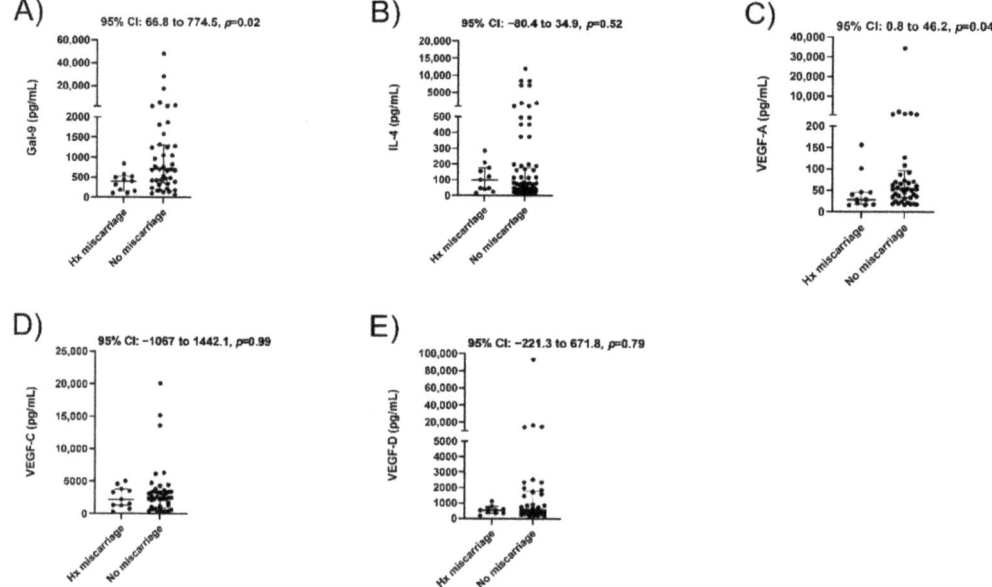

Figure 3. Maternal blood levels of immune tolerance and angiogenesis based on history (Hx) of miscarriage. Concentrations determined by ELISA for Galectin-9 (**A**), IL-4 (**B**), VEGF-A (**C**), VEGF-C (**D**), and VEGF-D (**E**). Data are displayed as the median with interquartile range along with 95% CI for the median difference between groups above each panel.

Table 3. Plasma concentrations in maternal blood from women with a history of miscarriage versus history of prior pregnancy with no history of miscarriage.

Plasma Concentrations (pg/mL)	History of Miscarriage (n = 11) Median (IQR)	History of Prior Pregnancy and No Miscarriage (n = 24) Median (IQR)	95% CI for the Median Difference between Groups †	p-Value
Gal-9	395.8 (156.4, 518.4)	761.0 (272.1, 1430.4)	−2.9 to 937.4	0.053
IL-4	99.3 (41.2, 176.0)	79.7 (28.3, 324.5)	−69.9 to 146.7	0.96
VEGF-A *	28.5 (17.0, 45.8)	51.5 (28.6, 280.5)	−2.9 to 71.7	0.08
VEGF-C	2205.6 (1293.3, 3790.2)	2327.3 (815.4, 3352.7)	−1365.4 to 1153.1	0.71
VEGF-D	548.5 (349.6, 788.9)	543.2 (314.2, 1780.6)	−256.3 to 582.0	0.90

† Difference calculated as history of prior pregnancy and no miscarriage group minus history of miscarriage group. * 3 patients had missing VEGF-A data; 2 with miscarriage prior to 12 weeks and 1 with viable gestation.

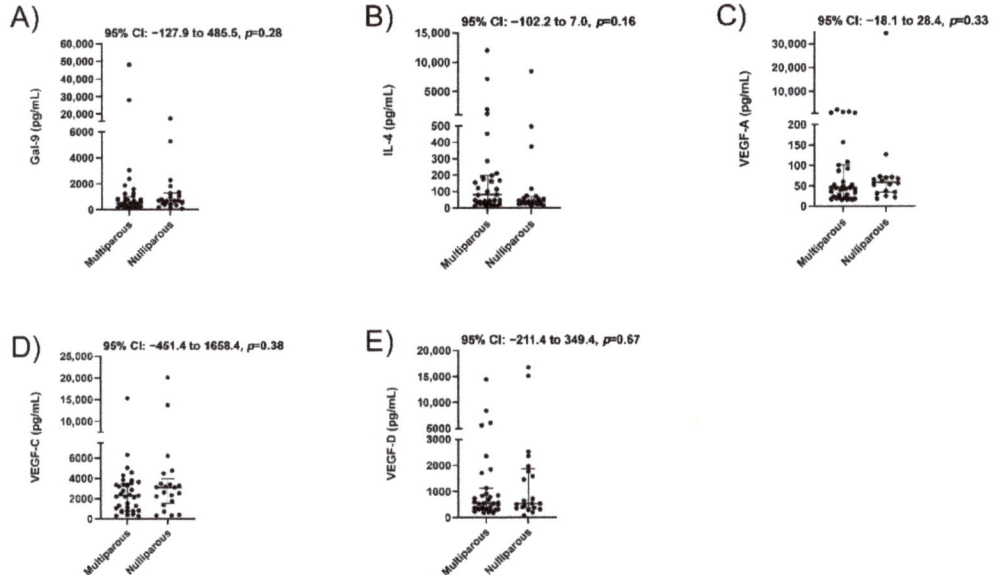

Figure 4. Plasma concentrations in maternal blood from women who are nulligravid (n = 21) versus women with prior pregnancy (n = 35). Concentrations of Galectin-9 (**A**), IL-4 (**B**), VEGF-A (**C**), VEGF-C (**D**), and VEGF-D (**E**) determined by ELISA. Data are displayed as median with interquartile range, along with 95% CI for the median difference between groups above each panel.

3.5. No Differences between Male and Female Fetuses

Lastly, we looked for differences in maternal blood protein concentrations by fetal sex among women with a live birth, as we had previously identified differences in maternal blood cytokines and angiogenic factors based on fetal sex [41]. We observed no significant differences between groups (n = 15 with a female live birth vs. n = 23 with a male live birth) in the concentrations for Gal-9 ($p = 0.74$) or IL-4 ($p = 0.50$) in maternal blood (Figure 5A,B). Additionally, there were no differences between VEGF-A (Figure 5C, $p = 0.30$), VEGF-C (Figure 5D, $p = 0.77$), or VEGF-D (Figure 5E, $p = 0.47$). Therefore, we suspect that fetal sex does not change levels of these cytokines and angiogenic factors in early pregnancy.

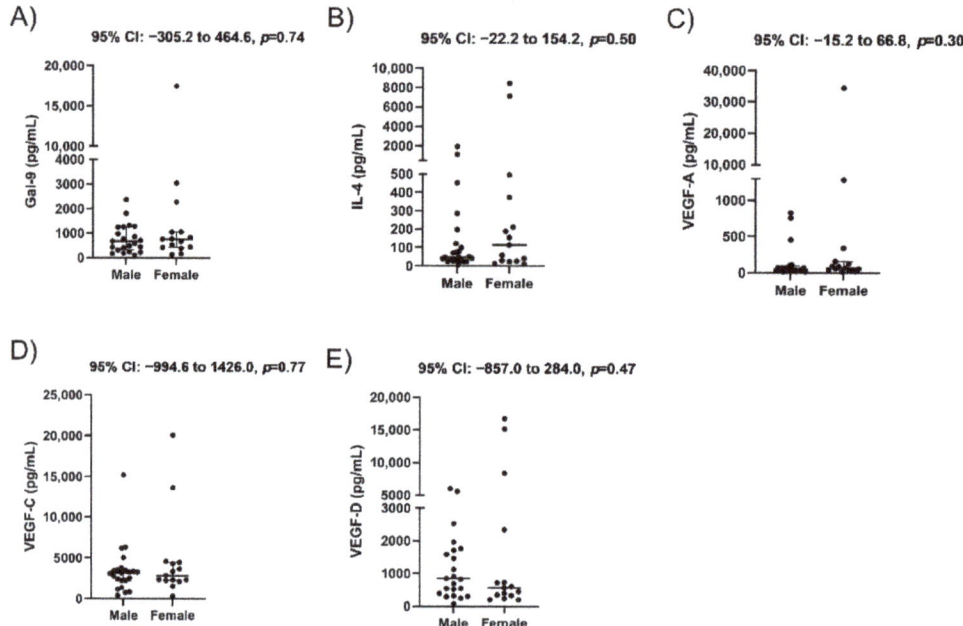

Figure 5. Maternal plasma concentrations based on fetal sex. Concentrations determined by ELISA for Galectin-9 (**A**), IL-4 (**B**), VEGF-A (**C**), VEGF-C (**D**), and VEGF-D (**E**) compared based on the sex of the fetus. Data are displayed as the median with interquartile range, along with 95% CI for the median difference between groups above each panel.

4. Discussion

The immune system is complex and composed of both innate and adaptive immunity, which protects against foreign antigens (i.e., non-self or pathogens). Gal-9 was selected for assessment of prognostic value based on previous studies that have demonstrated significantly reduced plasma and decidual Gal-9 concentrations among women experiencing a miscarriage compared to a viable pregnancy [22,28]. In the present study, we did not identify significantly lower concentrations of Gal-9 based on the current pregnancy outcomes (miscarriage or live birth). Reasons that our results differed from prior studies may include that prior studies did not report on the gestational age when the samples were collected or the timing in relation to the diagnosis of miscarriage. Additionally, they recruited women with spontaneous miscarriage or undergoing elective termination and, thus, the true pregnancy outcome is unknown. In the present study, Gal-9 was lower in women with a history of pregnancy loss, but not different based on whether this was a women's first pregnancy. This adds to the hypothesis that Gal-9 levels appear to have a role in pregnancy viability; however, its utility to identify increased risk for adverse pregnancy outcomes needs further assessment.

Cytokine expression profiles in the decidua appear to favor those produced by Th2 cells, including IL-4, which appears to be partially regulated by Gal-9 [10]. Reduced concentrations of IL-4 in the decidua of women experiencing a recurrent pregnancy loss compared to women with viable pregnancy choosing elective termination have previously been shown [42]; however, there have been limited previous evaluations of plasma cytokine profiles and pregnancy outcomes, which prompted our investigation. The present study did not show any difference in plasma IL-4 concentrations based on maternal pregnancy history nor current pregnancy outcomes. This finding is similar to the work by Marzi et al., which showed peripheral blood mononuclear cells (PBMC) production of IL-4 was not different in women with live births compared to women with a miscarriage or birth of a small for gestational age fetus; however, they obtained samples throughout all gestations of pregnancy [27]. Our findings differed from other studies that showed plasma IL-4 concentrations in early pregnancy were reduced in women with recurrent miscarriages compared to normal pregnancy, but levels measured in the miscarriage cohort occurred at the time of miscarriage diagnosis and not prospectively [22,28]. Based on the findings in our study, maternal blood IL-4 concentrations, obtained early in gestation, do not appear to be associated with the outcome of a pregnancy.

Angiogenesis is also of great importance during implantation and maintenance of pregnancy. VEGF and its receptors have been identified as key players in normal endometrial vascular remodeling and placentation in pregnancy, with increasing VEGF concentrations throughout the first trimester [36,39,43]. The current study demonstrated that lower blood concentrations of VEGF-C were seen in women who experienced either a miscarriage or pregnancy loss. This suggests that VEGF-C blood levels early in pregnancy may help identify pregnancies at higher risk for adverse outcome, but not be able to predict the timing of event. VEGF-A concentration was significantly decreased among women who experienced a prior miscarriage compared to women without a miscarriage history. These findings support prior work that also found serum levels of VEGF-A and -C obtained outside of pregnancy are decreased in women with a history of recurrent miscarriage compared to women with prior pregnancy and no miscarriage [43,44]. Additionally, this correlates with lower levels of VEGF expression in the decidua and chorionic villi in the first trimester seen in women who experienced recurrent pregnancy loss compared to elective termination [37,39]. These differences in VEGF concentrations highlight their important role in implantation and placental development.

The current study suggests VEGF plasma concentrations obtained in early pregnancy may be used to identify pregnancies at increased risk of miscarriage or fetal loss and provide a source for intervention. Scarpellini et al. demonstrated that in women with recurrent pregnancy loss, the administration of granulocyte colony stimulating factor (G-CSF) is associated with increased VEGF expression in trophoblasts; however, pregnant women between 8 and 12 weeks gestation without recurrent pregnancy loss and who did not receive G-CSF had higher expression levels of VEGF [45]. This study of G-CSF exposure and our current findings demonstrates the potential to identify interventions or therapies that improve the chance for successful pregnancies once better biomarkers and risk factors for miscarriage are understood.

In the present study, we also sought to explore if fetal sex altered maternal cytokine secretion, given exposure to a foreign Y chromosome, which may require an additional secretion of immune-suppressing proteins. We previously showed that mothers of male fetuses had increased plasma concentrations of VEGF-A and proinflammatory cytokines throughout pregnancy, although no difference in VEGF-D concentrations were seen between male and female offspring [41]. Placental expression for genes involved in the immune system and graft-versus-host interactions have also shown to be increased in the placentas of male compared to female fetuses born prematurely [46]. In the present study, however, we did not detect a difference in VEGF-A, -C, and -D blood concentrations. Additionally, neither Gal-9 nor IL-4 showed different expression levels based on fetal sex. Our sample was limited to only those with a live birth as genetic information to confirm the fetal sex was not present for any of the pregnancy losses. The lack of significant differences in angiogenic and immune tolerance proteins was an unexpected finding. Further evaluation of factors that do differ between mothers carrying male versus female offspring may allow for a deeper understanding of the interplay of the immune system, angiogenesis, and pregnancy viability.

While this study did meet the sample size for pregnancy losses required by our power calculation, it is still limited by the small numbers in the setting of a wider range of concentrations than anticipated. Additionally, samples were obtained during a 5-week range in the first trimester. Prior studies have shown plasma concentrations of proteins of interest in the study increase in pregnancy, but there is not strong evidence regarding the gestational age at which they plateau [24,27,28,35]. While there are known factors for pregnancy loss, this study was not able to include genetic information, assessment for uterine factors associated with increased miscarriage risk, or biochemical loss. Repeating the study with a pre-pregnancy measurement and then weekly measurements from 5 until 10 weeks gestation, with genetic testing in all pregnancies, would be of interest to better determine if a certain time point or pattern could be utilized to predict pregnancy outcomes and offer opportunities for intervention in those with unexplained losses. We did not observe meaningful correlations between the concentration levels and maternal age or gestational age at recruitment in our study. Therefore, we did not fit multivariable models adjusting for these covariates; however, this should be explored in larger studies especially if there is more heterogeneity in the maternal age and gestational age at recruitment. Lastly, there is a lack of racial and ethnic diversity in the population. A strength of this study, however, was collecting samples prospectively in women with confirmed intrauterine pregnancy and following the pregnancy in its entirety. Many previous prospective studies of pregnant women recruited patients at the time of miscarriage diagnosis or women undergoing elective termination, which could be responsible for differences in our study compared to others.

5. Conclusions

Successful pregnancy implantation and growth is complex. While chromosomal factors are known to be critical for pregnancy success, evidence suggests that angiogenic and immune marker expression also has a significant impact on the success or failure of a pregnancy. Among women with a viable early pregnancy, we found that reduced concentrations of Gal-9 and VEGF-A are more common among women with a prior miscarriage, while decreased VEGF-C expression in the first trimester suggested an increased risk of miscarriage or fetal loss. Further understanding and identification of altered biomarkers prior to or early in pregnancy that increase miscarriage risk is important. Developing thresholds and predictability of serum levels could lead to better pregnancy counseling and the development of potential therapeutic strategies to prevent pregnancy loss.

Supplementary Materials: The following are available online at https://www.mdpi.com/article/10.3390/jcm10163579/s1, Supplemental Figure S1: Correlations between plasma proteins, gestational age at recruitment, and maternal age. (A) Correlation between plasma proteins and maternal age. (B) Correlation between plasma proteins and gestational age at blood collection. Spearman rank coefficients are presented. All p-values were >0.05.

Author Contributions: Conceptualization, M.A.W., S.C.B., C.C.V.O., R.R., C.C.S. and E.A.L.E.; Data curation, M.A.W., S.C.B., A.L.W., B.F. and E.A.L.E.; Formal analysis, M.A.W., A.L.W. and E.A.L.E.; Funding acquisition, M.A.W., S.C.B. and E.A.L.E.; Investigation, M.A.W., S.C.B., C.C.V.O., B.F. and E.A.L.E.; Methodology, M.A.W., S.C.B., A.L.W., C.C.V.O., C.C.S. and E.A.L.E.; Project administration, C.C.V.O.; Resources, B.F. and E.A.L.E.; Supervision, C.C.S. and E.A.L.E.; Writing—original draft, M.A.W.; Writing—review and editing, A.L.W., R.R., C.C.S. and E.A.L.E. All authors have read and agreed to the published version of the manuscript.

Funding: This study was funded by the Mayo Clinic Department of Obstetrics and Gynecology (M.W. and S.B.) and the NICHD Building Interdisciplinary Research Careers in Women's Health (BIRCWH) K12 HD065987 (EE).

Institutional Review Board Statement: The study was conducted according to the guidelines of the Declaration of Helsinki and approved by the Institutional Review Board of Mayo Clinic (IRB 18-011413 24 June 2019 and 13-008482 17 June 2014). Informed consent was obtained from all subjects involved in this study.

Informed Consent Statement: Informed consent was obtained from all subjects involved in the study.

Data Availability Statement: De-identified data are available upon reasonable request by contacting the corresponding author.

Conflicts of Interest: The authors declare no conflict of interest.

References

1. Rossen, L.M.; Ahrens, K.A.; Branum, A.M. Trends in Risk of Pregnancy Loss Among US Women, 1990–2011. *Paediatr. Perinat. Epidemiol.* **2018**, *32*, 19–29. [CrossRef]
2. Cumming, G.; Klein, S.; Bolsover, D.; Lee, A.; Alexander, D.; MacLean, M.; Jurgens, J. The emotional burden of miscarriage for women and their partners: Trajectories of anxiety and depression over 13 months. *BJOG Int. J. Obstet. Gynaecol.* **2007**, *114*, 1138–1145. [CrossRef]
3. Bardos, J.; Hercz, D.; Friedenthal, J.; Missmer, S.A.; Williams, Z. A national survey on public perceptions of miscarriage. *Obstet. Gynecol.* **2015**, *125*, 1313–1320. [CrossRef] [PubMed]
4. Gug, C.; Rațiu, A.; Navolan, D.; Drăgan, I.; Groza, I.-M.; Păpurică, M.; Vaida, M.-A.; Mozoș, I.; Jurcă, M.C. Incidence and Spectrum of Chromosome Abnormalities in Miscarriage Samples: A Retrospective Study of 330 Cases. *Cytogenet. Genome. Res.* **2019**, *158*, 171–183. [CrossRef] [PubMed]
5. Petracchi, F.; Colaci, D.S.; Igarzabal, L.; Gadow, E. Cytogenetic analysis of first trimester pregnancy loss. *Int. J. Gynaecol. Obstet.* **2009**, *104*, 243–244. [CrossRef]
6. Tafuri, A.; Alferink, J.; Moller, P.; Hammerling, G.J.; Arnold, B.T. Cell awareness of paternal alloantigens during pregnancy. *Science* **1995**, *270*, 630–633. [CrossRef]
7. Munn, D.H.; Zhou, M.; Attwood, J.T.; Bondarev, I.; Conway, S.J.; Marshall, B.; Brown, C.; Mellor, A.L. Prevention of allogeneic fetal rejection by tryptophan catabolism. *Science* **1998**, *281*, 1191–1193. [CrossRef] [PubMed]
8. Mellor, A.L.; Munn, D.H. Immunology at the maternal-fetal interface: Lessons for T cell tolerance and suppression. *Annu. Rev. Immunol.* **2000**, *18*, 367–391. [CrossRef]
9. Aluvihare, V.R.; Kallikourdis, M.; Betz, A.G. Regulatory T cells mediate maternal tolerance to the fetus. *Nat. Immunol.* **2004**, *5*, 266–271. [CrossRef] [PubMed]
10. Saito, S.; Sasaki, Y.; Sakai, M. CD4(+)CD25high regulatory T cells in human pregnancy. *J. Reprod. Immunol.* **2005**, *65*, 111–120. [CrossRef]
11. Petroff, M.G. Immune interactions at the maternal-fetal interface. *J. Reprod. Immunol.* **2005**, *68*, 1–13. [CrossRef]
12. Riley, J.K. Trophoblast immune receptors in maternal-fetal tolerance. *Immunol. Investig.* **2008**, *37*, 395–426. [CrossRef] [PubMed]
13. Ueno, T.; Habicht, A.; Clarkson, M.R.; Albin, M.J.; Yamaura, K.; Boenisch, O.; Popoola, J.; Wang, Y.; Yagita, H.; Akiba, H.; et al. The emerging role of T cell Ig mucin 1 in alloimmune responses in an experimental mouse transplant model. *J. Clin. Investig.* **2008**, *118*, 742–751. [CrossRef]
14. Boenisch, O.; D'Addio, F.; Watanabe, T.; Elyaman, W.; Magee, C.N.; Yeung, M.Y.; Padera, R.F.; Rodig, S.J.; Murayama, T.; Tanaka, K.; et al. TIM-3: A novel regulatory molecule of alloimmune activation. *J. Immunol.* **2010**, *185*, 5806–5819. [CrossRef]
15. Sánchez-Fueyo, A.; Tian, J.; Picarella, D.; Domenig, C.; Zheng, X.X.; Sabatos, C.A.; Strom, T.B. Tim-3 inhibits T helper type 1-mediated auto- and alloimmune responses and promotes immunological tolerance. *Nat. Immunol.* **2003**, *4*, 1093–1101. [CrossRef] [PubMed]
16. Monney, L.; Sabatos, C.A.; Gaglia, J.L.; Ryu, A.; Waldner, H.; Chernova, T.; Manning, S.; Greenfield, E.A.; Coyle, A.J.; Sobel, R.A.; et al. Th1-specific cell surface protein Tim-3 regulates macrophage activation and severity of an autoimmune disease. *Nature* **2002**, *415*, 536–541. [CrossRef] [PubMed]
17. Hu, X.H.; Tang, M.X.; Mor, G.; Liao, A.H. Tim-3: Expression on immune cells and roles at the maternal-fetal interface. *J. Reprod. Immunol.* **2016**, *118*, 92–99. [CrossRef]
18. Zhu, C.; Anderson, A.C.; Schubart, A.; Xiong, H.; Imitola, J.; Khoury, S.; Zheng, X.X.; Strom, T.B.; Kuchroo, V.K. The Tim-3 ligand galectin-9 negatively regulates T helper type 1 immunity. *Nat. Immunol.* **2005**, *6*, 1245–1252. [CrossRef]
19. Meggyes, M.; Miko, E.; Polgar, B.; Bogar, B.; Farkas, B.; Illes, Z.; Szereday, L. Peripheral blood TIM-3 positive NK and CD8+ T cells throughout pregnancy: TIM-3/galectin-9 interaction and its possible role during pregnancy. *PLoS ONE* **2014**, *9*, e92371. [CrossRef]
20. Wang, S.-C.; Li, Y.-H.; Piao, H.-L.; Hong, X.-W.; Zhang, D.; Xu, Y.-Y.; Tao, Y.; Wang, Y.; Yuan, M.-M.; Li, D.-J.; et al. PD-1 and Tim-3 pathways are associated with regulatory CD8+ T-cell function in decidua and maintenance of normal pregnancy. *Cell Death Dis.* **2015**, *6*, e1738. [CrossRef]
21. Zhao, J.; Lei, Z.; Liu, Y.; Li, B.; Zhang, L.; Fang, H.; Song, C.; Wang, X.; Zhang, G.-M.; Feng, Z.-H.; et al. Human pregnancy up-regulates Tim-3 in innate immune cells for systemic immunity. *J. Immunol.* **2009**, *182*, 6618–6624. [CrossRef]
22. Li, Y.; Zhang, J.; Zhang, D.; Hong, X.; Tao, Y.; Wang, S.; Xu, Y.; Piao, H.; Yin, W.; Yu, M.; et al. Tim-3 signaling in peripheral NK cells promotes maternal-fetal immune tolerance and alleviates pregnancy loss. *Sci. Signal.* **2017**, *10*, eaah4323. [CrossRef]
23. Li, G.; Lu, C.; Gao, J.; Wang, X.; Wu, H.; Lee, C.; Xing, B.; Zhang, Q. Association between PD-1/PD-L1 and T regulate cells in early recurrent miscarriage. *Int. J. Clin. Exp. Pathol.* **2015**, *8*, 6512–6518.
24. Enninga, E.A.L.; Harrington, S.M.; Creedon, D.J.; Ruano, R.; Markovic, S.N.; Dong, H.; Dronca, R.S. Immune checkpoint molecules soluble program death ligand 1 and galectin-9 are increased in pregnancy. *Am. J. Reprod. Immunol.* **2018**, *79*, e12795. [CrossRef]
25. Kuchroo, V.K.; Meyers, J.H.; Umetsu, D.T.; DeKruyff, R.H. TIM family of genes in immunity and tolerance. *Adv. Immunol.* **2006**, *91*, 227–249. [CrossRef]
26. Ndhlovu, L.C.; Lopez-Vergès, S.; Barbour, J.D.; Jones, R.B.; Jha, A.; Long, B.R.; Schoeffler, E.C.; Fujita, T.; Nixon, D.; Lanier, L.L. Tim-3 marks human natural killer cell maturation and suppresses cell-mediated cytotoxicity. *Blood* **2012**, *119*, 3734–3743. [CrossRef] [PubMed]

27. Marzi, M.; Vigano, A.; Trabattoni, D.; Villa, M.L.; Salvaggio, A.; Clerici, M. Characterization of type 1 and type 2 cytokine production profile in physiologic and pathologic human pregnancy. *Clin. Exp. Immunol.* **1996**, *106*, 127–133. [CrossRef] [PubMed]
28. Li, J.; Li, F.-F.; Zuo, W.; Zhou, Y.; Hao, H.-Y.; Dang, J.; Jiang, M.; He, M.-Z.; Deng, D.-R. Up-regulated expression of Tim-3/Gal-9 at maternal-fetal interface in pregnant woman with recurrent spontaneous abortion. *J. Huazhong Univ. Sci. Technol. [Med. Sci.]* **2014**, *34*, 586–590. [CrossRef]
29. Li, Y.-H.; Zhou, W.-H.; Tao, Y.; Wang, S.-C.; Jiang, Y.-L.; Zhang, D.; Piao, H.-L.; Fu, Q.; Li, D.-J.; Du, M.-R. The Galectin-9/Tim-3 pathway is involved in the regulation of NK cell function at the maternal-fetal interface in early pregnancy. *Cell Mol. Immunol.* **2016**, *13*, 73–81. [CrossRef]
30. Fukui, A.; Kwak-Kim, J.; Ntrivalas, E.; Gilman-Sachs, A.; Lee, S.K.; Beaman, K. Intracellular cytokine expression of peripheral blood natural killer cell subsets in women with recurrent spontaneous abortions and implantation failures. *Fertil. Steril.* **2008**, *89*, 157–165. [CrossRef] [PubMed]
31. Rowe, A.J.; Wulff, C.; Fraser, H.M. Localization of mRNA for vascular endothelial growth factor (VEGF), angiopoietins and their receptors during the peri-implantation period and early pregnancy in marmosets (Callithrix jacchus). *Reproduction* **2003**, *126*, 227–238. [CrossRef]
32. Ahmed, A.; Li, X.F.; Dunk, C.; Whittle, M.J.; Rushton, D.I.; Rollason, T. Colocalisation of vascular endothelial growth factor and its Flt-1 receptor in human placenta. *Growth Factors* **1995**, *12*, 235–243. [CrossRef]
33. Cooper, J.C.; Sharkey, A.M.; McLaren, J.; Charnock-Jones, D.S.; Smith, S.K. Localization of vascular endothelial growth factor and its receptor, flt, in human placenta and decidua by immunohistochemistry. *J. Reprod. Fertil.* **1995**, *105*, 205–213. [CrossRef] [PubMed]
34. Sugino, N.; Kashida, S.; Karube-Harada, A.; Takiguchi, S.; Kato, H. Expression of vascular endothelial growth factor (VEGF) and its receptors in human endometrium throughout the menstrual cycle and in early pregnancy. *Reproduction* **2002**, *123*, 379–387. [CrossRef]
35. Evans, P.; Wheeler, T.; Anthony, F.; Osmond, C. Maternal serum vascular endothelial growth factor during early pregnancy. *Clin. Sci. (Lond.)* **1997**, *92*, 567–571. [CrossRef] [PubMed]
36. Jackson, M.R.; Carney, E.W.; Lye, S.J.; Ritchie, J.W. Localization of two angiogenic growth factors (PDECGF and VEGF) in human placentae throughout gestation. *Placenta* **1994**, *15*, 341–353. [CrossRef]
37. Vuorela, P.; Carpen, O.; Tulppala, M.; Halmesmaki, E. VEGF, its receptors and the tie receptors in recurrent miscarriage. *Mol. Hum. Reprod.* **2000**, *6*, 276–282. [CrossRef] [PubMed]
38. Col-Madendag, I.; Madendag, Y.; Altinkaya, S.O.; Bayramoglu, H.; Danisman, N. The role of VEGF and its receptors in the etiology of early pregnancy loss. *Gynecol. Endocrinol.* **2014**, *30*, 153–156. [CrossRef]
39. He, X.; Chen, Q. Reduced expressions of connexin 43 and VEGF in the first-trimester tissues from women with recurrent pregnancy loss. *Reprod. Biol. Endocrinol.* **2016**, *14*, 46. [CrossRef]
40. Harris, P.A.; Taylor, R.; Thielke, R.; Payne, J.; Gonzalez, N.; Conde, J.G. Research electronic data capture (REDCap)—A metadata-driven methodology and workflow process for providing translational research informatics support. *J. Biomed. Inform.* **2009**, *42*, 377–381. [CrossRef]
41. Enninga, E.A.; Nevala, W.K.; Creedon, D.J.; Markovic, S.N.; Holtan, S.G. Fetal sex-based differences in maternal hormones, angiogenic factors, and immune mediators during pregnancy and the postpartum period. *Am. J. Reprod. Immunol.* **2015**, *73*, 251–262. [CrossRef] [PubMed]
42. Logiodice, F.; Lombardelli, L.; Kullolli, O.; Haller, H.; Maggi, E.; Rukavina, D.; Piccinni, M.P. Decidual Interleukin-22-Producing CD4+ T Cells (Th17/Th0/IL-22+ and Th17/Th2/IL-22+, Th2/IL-22+, Th0/IL-22+), Which Also Produce IL-4, Are Involved in the Success of Pregnancy. *Int. J. Mol. Sci.* **2019**, *20*, 428. [CrossRef] [PubMed]
43. Bagheri, A.; Kumar, P.; Kamath, A.; Rao, P. A ssociation of angiogenic cytokines (VEGF-A and VEGF-C) and clinical characteristic in women with unexplained recurrent miscarriage. *Bratisl. Lek. Listy.* **2017**, *118*, 258–264. [CrossRef] [PubMed]
44. Gupta, P.; Deo, S.; Jaiswar, S.P.; Sankhwar, P.L. Case Control Study to Compare Serum Vascular Endothelial Growth Factor (VEGF) Level in Women with Recurrent Pregnancy Loss (RPL) Compared to Women with Term Pregnancy. *J. Obstet. Gynaecol. India* **2019**, *69* (Suppl. S2), 95–102. [CrossRef] [PubMed]
45. Scarpellini, F.; Klinger, F.G.; Rossi, G.; Sbracia, M. Immunohistochemical Study on the Expression of G-CSF, G-CSFR, VEGF, VEGFR-1, Foxp3 in First Trimester Trophoblast of Recurrent Pregnancy Loss in Pregnancies Treated with G-CSF and Controls. *Int. J. Mol. Sci.* **2019**, *21*, 285. [CrossRef]
46. Cvitic, S.; Longtine, M.; Hackl, H.; Wagner, K.; Nelson, M.D.; Desoye, G.; Hiden, U. The human placental sexome differs between trophoblast epithelium and villous vessel endothelium. *PLoS ONE* **2013**, *8*, e79233. [CrossRef]

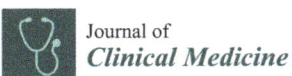

Article

Pre-Clinical Investigation of Cardioprotective Beta-Blockers as a Therapeutic Strategy for Preeclampsia

Natalie K. Binder [1,2,3,†], Teresa M. MacDonald [1,3,†], Sally A. Beard [1,2,3], Natasha de Alwis [1,2,3], Stephen Tong [1,3], Tu'uhevaha J. Kaitu'u-Lino [1,3,4] and Natalie J. Hannan [1,2,3,*]

1. Translational Obstetrics Group, Department of Obstetrics and Gynaecology, University of Melbourne, Mercy Hospital for Women, Heidelberg 3084, Australia; nkbinder@unimelb.edu.au (N.K.B.); teresa.macdonald@mercy.com.au (T.M.M.); sally.beard@unimelb.edu.au (S.A.B.); maryd2@student.unimelb.edu.au (N.d.A.); stong@unimelb.edu.au (S.T.); t.klino@unimelb.edu.au (T.J.K.-L.)
2. Therapeutics Discovery and Vascular Function Group, Department of Obstetrics and Gynaecology, University of Melbourne, Mercy Hospital for Women, Heidelberg 3084, Australia
3. Mercy Perinatal, Mercy Hospital for Women, Heidelberg 3084, Australia
4. Diagnostics Discovery and Reverse Translation, Department of Obstetrics and Gynaecology, University of Melbourne, Mercy Hospital for Women, Heidelberg 3084, Australia
* Correspondence: nhannan@unimelb.edu.au; Tel.: +61-3-8458-4371
† Equal contribution.

Abstract: Despite significant maternal and fetal morbidity, a treatment for preeclampsia currently remains an unmet need in clinical care. As too does the lifelong cardiovascular risks imparted on preeclampsia sufferers. Endothelial dysfunction and end-organ injury are synonymous with both preeclampsia and cardiovascular disease, including heart failure. We propose that beta-blockers, known to improve endothelial dysfunction in the treatment of cardiovascular disease, and specifically known to reduce mortality in the treatment of heart failure, may be beneficial in the treatment of preeclampsia. Here, we assessed whether the beta-blockers carvedilol, bisoprolol, and metoprolol could quench the release of anti-angiogenic factors, promote production of pro-angiogenic factors, reduce markers of inflammation, and reduce endothelial dysfunction using our in vitro pre-clinical preeclampsia models encompassing primary placental tissue and endothelial cells. Here, we show beta-blockers effected a modest reduction in secretion of anti-angiogenic soluble fms-like tyrosine kinase-1 and soluble endoglin and increased expression of pro-angiogenic placental growth factor, vascular endothelial growth factor and adrenomedullin in endothelial cells. Beta-blocker treatment mitigated inflammatory changes occurring after endothelial dysfunction and promoted cytoprotective antioxidant heme oxygenase-1. The positive effects of the beta-blockers were predominantly seen in endothelial cells, with a less consistent response seen in placental cells/tissue. In conclusion, beta-blockers show potential as a novel therapeutic approach in the treatment of preeclampsia and warrant further investigation.

Keywords: preeclampsia; beta-blocker; endothelial dysfunction; cardiovascular disease

1. Introduction

Preeclampsia is a serious pregnancy complication that affects 3–8% of all pregnancies. Because there are no effective medical therapies against the progression of preeclampsia aside from delivery, it remains a leading cause of maternal and perinatal deaths worldwide [1–3].

It is thought that preeclampsia develops after defective early trophoblast invasion and remodelling of the maternal spiral arterioles, causing significant oxidative stress [4,5]. Following this, excessive anti-angiogenic factors soluble fms-like tyrosine kinase-1 (sFlt-1) [6–9] and soluble endoglin (sENG) [10] are secreted into the maternal circulation [5,11–13]. These anti-angiogenic factors sequester circulating pro-angiogenic factors placental growth

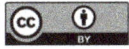

factor (PGF) and vascular endothelial growth factor (VEGF), reducing VEGF-mediated upregulation of endothelial nitric oxide [14]. Without an upregulation of endothelial nitric oxide, endothelin-1 (ET-1) production is likely uninhibited, and systemic inflammation and endothelial dysfunction ensues [15].

Endothelial dysfunction characterises preeclampsia and is a significant driver of the multi-organ injury clinically observed with the disease [16–19]. Circulating ET-1, a potent vasoconstrictor, is significantly increased in women with preeclampsia [20–23]. Increased ET-1 expression in the vasculature is also a marker of endothelial dysfunction. ET-1 receptor B (ETB) facilitates endothelium-mediated vasodilation by clearing ET-1 from circulation [24]. Vascular adhesion molecule (VCAM), another marker of endothelial dysfunction is also elevated with preeclampsia [25].

Considering the pathophysiology of preeclampsia, targeting the reduction of sFlt-1 and sENG production and release into the circulation has potential as a therapeutic strategy for the disease. A medical treatment that is safe in pregnancy, able to restore the angiogenic balance, improve endothelial function, and reduce inflammation, would likely prevent serious, long term damage to the maternal endothelium, and would represent a significant therapeutic advance. As such, we have developed a therapeutic testing pipeline to investigate whether existing drugs from other fields might be able to be repurposed to restore angiogenic balance and prevent endothelial dysfunction in preeclampsia [26–32].

Significantly, women who suffer preeclampsia are at increased risk of future cardiovascular disease, including a 4-fold increased risk of future heart failure [33]. Like preeclampsia, endothelial dysfunction and end-organ injury are also synonymous with heart failure and are associated with poorer prognosis [34–38]. The vasoactive peptide adrenomedullin (ADM) is a potent vasodilator with implications in both preeclampsia and cardiovascular disease [39,40]. In the management of heart failure, the beta-blockers carvedilol [41,42], bisoprolol [43], and metoprolol [44,45] have each been shown to reduce mortality to a similar extent [46]. As such, the use of any of them in treating patients with symptomatic heart failure constitutes standard therapy [47–49]. Beta-blockers while known to regulate blood pressure control, have also been shown to improve endothelial function when used in the treatment of cardiovascular disease [50]. While currently labetalol is the only beta-blocker used in the treatment of preeclampsia as an anti-hypertensive agent [51], in general many beta-blockers are considered safe in pregnancy based on their use in pregnant patients with cardiovascular disease [52]. The exception to this is atenolol, which is contraindicated given its association with small-for-gestational-age infants [52,53].

Given the relationship between preeclampsia, cardiovascular disease and heart failure at a pathophysiological level and in terms of subsequent lifetime risk, we hypothesised that the same beta-blockers able to modulate mortality risk in heart failure, might be of benefit in the treatment of preeclampsia. We therefore set out to evaluate the effects of carvedilol, bisoprolol, and metoprolol on the secretion of pro- and anti-angiogenic and inflammatory factors central to preeclampsia pathogenesis from placental and endothelial cells in vitro.

2. Materials and Methods

2.1. Tissue Collection

Ethical approval for this study was obtained from the Mercy Health Human Research Ethics Committee (R11/34). Women presenting to the Mercy Hospital for Women, Heidelberg, Australia, gave informed written consent for tissue collection. Placentas and umbilical cords were collected from normotensive term pregnancies ($\geq$37 weeks' gestation up to 41 weeks' gestation) at elective caesarean section, where a fetus of normal customised birth weight centile was delivered. Samples were excluded where pregnancies were associated with gestational diabetes mellitus requiring insulin, preeclampsia or hypertension, congenital infection, chromosomal or congenital abnormalities, or evidence of chorioamnionitis (confirmed by placental histopathology) (Table 1). Samples were collected within 30 min of delivery and washed in cold phosphate-buffered saline (PBS).

Table 1. Patient characteristics for term gestational tissue collection.

Characteristic	Number
Maternal Age, years (median (Q1, Q3))	33 (31, 38)
Fetal Sex (%)	
• Male	8 (73)
• Female	3 (27)
Maternal BMI (median (Q1, Q3))	22.7 (22.1, 25.4)
Smoker (%)	0
Birth Centile (%)	
• <25th	0 (0)
• 26th–50th	2 (18)
• 51st–75th	6 (55)
• 76th–97th	3 (27)
• >98th	0 (0)
Diabetes (%)	
• None	10 (91)
• GDM (diet)	1 (9)
Mode of delivery (%)	
• Elective caesarean (not in labour)	11 (100)

2.2. Primary Human Umbilical Vein Endothelial Cell (HUVEC) Isolation

HUVECs were isolated from three or four individual umbilical cords per experiment, as previously described [54]. Briefly, the umbilical cord vein was cannulated and flushed with PBS to wash out blood cells. Next, 10 mL of collagenase (1 mg/mL, Worthington Biochemical Corporation, Lakewood, NJ, USA was infused into the cord and incubated at 37 °C for 10 min. The dissociated HUVECs were recovered by pelleting and resuspension, followed by culture in M199 media (Life Technologies, Carlsbad, CA, USA) containing 10% fetal calf serum (Thermo Fisher Scientific, Waltham, MA, USA), 1% antibiotic-antimycotic (Life Technologies), 1% endothelial cell growth factor (Sigma, St. Louis, Missouri, United States) and 1% heparin (Sigma). Cells were used between passage 2 to 4 and cultured at 37 °C in 20% O_2 and 5% CO_2.

2.3. Primary Human Cytotrophoblast Isolation

Human cytotrophoblasts were isolated from three or four individual placentas per experiment, as previously described [55]. Primary cytotrophoblasts were cultured in DMEM GlutaMAX (Life Technologies) containing 10% fetal calf serum and 1% antibiotic-antimycotic on fibronectin (10 mg/mL; BD Biosciences, Franklin Lakes, New Jersey, United States) coated wells. Cells were plated and allowed to attach over 12–18 h before washing with dPBS (Life Technologies) to remove cell debris. Cells were cultured under 8% O_2, 5% CO_2 at 37 °C.

2.4. Isolation and Culture of Placental Explants

Placental explants were isolated from three or four individual placentas per experiment. Small pieces of villous tissue were cut from the mid-portion of the placenta to avoid the maternal and fetal surfaces. These were thoroughly washed with PBS then dissected into small fragments of 1–2 mm size and three pieces put into each well of a 24 well plate. Explants were allowed to equilibrate at 37 °C for 12–18 h under 8% O_2, 5% CO_2 in DMEM GlutaMAX containing 10% fetal calf serum and 1% antibiotic-antimycotic.

2.5. Beta-Blockers In Vitro Experiments

Our in vitro models of preeclampsia recapitulate important characteristics of the disease pathogenesis, providing the opportunity to test therapeutic ability to target several key aspects of the disease, including excess secretion of anti-angiogenic factors (sFlt and sENG) and vascular endothelial dysfunction. These in vitro models of preeclampsia form the basis of our therapeutic testing pipeline [26,32,56,57].

Isolated primary HUVECs, cytotrophoblasts, and placental explants were treated with three different beta-blockers; carvedilol (1 uM and 10 uM, Sigma), bisoprolol (1 uM, 10 uM, 100 uM, and 1 mM, Sigma), and metoprolol tartrate (1 uM, 10 uM, and 100 uM, Sigma) in triplicate wells and cultured for 24 h. Media and cellular RNA were then collected and analysed by ELISA or quantitative RT-PCR (qPCR), respectively.

Endothelial dysfunction was induced in isolated primary HUVECs with TNFα (1 ng/mL, Life Technologies) for two hours prior to treatment with the beta-blockers (doses as above) and cultured for a further 24 h. Cellular RNA was collected and analysed by qPCR.

For HUVEC and cytotrophoblast experiments, a cell viability assay was run concurrently (CellTiter 96 AQueous Non-Radioactive Cell Proliferation Assay, Promega, Madison, WI, USA), according to manufacturer's instructions.

2.6. ELISA

Concentrations of sFlt-1 and sENG were measured in HUVEC, cytotrophoblast and placental explant 24 h culture media using the DuoSet Human VEGF R1/Flt-1 and endoglin/CD105 ELISA kits, respectively (R&D Systems, Minneapolis, MN, USA). Optical density for ELISA was determined using a BioRad X-Mark microplate spectrophotometer (BioRad, Hercules, CA, USA), and protein concentrations calculated using BioRad Microplate manager 6 software.

2.7. Quantitative RT-PCR

Total RNA was extracted from isolated primary HUVECs, cytotrophoblasts and placental explants after drug treatment using the RNeasy mini kit (Qiagen, Valencia, CA, USA) and quantified using a NanoDrop ND 1000 spectrophotometer (NanoDrop Technologies Inc, Wilmington, DE, USA). RNA was converted to cDNA using the High-Capacity cDNA Reverse Transcription Kit (Applied Biosystems, Foster City, CA, USA) as per manufacturer guidelines. qPCR was performed using Taqman hydrolysis probes for *ENG* (Hs00923996_m1), *VCAM1* (Hs01003372_m1), *ET-1* (Hs00174961_m1), *NLRP3* (Hs00918082_m1), *IL1b* (Hs01555410_m1), *EDNRB* (Hs00240747_m1), *PTGS2* (Hs00153133_m1), *IL6* (Hs00985639_m1), *VEGF* (Hs00900055_m1), *PGF* (Hs00182176_m1), *HMOX1* (Hs01110250_m1) and *ADM* (Hs00181605_m1) on the CFX 384 (Biorad) using FAM-labelled Taqman universal PCR mastermix (Applied Biosystems) with the following run conditions: 50 °C for 2 min, 95 °C for 10 min, 95 °C for 15 s, 60 °C for 1 min (40 cycles). All data were normalized to a reference gene, *YWHAZ* (Hs01122454_m1), and the results graphed as fold change relative to control using the $2^{-\Delta\Delta CT}$ method. The sFlt-1 splice variants *i13* and *e15a* were measured with Fast SYBR Green Master mix (Applied Biosystems) using primers specific for each variant as previously published [58], using *YHWAZ* as the reference gene with the following run conditions: 95 °C for 20 s, 95 °C for 1 s, 60 °C for 20 s (40 cycles). All samples were run in technical duplicate.

2.8. Statistical Analysis

All in vitro experiments were performed with technical triplicates and repeated a minimum of three times using tissue or cells isolated from different placentas.

Data was tested for normal distribution and statistically analysed as appropriate. When three or more groups were compared a 1-way ANOVA (for parametric data) or Kruskal–Wallis test (for non-parametric data) was used. Post hoc analysis was carried out using either the Tukey (parametric) or Dunn's test (non-parametric). All data are expressed as mean ± SEM. p values < 0.05 were considered significant. Statistical analysis was performed using GraphPad Prism 8 software (GraphPad Software, La Jolla, CA, USA).

3. Results

3.1. Beta-Blocker Treatment Effects on the Secretion of Anti-Angiogenic Factors from Placental Cells/Tissue and Endothelial Cells

Treatment of primary HUVECs with the beta-blocker carvedilol significantly reduced the secretion of anti-angiogenic factor sFlt-1 (Figure 1A). The other two beta-blockers investigated, bisoprolol and metoprolol, did not affect sFlt-1 secretion from primary HUVECs. In primary human trophoblasts and placenta explants, all three beta-blockers had no effect on sFlt-1 secretion (Figure 1B,C, respectively).

Top dose metoprolol (1000 uM) resulted in a significant reduction in sENG secretion from primary HUVECs (Figure 1D), as did 100 uM bisoprolol in placental explants (Figure 1E).

3.2. Beta-Blocker Treatment Effects on the Expression of Anti-Angiogenic Factors in Placental Tissue and Endothelial Cells

In primary human placental explants, mRNA expression of the sFlt-1 isoforms, *sFlt-1-e15a* and *sFlt-1-i13* were not affected by treatment with any of the beta-blockers investigated (Figure 2A,B, respectively). Expression of *ENG* mRNA in primary HUVECs was significantly increased with top dose carvedilol (10 uM) and metoprolol (100 uM), but not bisoprolol at any dose (Figure 2C).

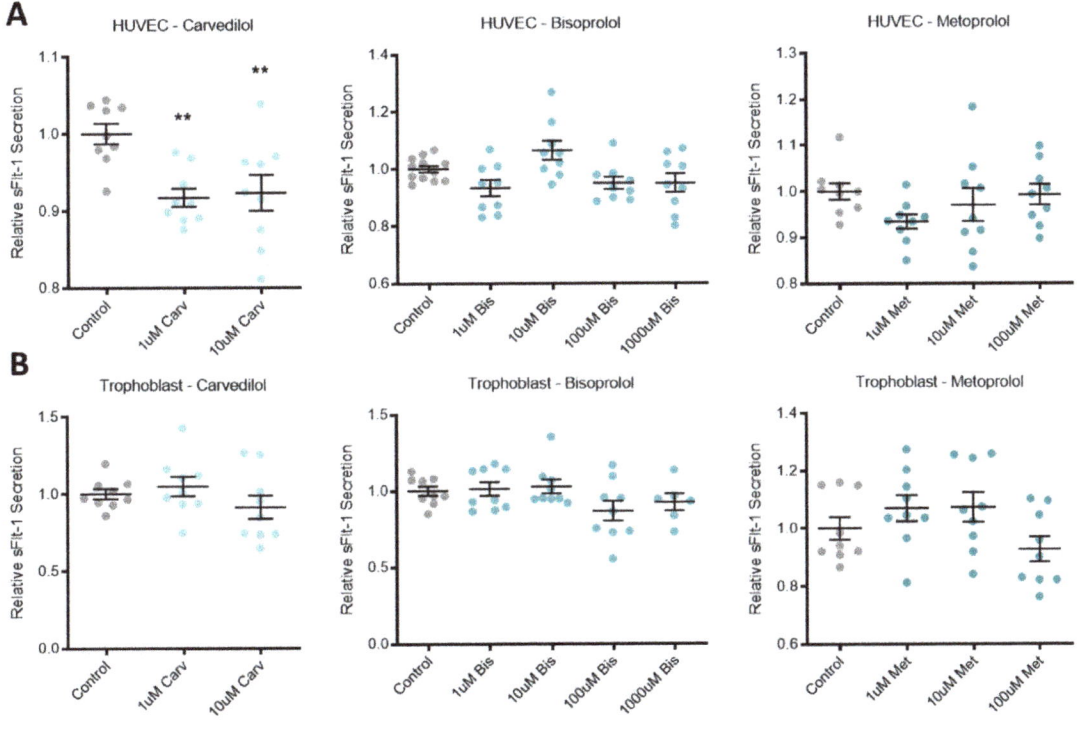

Figure 1. *Cont.*

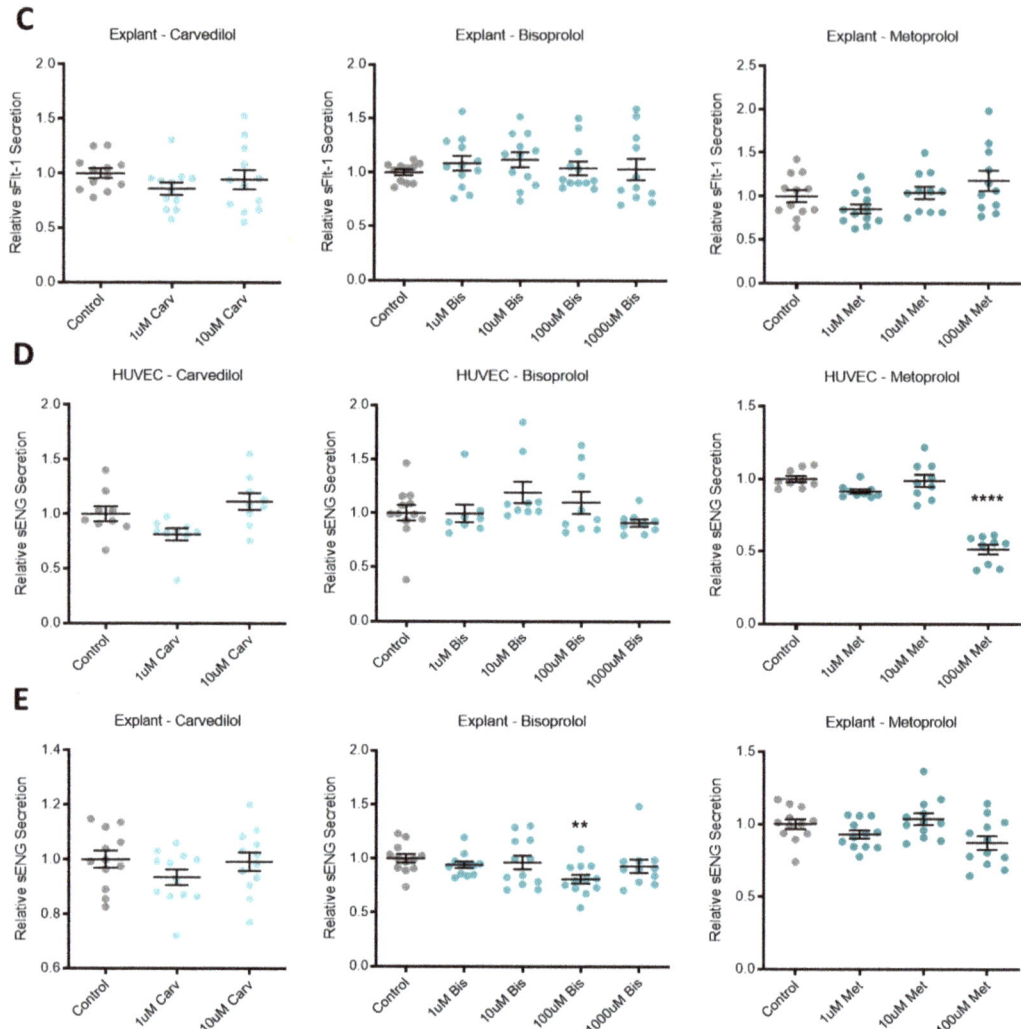

Figure 1. Beta-blockers had limited effect on secreted anti-angiogenic factors across different tissue types. Relative sFlt-1 secretion in HUVCEs (**A**) was significantly reduced with carvedilol (Carv) treatment, but not bisoprolol (Bis) treatment or metoprolol (Met) treatment. Relative sFlt-1 secretion was unchanged in trophoblasts (**B**) and explants (**C**) following beta-blocker treatment with Carv, Bis and Met. In HUVEC, relative sENG secretion (**D**) was decreased with treatment at the top dose of Met, but unchanged with Carv and Bis treatment. In explants, relative sENG secretion (**E**) was decreased with treatment at 100 uM Bis, but unchanged at the other doses or with Carv or Met. Data are mean ± SEM, expressed relative to control, n = 3–4, ** $p < 0.01$, **** $p < 0.0001$.

3.3. Beta-Blocker Treatment Effects on the Expression of Pro-Angiogenic Factors in Placental Tissue and Endothelial Cells

Expression of pro-angiogenic factors *VEGF*, *PGF*, and *ADM* were increased by different beta-blocker treatment of primary HUVECs. VEGF mRNA expression was upregulated by metoprolol (Figure 3A), *PGF* by carvedilol, bisoprolol and metoprolol (Figure 3C), and *ADM* by carvedilol and metoprolol (Figure 3E). Neither *VEGF* nor *PGF* mRNA expression was differentially regulated in primary human explants following beta-blocker treatment (Figure 3B,D, respectively).

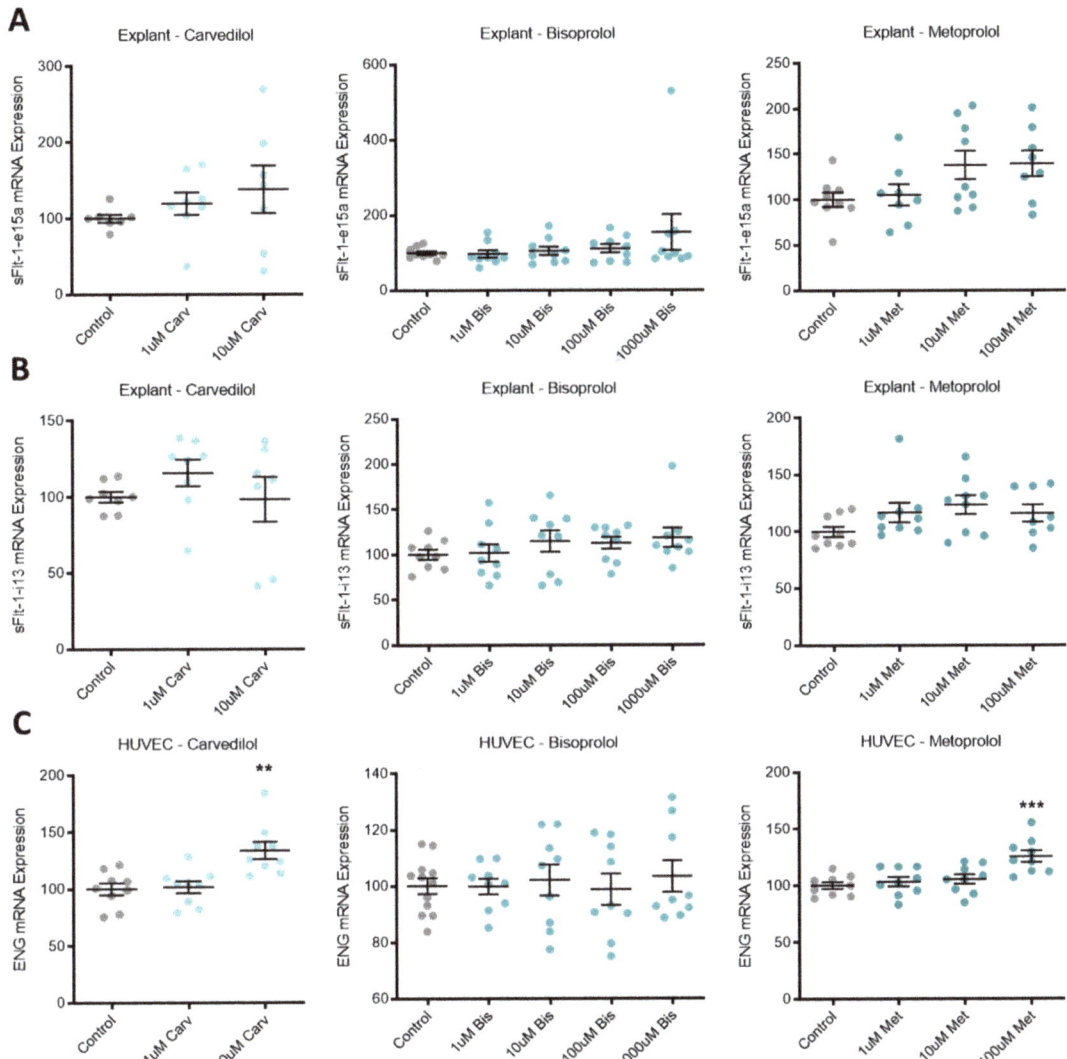

Figure 2. Endoglin mRNA is upregulated in HUVECs following beta-blocker treatment. Placental explant expression of sFlt-1 isoforms, sFlt-1-e15a (**A**) and sFlt-1-i13 (**B**) was not affected by treatment with beta-blockers carvedilol (Carv), bisoprolol (Bis), or metoprolol (Met). HUVEC expression of ENG mRNA (**C**) was significantly increased with top dose Carv and Met, but not Bis. Data are mean ± SEM, expressed as a percentage of control, $n = 3-4$, ** $p < 0.01$, *** $p < 0.001$.

3.4. Beta-Blocker Treatment Effects on the Expression of Inflammatory Mediators in Endothelial Cells

Expression of inflammatory mediator *IL-1b* in HUVECs was not affected by beta-blocker treatment (Figure 4A). Additionally, in primary cultured HUVECs, beta-blocker treatment with top doses of carvedilol, bisoprolol, and metoprolol significantly increased mRNA expression of *PTGS2* (Figure 4E).

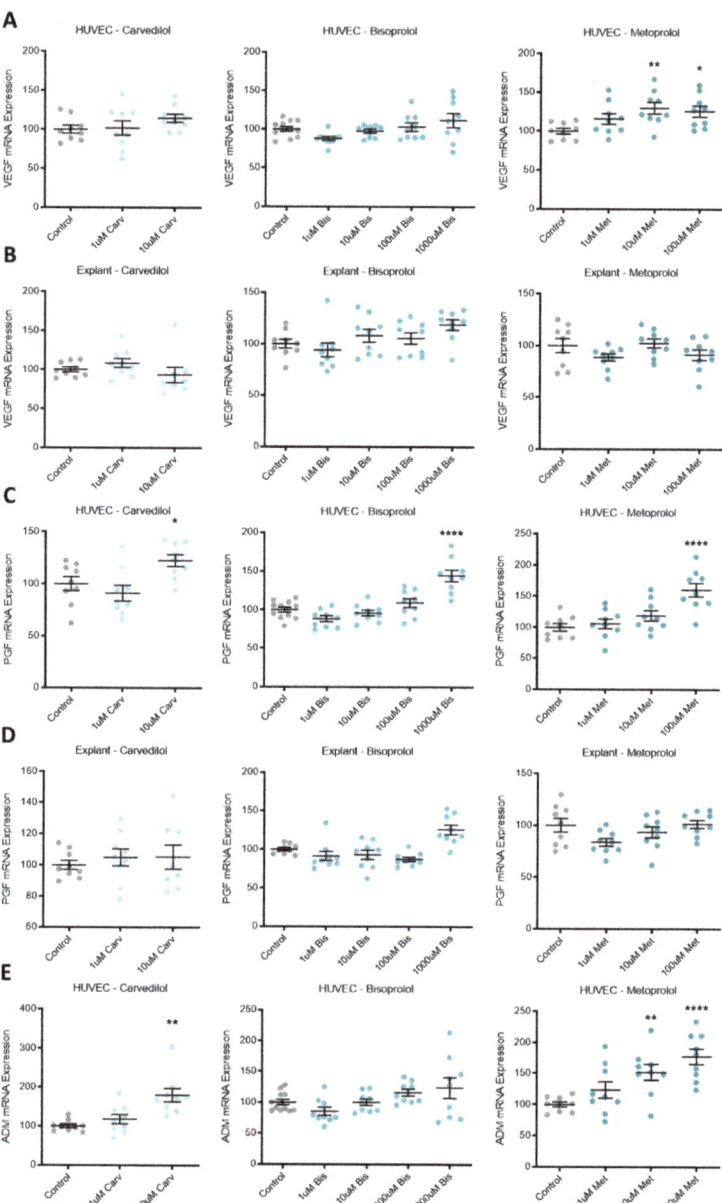

Figure 3. Pro-angiogenic factors upregulated following beta-blocker treatment of HUVECs, but not explants. VEGF mRNA expression in HUVECs (**A**) was significantly increased with metoprolol (Met) treatment, but not carvedilol (Carv) or bisoprolol (Bis). PGF mRNA expression in HUVECs (**C**) was significantly increased with the top dose of Carv, Bis, and Met. ADM mRNA expression in HUVECs (**E**) was significantly increased with top dose Carv treatment and Met treatment, but not Bis. VEGF and PGF mRNA expression were unchanged in placental explants following beta-blocker treatment (**B,D**, respectively). Data are mean ± SEM, expressed as a percentage of control, $n = 3$–4, * $p < 0.05$, ** $p < 0.01$, **** $p < 0.0001$.

When TNFα was added to HUVECs to induce endothelial dysfunction, *IL-1b* expression was significantly increased from control levels and decreased with doses of bisoprolol and metoprolol, but not carvedilol (Figure 4B). TNFα induced endothelial dysfunction also significantly increased mRNA levels of *IL-6* (Figure 4C), *NLRP3* (Figure 4D) and *PTGS2* (Figure 4F). Beta-blocker treatment with top dose carvedilol, bisoprolol, and metoprolol significantly decreased induced *IL-6* expression (Figure 4C). *NLRP3* mRNA expression was not affected by beta-blocker treatment (Figure 4D). *PTGS2* expression increased with top dose carvedilol, decreased with 100 uM bisoprolol, and was unaffected by metoprolol (Figure 4F).

3.5. Beta-Blocker Treatment Effects on Antioxidant HO-1

Expression of the antioxidant enzyme *HO-1* was significantly increased in HUVECs following top dose treatment with carvedilol, bisoprolol, and metoprolol (Figure 5).

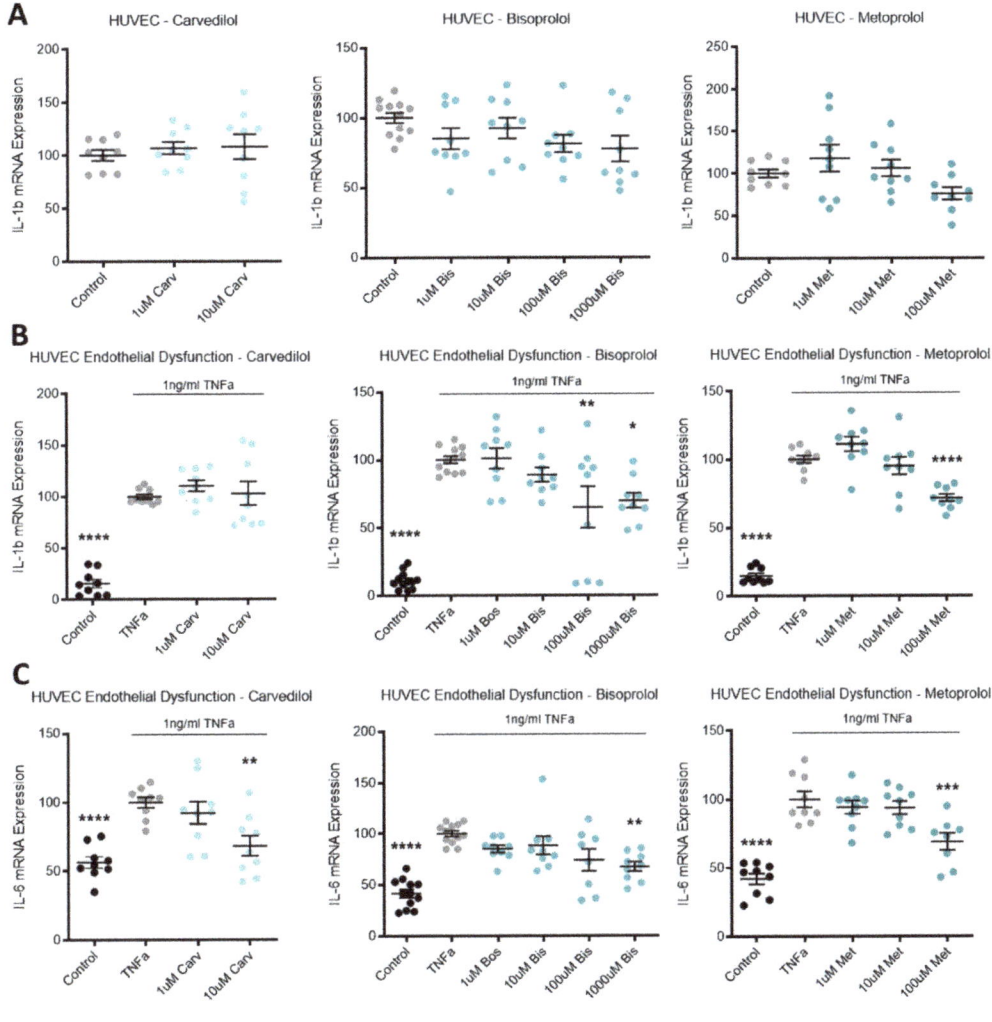

Figure 4. *Cont.*

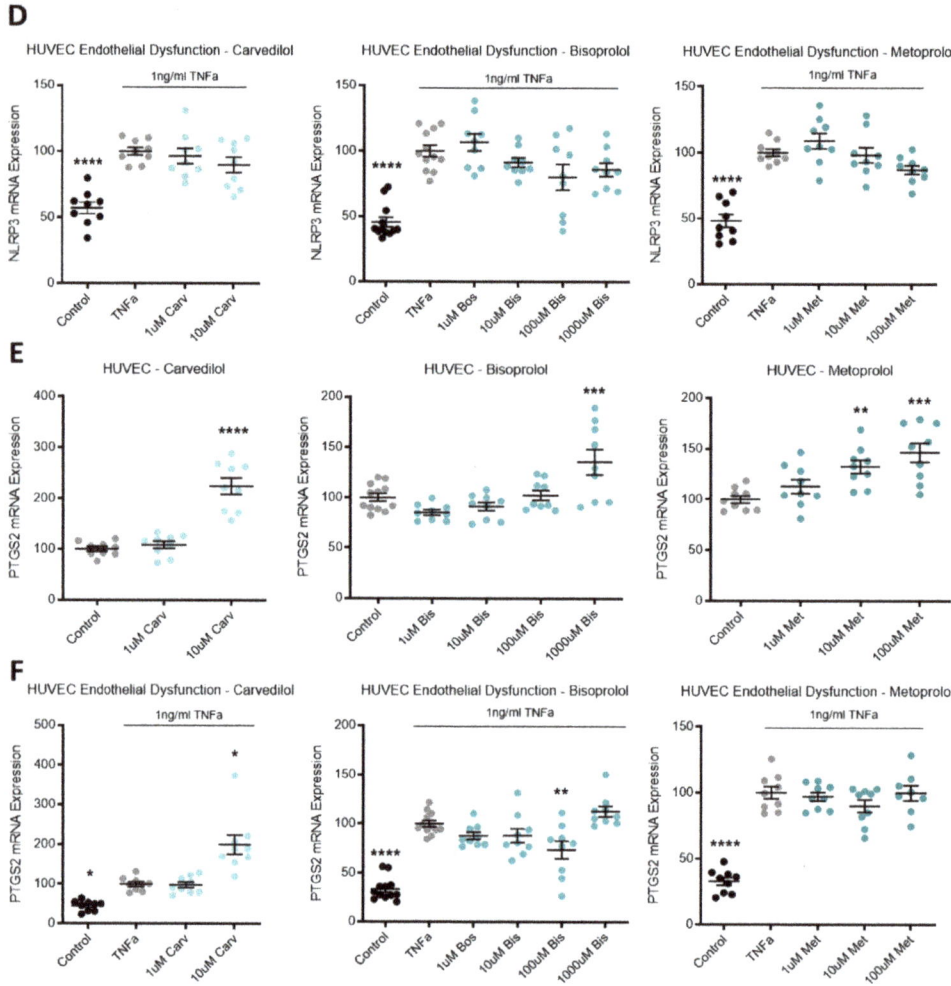

Figure 4. Inflammatory markers are altered following beta-blocker treatment. Expression of IL-1b mRNA in HUVECs (**A**) was not affected by treatment with beta-blockers carvedilol (Carv), bisoprolol (Bis), or metoprolol (Met). When TNFα is added to HUVECs to induce endothelial dysfunction, IL-1b expression is significantly increased from control levels (**B**) and decreases with doses of Bis and Met, but not Carv. TNFα induced endothelial dysfunction also significantly increases mRNA levels of IL-6 (**C**) and NLRP3 (**D**). Beta-blocker treatment with top dose Carv, Bis, and Met significantly decreases induced IL-6 expression (**C**). NLRP3 mRNA expression was not affected by beta-blockers treatment (**D**). Expression of PTGS2 mRNA in HUVECs (**E**) was significantly increased following top dose beta-blocker treatment with Carv, Bis, and Met. PTGS2 expression is significantly induced with TNFα (endothelial dysfunction) (**F**), which is further increased with top dose Carv, decreased with 100 uM Bis, and unaffected by Met. Data are mean ± SEM, expressed as a percentage of control (HUVEC) or TNFα control (endothelial dysfunction), $n = 3$–4, * $p < 0.05$, ** $p < 0.01$, *** $p < 0.001$, **** $p < 0.0001$.

3.6. Beta-Blocker Treatment Effects on Endothelial Dysfunction Markers

TNFα was used to induce endothelial dysfunction in primary cultured HUVECs. Compared to the no-TNFα control, TNFα significantly upregulated *VCAM* mRNA (Figure 6A). The top dose of each beta-blocker, carvedilol, bisoprolol, and metoprolol, significantly reduced *VCAM* mRNA expression (Figure 6A). In the same model of endothelial dysfunction, *ET-1* and its receptor, endothelin-1 receptor B (*ETB*), mRNA expression was not affected by beta-blocker treatment (Figure 6B,C, respectively).

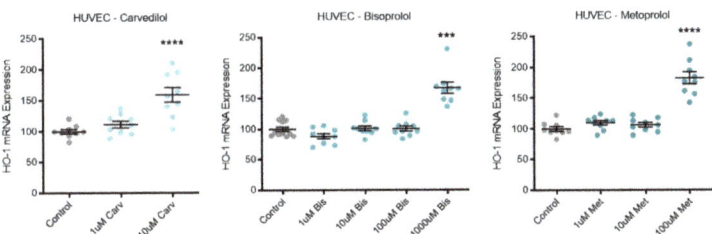

Figure 5. Antioxidant HO-1 is increased with beta-blocker treatment. Expression of HO-1 mRNA is significantly increased in HUVECs following top dose beta-blocker treatment with carvedilol (Carv), bisoprolol (Bis), and metoprolol (Met). Data are mean ± SEM, expressed as a percentage of control, $n = 3–4$, *** $p < 0.001$, **** $p < 0.0001$.

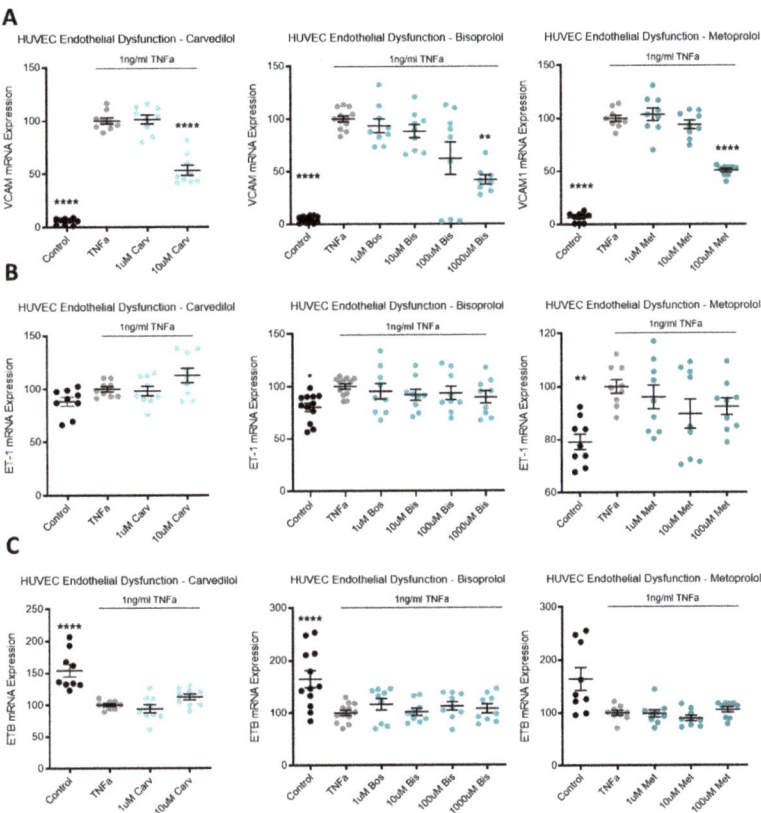

Figure 6. In a model of endothelial dysfunction, VCAM mRNA expression is decreased with beta-blocker treatment. In HUVECs treated with TNFα to induce endothelial dysfunction (**A**), VCAM mRNA is significantly reduced with top dose beta-blockers, carvedilol (Carv), bisoprolol (Bis), and metoprolol (Met). In the same model, ET-1 mRNA (**B**) and ETB mRNA (**C**) expression are not affected by Carv, Bis, or Met. Data are mean ± SEM, expressed as a percentage of TNFα control, $n = 3–4$, * $p < 0.05$, ** $p < 0.01$, **** $p < 0.0001$.

4. Discussion

We report that beta-blockers that successfully reduce mortality in heart failure, also exert effects consistent with a reduction in endothelial dysfunction in models of preeclampsia. Through our suite of in vitro studies, carvedilol, bisoprolol, and metoprolol demonstrated a modest improvement in angiogenic balance, and significant improvement in various markers of vasoactivity, inflammation, and endothelial dysfunction. Treatments that address endothelial dysfunction in preeclampsia represent a significant knowledge gap in our pursuit of preeclampsia therapeutics. While beta-blockers have exhibited a positive effect on endothelial dysfunction in a cardiovascular disease setting, the actions of beta-blockers in gestational tissues presents novel findings.

Most therapeutics being investigated for the treatment of preeclampsia are concerned with lowering excessive placental secretion of anti-angiogenic factors sFlt-1 and sENG. Here, beta-blockers had no effect on placental (isolated trophoblasts and placental explant) secretion of sFlt-1, and only a modest reduction in sENG secretion from placental explants with bisoprolol. This was seen at both the protein and RNA level. There was also no change in the expression of pro-angiogenic *VEGF* or *PGF* in placental explants following beta-blocker treatment. In isolated primary HUVECs, beta-blockers did help restore the angiogenic balance somewhat. They decreased sFlt-1 (carvedilol) and sENG (metoprolol) secretion, and increased *VEGF* (metoprolol), *ADM* (carvedilol and metoprolol), and *PGF* (carvedilol, bisoprolol, and metoprolol), expression. This is significant given that PGF is almost ubiquitously low in cases of, and even preceding the development of, preeclampsia [59,60]. If angiogenic balance could be restored with such a therapy, this might offer an important step forward in the treatment of preeclampsia, especially as these drugs are also used for blood pressure control. Given they exert the additional benefit of reducing injury to the endothelium this could be an important consideration for post-partum therapies also.

Aside from restoring the angiogenic balance, decreasing inflammation is also desirable in a therapeutic to treat preeclampsia. In isolated primary HUVECs, the beta-blockers did not significantly reduce expression of the inflammatory mediator, interleukin (IL)-1b. However, importantly when disease was modelled whereby HUVEC were stimulated with TNFα to induce endothelial dysfunction (and a state of inflammation), beta-blockers were able to significantly reduce *IL-1b* (bisoprolol and metoprolol) and *IL-6* (carvedilol, bisoprolol, and metoprolol), but they had no effect on the critical regulator of the inflammasome, *NLRP3*. Interestingly, in isolated primary HUVECs all three beta-blockers, carvedilol, bisoprolol, and metoprolol increased expression of *PTGS2*, which encodes cyclooxygenase 2 (COX2), an enzyme largely recognised to be pro-inflammatory. However, there is significant evidence to show that COX2 is bimodal; with its first peak initially driving inflammation, and its second peak (almost 4-fold greater in magnitude) coinciding with a resolution in inflammation [61]. Compared to normotensive controls, COX2 is decreased in the placenta [62] and circulation [63] of women with preeclampsia. Further, therapeutic inhibition of COX2 is associated with adverse cardiac events [64] and delayed inflammation resolution [61], suggesting beta-blocker treatment, by increasing *PTGS2* expression may be both beneficial in the treatment of preeclampsia and also the long-term increased cardiovascular risks the disease imposes. However, this is less clear in the case of endothelial dysfunction, where following TNFα stimulation of HUVECs, carvedilol increased *PTGS2* expression while bisoprolol decreased it. Further investigation is warranted to elicit the mechanisms at play behind some of the different responses seen to the three different drugs throughout our experiments.

Looking further into the endothelial dysfunction model, all three beta-blockers significantly reduced expression of vascular cell adhesion molecule 1 (*VCAM*), a critical factor in the inflammatory process involved in the recruitment and migration of leukocytes [65], and marker of endothelial dysfunction. Unfortunately, beta-blockers did not reduce vasoconstrictor *ET-1* expression, nor upregulate its receptor, *ETB*, that acts as a vasodilator by removing ET-1 from circulation [24]. Given the potency of ET-1 as a vasoconstrictor, as well as being a biomarker of endothelial dysfunction and its intricate association with both preeclampsia and cardiovascular disease and heart failure, we expected that the cardioprotective beta-blockers may have reduced its expression. Importantly however, ADM, as well as having pro-angiogenic and anti-inflammatory effects, is also vasoactive, acting as a potent vasodilator and is significantly upregulated by both carvedilol and metoprolol. Interestingly, ADM is upregulated in instances of congestive heart failure and myocardial infarction, as a compensatory mechanism to protect the vasculature [66–68].

In addition, treatment with all three beta-blockers demonstrated an increase in the expression of the cytoprotective antioxidant enzyme heme-oxygenase-1 (*HO-1*). HO-1 is an important enzyme regulated by nuclear factor (erythroid-derived 2)-like 2 (NRF2), that as well as protecting cells from programmed cell death, also inhibits the pathogenesis of inflammatory disease [69]. Given the inflammatory nature of preeclampsia, upregulation of HO-1 is a valuable characteristic of any potential therapeutic.

Our findings suggest that there may be merit in evaluating the beta-blockers carvedilol, bisoprolol, and metoprolol further for their potential in treating or preventing preeclampsia; or in decreasing the lifelong cardiovascular risk incurred by women who suffer the disease. This study suggests that any therapeutic benefits that they display are more likely due to increased endothelial expression of the important pro-angiogenic factors *PGF*, *VEGF* and *ADM*, and through mitigation of inflammatory changes that occur subsequent to endothelial dysfunction, rather than through regulation of placental anti-angiogenic factor secretion, which was only modestly affected at best. Moreover, the effects of the beta-blockers are primarily seen in endothelial cells, with a less consistent response seen in placental tissue.

To our knowledge, this is the first study to investigate the effects of carvedilol, bisoprolol, and metoprolol on sFlt-1, sENG and PGF secretion and expression. Despite this novelty, our results in regard to the beta-blockers' anti-inflammatory properties and reduction in endothelial dysfunction are supported by previous studies from the cardiovascular field in which the drugs have had comparisons made. While we saw many similarities in the responses to the beta-blocker treatments, some of the differences demonstrated may plausibly be due to the different types of beta-blockers that carvedilol, bisoprolol and metoprolol represent. Carvedilol, a third generation non-selective beta-blocker has been found to demonstrate improved endothelial function [70] through antioxidant effects [71,72]; but the molecular mechanisms still require clarification [71,73]. Unlike carvedilol, bisoprolol is a second generation beta-1 selective beta-blocker. Despite these differences, carvedilol has not been shown to have benefit over bisoprolol in lowering oxidant stress [38]. Like carvedilol, bisoprolol has been found to improve endothelial function when used in the context of cardiovascular diseases; these include hypertension and angina [74,75]. Metoprolol is similar to bisoprolol in that it is also a selective beta-1 receptor blocker. Metoprolol has also been shown to benefit endothelial function and to have antioxidant properties in cardiovascular disease [76,77]. Given that all three beta-blockers significantly increased *HO-1* expression in this model, we may infer that carvedilol, bisoprolol and metoprolol may all act to increase endogenous antioxidant defences and thus may be of benefit in the treatment of preeclampsia. Metoprolol is available as both an immediate release (metoprolol tartrate—used in this study) and sustained release (metoprolol succinate) formulation. While the active ingredient remains the same, further investigation of sustained release metoprolol succinate, which has been shown to reduce mortality in heart failure [44,45] would be of great interest.

A further consideration is that safety data in pregnancy would be required for all of these medications if they were to be used to treat preeclampsia. Currently all three medications are classified as TGA category C—much like labetalol, a beta-blocker frequently used to treat hypertension in pregnancy. Promisingly however, carvedilol and metoprolol are considered safe in pregnancy based on their use in pregnant women with other cardiovascular diseases including heart failure [52], and the only beta-blocker which is actively contraindicated in pregnancy is atenolol [52]; it has been associated with small-for-gestational-age infants [53].

In conclusion, we have presented evidence for beta-blockers as potential therapeutics for preeclampsia, with the idea that along with mitigating some of the hallmarks of endothelial dysfunction associated with preeclampsia, these benefits may extend to combating the increased lifelong cardiovascular risks to which these women are subjected. Further evaluation of beta-blockers using whole vessel myography as well as animal models of preeclampsia are required prior to clinical safety and efficacy studies.

Author Contributions: Conceptualisation, N.J.H. and T.M.M.; methodology, N.J.H., N.K.B. and S.A.B.; validation, N.K.B., S.A.B. and N.d.A.; formal analysis, N.K.B. and S.A.B.; investigation, S.A.B. and N.d.A.; resources, N.J.H., T.J.K.-L. and S.T.; data curation, N.K.B., T.M.M. and N.J.H.; writing—original draft preparation, N.K.B., T.M.M. and N.J.H.; writing—review and editing, N.K.B., T.M.M. and N.J.H.; supervision, N.J.H., T.J.K.-L. and S.T.; project administration, N.K.B., S.A.B. and N.J.H.; funding acquisition, N.J.H., T.J.K.-L. and S.T. All authors have read and agreed to the published version of the manuscript.

Funding: The NHMRC provided salary support (T.J.K.-L.; #1159261, S.T.; #1136418, and N.J.H.; #1146128). The funders had no role in study design, data collection, analysis, or decision to publish.

Institutional Review Board Statement: Ethical approval for this study was obtained from the Mercy Health Human Research Ethics Committee (R11/34).

Informed Consent Statement: Women presenting to the Mercy Hospital for Women, Heidelberg, Australia, gave informed written consent for tissue collection. The study was conducted in accordance with the Declaration of Helsinki of 1975.

Data Availability Statement: The data presented in this study are available on request from the corresponding author. The data are not publicly available due to patient privacy.

Acknowledgments: We would like to thank the research midwives, Gabrielle Pell, Genevieve Christophers and Rachel Murdoch, Mercy Hospital for Women Obstetrics and Midwifery staff and patients for participating in this research.

Conflicts of Interest: The authors report no conflict of interest.

References

1. Vest, A.R.; Cho, L.S. Hypertension in pregnancy. *Curr. Atheroscler. Rep.* **2014**, *16*, 395. [CrossRef]
2. Redman, C.W.; Sargent, I.L. Latest advances in understanding preeclampsia. *Science* **2005**, *308*, 1592–1594. [CrossRef]
3. Sibai, B.; Dekker, G.; Kupferminc, M. Pre-eclampsia. *Lancet* **2005**, *365*, 785–799. [CrossRef]
4. Labarrere, C.A.; DiCarlo, H.L.; Bammerlin, E.; Hardin, J.W.; Kim, Y.M.; Chaemsaithong, P.; Haas, D.M.; Kassab, G.S.; Romero, R. Failure of physiologic transformation of spiral arteries, endothelial and trophoblast cell activation, and acute atherosis in the basal plate of the placenta. *Am. J. Obstet. Gynecol.* **2017**, *216*, 287.e1–287.e16. [CrossRef]
5. Redman, C.W.; Staff, A.C. Preeclampsia, biomarkers, syncytiotrophoblast stress, and placental capacity. *Am. J. Obstet. Gynecol.* **2015**, *213* (Suppl. S4), S9.e1–S9.e4. [CrossRef] [PubMed]
6. Maynard, S.; Min, J.Y.; Merchan, J.; Lim, K.H.; Li, J.; Mondal, S.; Libermann, T.A.; Morgan, J.P.; Sellke, F.W.; Stillman, I.E.; et al. Excess placental soluble fms-like tyrosine kinase 1 (sFlt-1) may contribute to endothelial dysfunction, hypertension, and proteinuria in pre-eclampsia. *J. Clin. Investig.* **2003**, *111*, 649–658. [CrossRef] [PubMed]
7. Maynard, S.E.; Karumanchi, S.A. Angiogenic Factors and Preeclampsia. *Semin. Nephrol.* **2011**, *31*, 33–46. [CrossRef]
8. Nagamatsu, T.; Fujii, T.; Kusumi, M.; Zou, L.; Yamashita, T.; Osuga, Y.; Momoeda, M.; Kozuma, S.; Taketani, Y. Cytotrophoblasts Up-Regulate Soluble Fms-Like Tyrosine Kinase-1 Expression under Reduced Oxygen: An Implication for the Placental Vascular Development and the Pathophysiology of Preeclampsia. *Endocrinology* **2004**, *145*, 4838–4845. [CrossRef]
9. Holme, A.M.; Roland, M.C.; Henriksen, T.; Michelsen, T.M. In vivo uteroplacental release of placental growth factor and soluble Fms-like tyrosine kinase-1 in normal and preeclamptic pregnancies. *Am. J. Obstet. Gynecol.* **2016**, *215*, 782.e1–782.e9. [CrossRef]
10. Venkatesha, S.; Toporsian, M.; Lam, C.; Hanai, J.; Mammoto, T.; Kim, Y.M.; Bdolah, Y.; Lim, K.H.; Yuan, H.T.; Libermann, T.A.; et al. Soluble endoglin contributes to the pathogenesis of preeclampsia. *Nat. Med.* **2006**, *12*, 642–649. [CrossRef] [PubMed]
11. Kim, M.Y.; Buyon, J.P.; Guerra, M.M.; Rana, S.; Zhang, D.; Laskin, C.A.; Petri, M.; Lockshin, M.D.; Sammaritano, L.R.; Branch, D.W.; et al. Angiogenic factor imbalance early in pregnancy predicts adverse outcomes in patients with lupus and antiphospholipid antibodies: Results of the PROMISSE study. *Am. J. Obstet. Gynecol.* **2016**, *214*, 108.e1–108.e14. [CrossRef]
12. Lee, M.S.; Cantonwine, D.; Little, S.E.; McElrath, T.F.; Parry, S.I.; Lim, K.-H.; Wilkins-Haug, L.E. Angiogenic markers in pregnancies conceived through in vitro fertilization. *Am. J. Obstet. Gynecol.* **2015**, *213*, 212.e1–212.e8. [CrossRef]

13. Faupel-Badger, J.; McElrath, T.F.; Lauria, M.; Houghton, L.C.; Lim, K.-H.; Parry, S.; Cantonwine, D.; Lai, G.; Karumanchi, S.A.; Hoover, R.N.; et al. Maternal circulating angiogenic factors in twin and singleton pregnancies. *Am. J. Obstet. Gynecol.* **2015**, *212*, 636.e1–636.e8. [CrossRef]
14. Burke, S.D.; Zsengeller, Z.; Khankin, E.; Lo, A.S.; Rajakumar, A.; Dupont, J.J.; McCurley, A.; Moss, M.E.; Zhang, D.; Clark, C.D.; et al. Soluble fms-like tyrosine kinase 1 promotes angiotensin II sensitivity in preeclampsia. *J. Clin. Investig.* **2016**, *126*, 2561–2574. [CrossRef] [PubMed]
15. Verdonk, K.; Saleh, L.; Lankhorst, S.; Smilde, J.I.; van Ingen, M.M.; Garrelds, I.M.; Friesema, E.C.; Russcher, H.; Meiracker, A.H.V.D.; Visser, W.; et al. Association Studies Suggest a Key Role for Endothelin-1 in the Pathogenesis of Preeclampsia and the Accompanying Renin–Angiotensin–Aldosterone System Suppression. *Hypertension* **2015**, *65*, 1316–1323. [CrossRef]
16. Powe, C.E.; Levine, R.J.; Karumanchi, S.A. Preeclampsia, a disease of the maternal endothelium: The role of antiangiogenic factors and implications for later cardiovascular disease. *Circulation* **2011**, *123*, 2856–2869. [CrossRef]
17. Young, B.C.; Levine, R.J.; Karumanchi, S.A. Pathogenesis of Preeclampsia. *Annu. Rev. Pathol. Mech. Dis.* **2010**, *5*, 173–192. [CrossRef]
18. Chaiworapongsa, T.; Chaemsaithong, P.; Yeo, L.; Romero, R. Pre-eclampsia part 1: Current understanding of its pathophysiology. *Nat. Rev. Nephrol.* **2014**, *10*, 466–480. [CrossRef]
19. O'Gorman, N.N.; Wright, D.; Poon, L.L.; Rolnik, D.L.; Syngelaki, A.A.; Wright, A.A.; Akolekar, R.R.; Cicero, S.S.; Janga, D.D.; Jani, J.; et al. Accuracy of competing-risks model in screening for pre-eclampsia by maternal factors and biomarkers at 11–13 weeks' gestation. *Ultrasound Obstet. Gynecol.* **2017**, *49*, 751–755. [CrossRef] [PubMed]
20. Rust, O.A.; Bofill, J.A.; Zappe, D.H.; Hall, J.E.; Burnett, J.C., Jr.; Martin, J.N., Jr. The origin of endothelin-1 in patients with severe preeclampsia. *Obstet. Gynecol.* **1997**, *89*, 754–757. [CrossRef]
21. Lu, Y.-P.; Hasan, A.A.; Zeng, S.; Hocher, B. Plasma ET-1 Concentrations Are Elevated in Pregnant Women with Hypertension-Meta-Analysis of Clinical Studies. *Kidney Blood Press. Res.* **2017**, *42*, 654–663. [CrossRef] [PubMed]
22. Taylor, R.N.; Varma, M.; Teng, N.N.; Roberts, J.M. Women with Preeclampsia have Higher Plasma Endothelin Levels than Women with Normal Pregnancies. *J. Clin. Endocrinol. Metab.* **1990**, *71*, 1675–1677. [CrossRef]
23. Bernardi, F.; Constantino, L.; Machado, R.; Petronilho, F.; Pizzol, F.D. Plasma nitric oxide, endothelin-1, arginase and superoxide dismutase in pre-eclamptic women. *J. Obstet. Gynaecol. Res.* **2008**, *34*, 957–963. [CrossRef]
24. Ekelund, U.; Adner, M.; Edvinsson, L.; Mellander, S. Effects of selective ETB-receptor stimulation on arterial, venous and capillary functions in cat skeletal muscle. *Br. J. Pharmacol.* **1994**, *112*, 887–894. [CrossRef] [PubMed]
25. Austgulen, R.; Lien, E.; Vince, G.; Redman, C.W. Increased maternal plasma levels of soluble adhesion molecules (ICAM-1, VCAM-1, E-selectin) in preeclampsia. *Eur. J. Obstet. Gynecol. Reprod. Biol.* **1997**, *71*, 53–58. [CrossRef]
26. Onda, K.; Tong, S.; Beard, S.; Binder, N.; Muto, M.; Senadheera, S.N.; Parry, L.; Dilworth, M.; Renshall, L.; Brownfoot, F.; et al. Proton Pump Inhibitors Decrease Soluble fms-Like Tyrosine Kinase-1 and Soluble Endoglin Secretion, Decrease Hypertension, and Rescue Endothelial Dysfunction. *Hypertension* **2017**, *69*, 457–468. [CrossRef]
27. Binder, N.K.; Brownfoot, F.C.; Beard, S.; Cannon, P.; Nguyen, T.V.; Tong, S.; Kaitu'U-Lino, T.J.; Hannan, N.J. Esomeprazole and sulfasalazine in combination additively reduce sFlt-1 secretion and diminish endothelial dysfunction: Potential for a combination treatment for preeclampsia. *Pregnancy Hypertens.* **2020**, *22*, 86–92. [CrossRef]
28. Brownfoot, F.C.; Hannan, N.; Cannon, P.; Nguyen, V.; Hastie, R.; Parry, L.J.; Senadheera, S.; Tuohey, L.; Tong, S.; Kaitu'U-Lino, T.J. Sulfasalazine reduces placental secretion of antiangiogenic factors, up-regulates the secretion of placental growth factor and rescues endothelial dysfunction. *EBioMedicine* **2019**, *41*, 636–648. [CrossRef]
29. Brownfoot, F.C.; Hastie, R.; Hannan, N.; Cannon, P.; Tuohey, L.; Parry, L.; Senadheera, S.; Illanes, S.; Kaitu'U-Lino, T.J.; Tong, S. Metformin as a prevention and treatment for preeclampsia: Effects on soluble fms-like tyrosine kinase 1 and soluble endoglin secretion and endothelial dysfunction. *Am. J. Obstet. Gynecol.* **2016**, *214*, 356.e1–356.e15. [CrossRef] [PubMed]
30. Brownfoot, F.C.; Tong, S.; Hannan, N.; Binder, N.K.; Walker, S.P.; Cannon, P.; Hastie, R.; Onda, K.; Kaitu'U-Lino, T.J. Effects of Pravastatin on Human Placenta, Endothelium, and Women With Severe Preeclampsia. *Hypertension* **2015**, *66*, 687–697. [CrossRef]
31. de Alwis, N.; Beard, S.; Mangwiro, Y.T.; Binder, N.K.; Kaitu'U-Lino, T.J.; Brownfoot, F.C.; Tong, S.; Hannan, N.J. Pravastatin as the statin of choice for reducing pre-eclampsia-associated endothelial dysfunction. *Pregnancy Hypertens.* **2020**, *20*, 83–91. [CrossRef]
32. Kaitu'U-Lino, T.J.; Brownfoot, F.C.; Beard, S.; Cannon, P.; Hastie, R.; Nguyen, T.V.; Binder, N.K.; Tong, S.; Hannan, N.J. Combining metformin and esomeprazole is additive in reducing sFlt-1 secretion and decreasing endothelial dysfunction–implications for treating preeclampsia. *PLoS ONE* **2018**, *13*, e0188845. [CrossRef] [PubMed]
33. Wu, P.; Haththotuwa, R.; Kwok, C.S.; Babu, A.; Kotronias, R.A.; Rushton, C.; Zaman, A.; Fryer, A.A.; Kadam, U.; Chew-Graham, C.A.; et al. Preeclampsia and Future Cardiovascular Health: A Systematic Review and Meta-Analysis. *Circ. Cardiovasc. Qual. Outcomes* **2017**, *10*, e003497. [CrossRef]
34. Zuchi, C.; Tritto, I.; Carluccio, E.; Mattei, C.; Cattadori, G.; Ambrosio, G. Role of endothelial dysfunction in heart failure. *Heart Fail. Rev.* **2020**, *25*, 21–30. [CrossRef]
35. Franssen, C.; Chen, S.; Unger, A.; Korkmaz, H.I.; de Keulenaer, G.W.; Tschöpe, C.; Leite-Moreira, A.F.; Musters, R.; Niessen, H.W.; Linke, W.A.; et al. Myocardial Microvascular Inflammatory Endothelial Activation in Heart Failure With Preserved Ejection Fraction. *JACC Heart Fail.* **2016**, *4*, 312–324. [PubMed]

36. Paulus, W.J.; Tschöpe, C. A novel paradigm for heart failure with preserved ejection fraction: Comorbidities drive myocardial dysfunction and remodeling through coronary microvascular endothelial inflammation. *J. Am. Coll. Cardiol.* **2013**, *62*, 263–271. [CrossRef] [PubMed]
37. Harjola, V.-P.; Mullens, W.; Banaszewski, M.; Bauersachs, J.; Brunner-La Rocca, H.P.; Chioncel, O.; Collins, S.P.; Doehner, W.; Filippatos, G.S.; Flammer, A.J.; et al. Organ dysfunction, injury and failure in acute heart failure: From pathophysiology to diagnosis and management. A review on behalf of the Acute Heart Failure Committee of the Heart Failure Association (HFA) of the European Society of Cardiology (ESC). *Eur. J. Heart Fail.* **2017**, *19*, 821–836. [CrossRef] [PubMed]
38. Chin, B.S.; Gibbs, C.R.; Blann, A.D.; Lip, G.Y. Neither carvedilol nor bisoprolol in maximally tolerated doses has any specific advantage in lowering chronic heart failure oxidant stress: Implications for beta-blocker selection. *Clin. Sci.* **2003**, *105*, 507–512. [CrossRef]
39. Boć-Zalewska, A.; Seremak-Mrozikiewicz, A.; Barlik, M.; Kurzawińska, G.; Drews, K. The possible role of adrenomedullin in the etiology of gestational hypertension and preeclampsia. *Ginekol. Polska* **2011**, *82*, 178–184.
40. van Lier, D.; Pickkers, P. Circulating biomarkers to assess cardiovascular function in critically ill. *Curr. Opin. Crit. Care* **2021**, *27*, 261–268.
41. Packer, M.; Coats, A.S.; Fowler, M.B.; Katus, H.A.; Krum, H.; Mohacsi, P.; Rouleau, J.L.; Tendera, M.; Castaigne, A.; Roecker, E.B.; et al. Effect of Carvedilol on Survival in Severe Chronic Heart Failure. *N. Engl. J. Med.* **2001**, *344*, 1651–1658. [CrossRef]
42. Packer, M.; Bristow, M.R.; Cohn, J.N.; Colucci, W.; Fowler, M.B.; Gilbert, E.M.; Shusterman, N.H. The Effect of Carvedilol on Morbidity and Mortality in Patients with Chronic Heart Failure. *N. Engl. J. Med.* **1996**, *334*, 1349–1355. [CrossRef]
43. The Cardiac Insufficiency Bisoprolol Study II (CIBIS-II): A randomised trial. *Lancet* **1999**, *353*, 9–13. [CrossRef]
44. Effect of metoprolol CR/XL in chronic heart failure: Metoprolol CR/XL Randomised Intervention Trial in Congestive Heart Failure (MERIT-HF). *Lancet* **1999**, *353*, 2001–2007. [CrossRef]
45. Hjalmarson, Å.; Goldstein, S.; Fagerberg, B.; Wedel, H.; Waagstein, F.; Kjekshus, J.; Wikstrand, J.; El Allaf, D.; Vítovec, J.; Aldershvile, J.; et al. Effects of Controlled-Release Metoprolol on Total Mortality, Hospitalizations, and Well-being in Patients With Heart Failure. *JAMA* **2000**, *283*, 1295–1302. [CrossRef] [PubMed]
46. Fröhlich, H.; Torres, L.; Täger, T.; Schellberg, D.; Corletto, A.; Kazmi, S.; Goode, K.; Grundtvig, M.; Hole, T.; Katus, H.A.; et al. Bisoprolol compared with carvedilol and metoprolol succinate in the treatment of patients with chronic heart failure. *Clin. Res. Cardiol.* **2017**, *106*, 711–721. [CrossRef]
47. Ponikowski, P.; Voors, A.A.; Anker, S.D.; Bueno, H.; Cleland, J.G.; Coats, A.J.; Falk, V.; González-Juanatey, J.R.; Harjola, V.P.; Jankowska, E.A.; et al. 2016 ESC Guidelines for the diagnosis and treatment of acute and chronic heart failure: The Task Force for the diagnosis and treatment of acute and chronic heart failure of the European Society of Cardiology (ESC). Developed with the special contribution of the Heart Failure Association (HFA) of the ESC. *Eur. J. Heart Fail.* **2016**, *18*, 891–975.
48. Packer, M.; Cohn, J.N.; Abraham, W.T.; Colucci, W.S.; Fowler, M.B.; Greenberg, B.H.; Leier, C.V.; Massie, B.M.; Young, J.B.; Aaronson, K.D.; et al. Consensus recommendations for the management of chronic heart failure: Introduction. *Am. J. Cardiol.* **1999**, *83*, 1a–38a. [CrossRef]
49. Heart Failure Society of America (HFSA). HFSA guidelines for management of patients with heart failure caused by left ventricular systolic dysfunction-pharmacological approaches. *J. Card. Fail.* **1999**, *5*, 357–382. [CrossRef]
50. Peller, M.; Ozierański, K.; Balsam, P.; Grabowski, M.; Filipiak, K.J.; Opolski, G. Influence of beta-blockers on endothelial function: A meta-analysis of randomized controlled trials. *Cardiol. J.* **2015**, *22*, 708–716. [CrossRef] [PubMed]
51. Lowe, S.A.; Bowyer, L.; Lust, K.; McMahon, L.P.; Morton, M.; North, R.A.; Paech, M.; Said, J.M. SOMANZ guidelines for the management of hypertensive disorders of pregnancy 2014. *Aust. N. Z. J. Obstet. Gynecol.* **2015**, *55*, e1–e29. [CrossRef]
52. Halpern, D.G.; Weinberg, C.R.; Pinnelas, R.; Mehta-Lee, S.; Economy, K.E.; Valente, A.M. Use of Medication for Cardiovascular Disease During Pregnancy: JACC State-of-the-Art Review. *J. Am. Coll. Cardiol.* **2019**, *73*, 457–476. [CrossRef]
53. Bellos, I.; Pergialiotis, V.; Papapanagiotou, A.; Loutradis, D.; Daskalakis, G. Comparative efficacy and safety of oral antihypertensive agents in pregnant women with chronic hypertension: A network metaanalysis. *Am. J. Obstet. Gynecol.* **2020**, *223*, 525–537. [CrossRef]
54. Brownfoot, F.; Hannan, N.; Onda, K.; Tong, S.; Kaitu'U-Lino, T. Soluble endoglin production is upregulated by oxysterols but not quenched by pravastatin in primary placental and endothelial cells. *Placenta* **2014**, *35*, 724–731. [CrossRef]
55. Kaitu'U-Lino, T.J.; Tong, S.; Beard, S.; Hastie, R.; Tuohey, L.; Brownfoot, F.; Onda, K.; Hannan, N. Characterization of protocols for primary trophoblast purification, optimized for functional investigation of sFlt-1 and soluble endoglin. *Pregnancy Hypertens.* **2014**, *4*, 287–295. [CrossRef]
56. Brownfoot, F.; Binder, N.; Hastie, R.; Harper, A.; Beard, S.; Tuohey, L.; Keenan, E.; Tong, S.; Hannan, N. Nicotinamide and its effects on endothelial dysfunction and secretion of antiangiogenic factors by primary human placental cells and tissues. *Placenta* **2021**, *109*, 28–31. [CrossRef] [PubMed]
57. Onda, K.; Tong, S.; Nakahara, A.; Kondo, M.; Monchusho, H.; Hirano, T.; Kaitu'u-Lino, T.; Beard, S.; Binder, N.; Tuohey, L.; et al. Sofalcone upregulates the nuclear factor (erythroid-derived 2)-like 2/heme oxygenase-1 pathway, reduces soluble fms-like tyrosine kinase-1, and quenches endothelial dysfunction: Potential therapeutic for preeclampsia. *Hypertension* **2015**, *65*, 855–862. [CrossRef]

58. Whitehead, C.; Palmer, K.; Nilsson, U.; Gao, Y.; Saglam, B.; Lappas, M.; Tong, S. Placental expression of a novel primate-specific splice variant of sFlt-1 is upregulated in pregnancies complicated by severe early onset pre-eclampsia. *BJOG Int. J. Obstet. Gynaecol.* **2011**, *118*, 1268–1271. [CrossRef]
59. Macdonald, T.M.; Tran, C.; Kaitu'U-Lino, T.J.; Brennecke, S.P.; Hiscock, R.J.; Hui, L.; Dane, K.M.; Middleton, A.L.; Cannon, P.; Walker, S.P.; et al. Assessing the sensitivity of placental growth factor and soluble fms-like tyrosine kinase 1 at 36 weeks' gestation to predict small-for-gestational-age infants or late-onset preeclampsia: A prospective nested case-control study. *BMC Pregnancy Childbirth* **2018**, *18*, 354. [CrossRef]
60. Chau, K.; Hennessy, A.; Makris, A. Placental growth factor and pre-eclampsia. *J. Hum. Hypertens.* **2017**, *31*, 782–786. [CrossRef]
61. Gilroy, D.; Colvillenash, P.R.; Willis, D.K.; Chivers, J.; Paulclark, M.J.; Willoughby, D. Inducible cyclooxygenase may have anti-inflammatory properties. *Nat. Med.* **1999**, *5*, 698–701. [CrossRef]
62. Zhang, N.; Chang, X.; Bai, J.; Chen, Z.-J.; Li, W.-P.; Zhang, C. The Study of Cyclooxygenase 2 in Human Decidua of Preeclampsia. *Biol. Reprod.* **2016**, *95*, 56. [CrossRef]
63. Cui, L.; Shu, C.; Liu, Z.; Tong, W.; Cui, M.; Wei, C.; Tang, J.J.; Liu, X.; Hai, H.; Jiang, J.; et al. Serum protein marker panel for predicting preeclampsia. *Pregnancy Hypertens.* **2018**, *14*, 279–285. [CrossRef]
64. Rajakariar, R.; Yaqoob, M.M.; Gilroy, D.W. COX-2 in inflammation and resolution. *Mol. Interv.* **2006**, *6*, 199–207. [CrossRef]
65. Liao, J.K. Linking endothelial dysfunction with endothelial cell activation. *J. Clin. Investig.* **2013**, *123*, 540–541. [CrossRef]
66. Kobayashi, K.; Kitamura, K.; Etoh, T.; Nagatomo, Y.; Takenaga, M.; Ishikawa, T.; Imamura, T.; Koiwaya, Y.; Eto, T. Increased plasma adrenomedullin levels in chronic congestive heart failure. *Am. Heart J.* **1996**, *131*, 994–998. [CrossRef]
67. Nagaya, N.; Nishikimi, T.; Uematsu, M.; Yoshitomi, Y.; Miyao, Y.; Miyazaki, S.; Goto, Y.; Kojima, S.; Kuramochi, M.; Matsuo, H.; et al. Plasma adrenomedullin as an indicator of prognosis after acute myocardial infarction. *Heart* **1999**, *81*, 483–487. [CrossRef] [PubMed]
68. Miyao, Y.; Nishikimi, T.; Goto, Y.; Miyazaki, S.; Daikoku, S.; Morii, I.; Matsumoto, T.; Takishita, S.; Miyata, A.; Matsuo, H.; et al. Increased plasma adrenomedullin levels in patients with acute myocardial infarction in proportion to the clinical severity. *Heart* **1998**, *79*, 39–44. [CrossRef] [PubMed]
69. Gozzelino, R.; Jeney, V.; Soares, M. Mechanisms of Cell Protection by Heme Oxygenase-1. *Annu. Rev. Pharmacol. Toxicol.* **2010**, *50*, 323–354. [CrossRef] [PubMed]
70. Bank, A.J.; Kelly, A.S.; Thelen, A.M.; Kaiser, D.R.; Gonzalez-Campoy, J.M. Effects of Carvedilol Versus Metoprolol on Endothelial Function and Oxidative Stress in Patients With Type 2 Diabetes Mellitus. *Am. J. Hypertens.* **2007**, *20*, 777–783. [CrossRef]
71. Silva, I.V.G.; De Figueiredo, R.C.; Rios, D.R.A. Effect of Different Classes of Antihypertensive Drugs on Endothelial Function and Inflammation. *Int. J. Mol. Sci.* **2019**, *20*, 3458. [CrossRef] [PubMed]
72. Matsuda, Y.; Akita, H.; Terashima, M.; Shiga, N.; Kanazawa, K.; Yokoyama, M. Carvedilol improves endothelium-dependent dilatation in patients with coronary artery disease. *Am. Heart J.* **2000**, *140*, 753–759. [CrossRef]
73. Virdis, A.; Ghiadoni, L.; Taddei, S. Effects of Antihypertensive Treatment on Endothelial Function. *Curr. Hypertens. Rep.* **2011**, *13*, 276–281. [CrossRef] [PubMed]
74. Lin, Z.P.; Dong, M.; Liu, J. Bisoprolol improved endothelial function and myocardium survival of hypertension with stable angina: A randomized double-blinded trial. *Eur. Rev. Med. Pharmacol. Sci.* **2013**, *17*, 794–801.
75. Grigor'Eva, N.I.; Sharabrin, E.G.; Kuznetsov, A.N.; Mazalov, K.V.; Kontorshchikova, K.N.; Koroleva, E.F. Effects of beta 1-adrenoblocker bisoprolol on endothelial dysfunction in patients with stable angina pectoris in combination with chronic obstructive pulmonary disease. *Ter. Arkhiv* **2009**, *81*, 28–31.
76. Yan, L.; Dong, Y.-F.; Qing, T.-L.; Deng, Y.-P.; Han, X.; Shi, W.-J.; Li, J.-F.; Gao, F.-Y.; Zhang, X.-F.; Tian, Y.-J.; et al. Metoprolol rescues endothelial progenitor cell dysfunction in diabetes. *PeerJ* **2020**, *8*, e9306. [CrossRef]
77. Majidinia, M.; Rasmi, Y.; Ansari, M.H.K.; Seyed-Mohammadzad, M.; Saboory, E.; Shirpoor, A. Metoprolol Improves Endothelial Function in Patients with Cardiac Syndrome X. *Iran. J. Pharm. Res.* **2016**, *15*, 561–566.

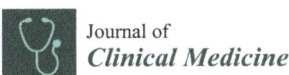

Article

The Inflammatory Milieu of Amniotic Fluid Increases with Chorio-Deciduitis Grade in Inflammation-Restricted to Choriodecidua, but Not Amnionitis, of Extra-Placental Membranes

Joon Hyung Lee [1], Chan-Wook Park [1,2,*], Kyung Chul Moon [3], Joong Shin Park [1] and Jong Kwan Jun [1,2]

[1] Department of Obstetrics and Gynecology, Seoul National University College of Medicine, Seoul 03080, Korea; kontractubex12@gmail.com (J.H.L.); jsparkmd@snu.ac.kr (J.S.P.); jhs0927@snu.ac.kr (J.K.J.)
[2] Medical Research Center, Institute of Reproductive Medicine and Population, Seoul National University, Seoul 03080, Korea
[3] Department of Pathology, Seoul National University College of Medicine, Seoul 03080, Korea; blue7270@gmail.com
* Correspondence: hwpark0803@gmail.com; Tel.: +82-2-2072-0635

Abstract: No information exists about whether intra-amniotic inflammatory response increases with a chorio-deciduitis grade in the context of both inflammation-restricted to chorio-decidua and amnionitis of extra-placental membranes among spontaneous preterm births. The objective of current study is to examine this issue. A study population included 195 singleton pregnant women with chorio-deciduitis, and who spontaneously delivered at preterm (21.6~35.7 weeks) within 7 days of amniocentesis. We examined intra-amniotic inflammatory response according to the chorio-deciduitis grade in the context of inflammation restricted to chorio-decidua and amnionitis of extra-placental membranes. Intra-amniotic inflammatory response was measured by MMP-8 concentration (ng/mL) and WBC-count (cells/mm^3) in amniotic-fluid (AF). Inflammation restricted to chorio-decidua and amnionitis were present in 47.7% (93/195) and 52.3% (102/195) of cases, respectively. Median AF MMP-8 concentration and WBC-count significantly increased with chorio-deciduitis grade in the context of inflammation restricted to chorio-decidua. However, there was no significant difference in median AF MMP-8 concentration and WBC-count between chorio-deciduitis grade-1 and grade-2 in the context of amnionitis. The inflammatory milieu of AF increases with chorio-deciduitis grade in inflammation-restricted to chorio-decidua, but not amnionitis, of extra-placental membranes. This finding suggests that a chorio-deciduitis grade may have little effect on the intensification of intra-amniotic inflammatory response in the context of amnionitis of extra-placental membranes.

Keywords: chorio-deciduitis; grade; amnionitis; acute histologic chorioamnionitis; intra-amniotic inflammatory response

1. Introduction

Ascending intrauterine infection is a major pathophysiology of spontaneous preterm birth (PTB) [1–13]. It is well-known that intrauterine infection from the vaginal and cervical canals ascends to chorio-decidua (CD) and amnion in extra-placental membranes (EPM) [6–9], finally leading to fetal infection [1–15]. This traditional concept of ascending intrauterine infection suggests that the progression of intra-uterine infection is likely to cause the inflammatory responses of biological fluid (i.e., amniotic fluid (AF) and umbilical cord blood). Indeed, the previous studies demonstrated that intra-amniotic inflammatory response (IAIR) is significantly more intense in inflammation beyond CD (i.e., amnion or chorionic plate) than in inflammation restricted to CD [16–19]. Therefore, inflammation restricted to CD is known to be an early stage acute histologic chorioamnionitis (acute-HCA) while inflammation in the compartments beyond CD (i.e., amnion) is an advanced stage acute-HCA. This finding was reaffirmed by other previous studies as follows: (1) IAIR was more severe in patients with amnionitis than in those with only chorionitis [20–23]; (2) IAIR was more intense when inflammation was present in both chorionic plate and CD than when it was restricted to CD only, which was exposed to the cervical canal in placenta previa [24]. Moreover, IAIR increased according to the progression of inflammation in the detailed subdivisions of each placental compartment (i.e., EPM [25–29], umbilical cord [30], and chorionic plate [31]).

Although the intensity of IAIR increases with the total grade of acute-HCA [32], there is a paucity of information about which is more important between staging or grading in acute-HCA for the intensity of IAIR. In this regard, we previously demonstrated that advanced stage (i.e., inflammation in the compartments beyond CD) is associated with higher AF matrix metalloprotease-8 (MMP-8) concentrations and white blood cell (WBC) counts than early stage (i.e., inflammation restricted to CD) in the same context of acute-HCA total grade 2 [33]. However, no information exists about whether the inflammatory milieu of AF increases with chorio-deciduitis grade in the context of both inflammation restricted to CD and amnionitis of EPM. Based on the more importance of staging than grading, it is plausible that IAIR is not influenced by an increase of grade in chorio-deciduitis as a less advanced inflammation in the same context of amnionitis. The hypothesis of this study is that the inflammatory milieu of AF increases with chorio-deciduitis grade in inflammation restricted to CD, but not amnionitis, of EPM. The objective of the study is to examine this issue.

2. Materials and Methods

2.1. Study Design and Patient Population

This is a retrospective cohort study. Study population included 195 singleton pregnant women that met the following criteria: (1) delivered at Seoul National University Hospital between January 1993 and March 2007; (2) gestational age (GA) at delivery between 21.6 weeks and 35.7 weeks; (3) spontaneous PTB due to either preterm labor and intact membranes (PTL) or preterm premature rupture of membranes (preterm-PROM); (4) placental histology showing chorio-deciduitis; (5) no major fetal anomaly; and (6) delivered within 7 days of amniocentesis. This criterion of amniocentesis-to-delivery interval was used to preserve a meaningful temporal relationship between the results of AF and placental histopathologic findings. At our institution, amniocentesis for the retrieval of AF was routinely offered to all patients who were admitted with the diagnosis of either PTL or preterm-PROM for the identification of intra-amniotic infection or inflammation. Moreover, placental histologic examination was routinely offered and performed for all pregnant women who delivered at preterm due to either PTL or preterm-PROM. PTL and preterm-PROM were diagnosed with previously published criteria [34,35]. Written informed consent was gained from all study population. The Institutional Review Board of our institute specifically approved the current study (IRB number: 1909-120-106).

2.2. Clinical Characteristics and Pregnancy Outcomes

Clinical characteristics and pregnancy outcomes were obtained from a medical record review. Data included maternal age, parity, cause of preterm delivery, GA at amniocentesis and delivery, birth weight, gender of newborn, delivery mode, 1-min Apgar score, 5-min Apgar score, amniocentesis-to-delivery interval, antenatal use of antibiotics, gestational diabetes mellitus and suspected or proven early onset neonatal sepsis.

2.3. Diagnosis of Chorio-Deciduitis and Amnionitis

Placental tissue samples for pathologic examination included EPM (i.e., CD and amnion), chorionic plate and umbilical cord. These samples were fixed in 10% neutral buffered formalin and embedded in paraffin. Sections of prepared tissue blocks were stained with hematoxylin and eosin (H&E). Several pathologists were blinded to the clinical information related to placental tissues and examined the placental histopathology immediately after delivery. However, placental histo-pathologic examination was independently verified by a single pathologist (K.C.M.) who was also blinded to the clinical information between the year of 2017 and 2018. Grade 1 (mild) chorio-deciduitis was diagnosed in the presence of a least 1 focus of >5 neutrophils in the CD, and grade 2 (severe) chorio-deciduitis was diagnosed in the presence of diffuse neutrophilic infiltration in the CD; and amnionitis was diagnosed in the presence of at least 1 focus of >5 neutrophils in the amnion according to the criteria previously published [36].

2.4. The Studies of Amniotic Fluid (AF)

AF was cultured for aerobic and anaerobic bacteria, and genital mycoplasmas (*Ureaplasma urealyticum* and *Mycoplasma hominis*) and analyzed for WBC count according to the methods previously described [34,35]. The remaining fluid was centrifuged and stored in polypropylene tubes at −70 °C. MMP-8 concentrations in stored AF were measured with a commercially available enzyme-linked immunosorbent assay (Amersham Pharmacia Biotech, Inc., Little Chalfont, Bucks). The sensitivity of the test was <0.3 ng/mL. Both intra- and inter-assay coefficients of variation were <10%. Details about this assay and its performance were previously described [37]. IAIR was measured by MMP-8 concentration and WBC count in AF.

2.5. Early Onset Neonatal Sepsis

Early onset neonatal sepsis was diagnosed in the presence of a positive blood culture result within 3 days after birth. Early onset neonatal sepsis was suspected in the absence of a positive culture when two or more of the following criteria were present: (1) WBC count of <5000 cells/mm^3; (2) polymorphonuclear leukocyte count of <1800 cells/mm^3; and (3) I/T ratio (ratio of bands to total neutrophils) >0.2. These criteria have been previously used in the pediatric and obstetric literature [20]. Ten newborns were excluded from the assessment of early onset neonatal sepsis because they died immediately after birth due to extremely prematurity.

2.6. Statistical Analysis

Mann–Whitney U test was used for the comparison of continuous variables (Tables 1 and 2, Figures 1 and 2). Comparisons of proportions were performed with the Fisher's exact test (Tables 1 and 2, Figure 3). Statistical significance was defined as a $p < 0.05$.

Table 1. Clinical characteristics and pregnancy outcomes according to chorio-deciduitis grade in the context of inflammation restricted to chorio-decidua (CD).

	Chorio-Deciduitis Grade 1	Chorio-Deciduitis Grade 2	p †
Inflammation restricted to CD (n = 93)	(n = 74)	(n = 19)	
Maternal age, years (mean ± SD)	30.0 ± 4.6	31.1 ± 3.3	0.230
Nulliparity	51.4% (38/74)	68.4% (13/19)	0.207
Causes of preterm birth			0.071
PTL	44.6% (33/74)	21.1% (4/19)	
Preterm-PROM	55.4% (41/74)	78.9% (15/19)	
GA at amniocentesis, (weeks) median, range	32.9 (23.0, 35.6)	32.6 (23.0, 35.6)	0.277
GA at delivery, (weeks) median, range	33.1 (23.4, 35.7)	32.7 (23.3, 35.7)	0.466
Amniocentesis-to-delivery interval, (hours) median, range	19.20 (0.01, 159.80)	53.30 (0.01, 152.80)	0.053

Table 1. Cont.

	Chorio-Deciduitis Grade 1	Chorio-Deciduitis Grade 2	p [†]
Birth weight, g (mean ± SD)	1854 ± 645	1691 ± 643	0.282
Male newborn	58.1% (43/74)	57.9% (11/19)	1.000
Cesarean section	33.8% (25/74)	36.8% (7/19)	0.793
Apgar score at 1 min <7	45.9% (34/74)	47.4% (9/19)	1.000
Apgar score at 5 min <7	28.4% (21/74)	15.8% (3/19)	0.381
Gestational diabetes mellitus	1.4% (1/74)	0% (0/19)	1.000
Antenatal use of antibiotics [††]	60.3% (44/73)	84.2% (16/19)	0.061
Suspected early onset neonatal sepsis [‡]	8.6% (6/70)	10.5% (2/19)	0.677
Proven early onset neonatal sepsis [‡]	2.9% (2/70)	10.5% (2/19)	0.199
Suspected or proven early onset neonatal sepsis [‡]	10.0% (7/70)	21.1% (4/19)	0.239

[†] Mann–Whitney U test was used for the comparison of continuous variables and Fisher's exact test was used for the comparison of proportions; [††] Of 93 cases, 92 patients were included in this analysis because the information about antenatal use of antibiotics in medical record was omitted in one patient; [‡] Four neonates were excluded from the analysis in the evaluation of early onset neonatal sepsis because they died shortly after delivery as a result of extremely prematurity and thus could not be evaluated with respect to the presence or absence of early onset neonatal sepsis; NS, not significant; GA, gestational age; PTL, preterm labor and intact membranes; Preterm-PROM, preterm premature rupture of membranes; CD, chorio-decidua.

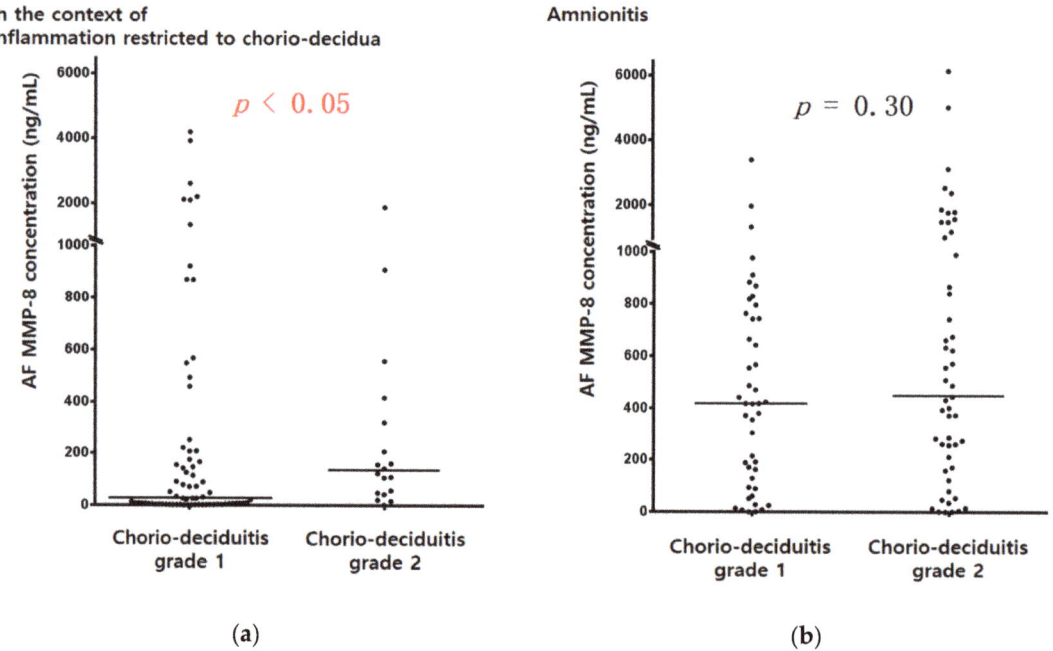

Figure 1. AF MMP-8 concentrations (ng/mL) according to chorio-deciduitis grade in the context of inflammation restricted to CD (a) (median, range; chorio-deciduitis grade 1: 26.0, (0.3, 4202.7); chorio-deciduitis grade 2: 131.9, (1.0, 1873.5); $p < 0.05$) and amnionitis (b) (median, range; chorio-deciduitis grade 1: 416.8, (0.3, 3392.0); chorio-deciduitis grade 2: 441.1, (0.4, 6142.6); Mann–Whitney U test, $p = 0.30$). Of 195 cases which met the entry for this study, 186 patients had an AF MMP-8 concentration; however, 9 patients did not have an AF MMP-8 concentration because of the limited amount of the remaining AF.

Table 2. Clinical characteristics and pregnancy outcomes according to chorio-deciduitis grade in the context of amnionitis.

Amnionitis (n = 102)	Chorio-Deciduitis Grade 1 (n = 49)	Chorio-Deciduitis Grade 2 (n = 53)	p [†]
Maternal age, years (mean ± SD)	30.4 ± 4.5	30.9 ± 4.6	0.573
Nulliparity	36.7% (18/49)	39.6% (21/53)	0.840
Causes of preterm birth			0.420
PTL	44.9% (22/49)	35.8% (19/53)	
Preterm-PROM	55.1% (27/49)	64.2% (34/53)	
GA at amniocentesis, (weeks) median, range	30.4 (24.1, 35.1)	29.1 (21.6, 35.1)	0.135
GA at delivery, (weeks) median, range	31.1 (24.1, 35.3)	29.3 (21.6, 35.7)	0.108
Amniocentesis-to-delivery interval, (h) median, range	32.80 (0.01, 163.70)	14.10 (0.01, 161.70)	0.503
Birth weight, g (mean ± SD)	1524 ± 501	1421 ± 584	0.260
Male newborn	46.9% (23/49)	39.6% (21/53)	0.549
Cesarean section	30.6% (15/49)	22.6% (12/53)	0.379
Apgar score at 1 min <7	61.2% (30/49)	64.2% (34/53)	0.839
Apgar score at 5 min <7	36.7% (18/49)	39.6% (21/53)	0.840
Gestational diabetes mellitus	2.0% (1/49)	5.7% (3/53)	0.619
Antenatal use of antibiotics [††]	79.2% (38/48)	78.8% (41/52)	1.000
Suspected early onset neonatal sepsis [‡]	25.0% (12/48)	20.8% (10/48)	0.809
Proven early onset neonatal sepsis [‡]	6.2% (3/48)	6.2% (3/48)	1.000
Suspected or proven early onset neonatal sepsis [‡]	31.2% (15/48)	27.1% (13/48)	0.823

[†] Mann–Whitney U test was used for the comparison of continuous variables and Fisher's exact test was used for the comparison of proportions; [††] Of 102 cases, 100 patients were included in this analysis because the information about antenatal use of antibiotics in medical record was omitted in two patients; [‡] Six neonates were excluded from the analysis in the evaluation of early onset neonatal sepsis because they died shortly after delivery as a result of extremely prematurity and thus could not be evaluated with respect to the presence or absence of early onset neonatal sepsis; NS, not significant; GA, gestational age; PTL, preterm labor and intact membranes; Preterm-PROM, preterm premature rupture of membranes; CD, chorio-decidua.

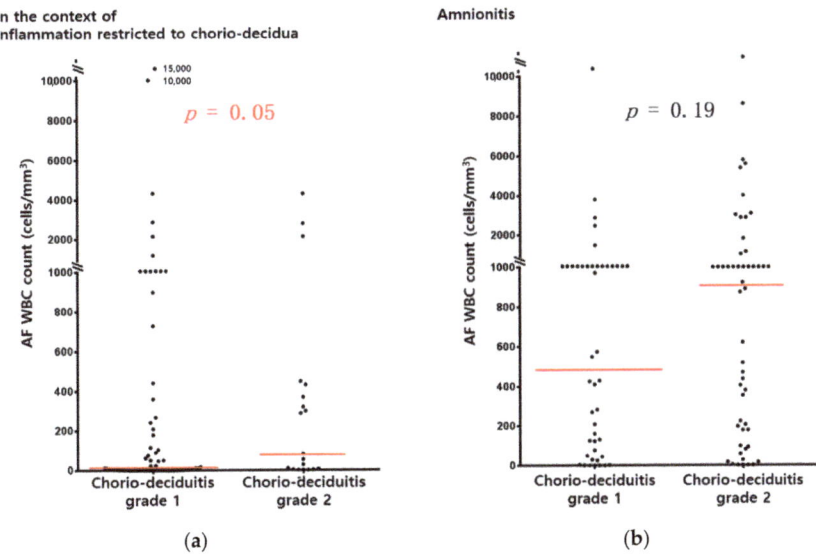

Figure 2. AF WBC counts (cells/mm^3) according to chorio-deciduitis grade in the context of inflammation restricted to CD (a) (median, range; chorio-deciduitis grade 1: 9, (0, 15,000); chorio-deciduitis grade 2: 83 (1, 4300); p = 0.05) and amnionitis (b) (median, range; chorio-deciduitis grade 1: 490, (0, 13,428); chorio-deciduitis grade 2: 909 (0, 19,764); Mann–Whitney U test, p = 0.19). Of 195 cases which met the entry for this study, 185 patients had an AF WBC count; however, 10 patients did not have an AF WBC count because of the limited amount of AF.

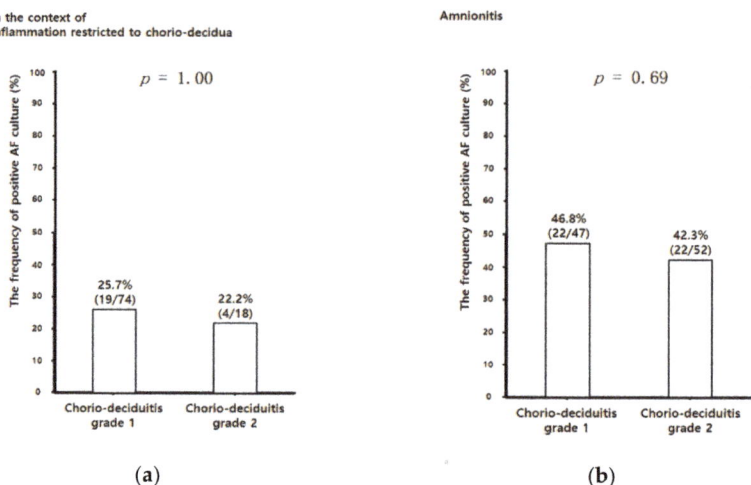

Figure 3. The frequency of positive AF culture according to chorio-deciduitis grade in the context of inflammation restricted to CD (**a**) (chorio-deciduitis grade 1: 25.7% (19/74); chorio-deciduitis grade 2: 22.2% (4/18); $p = 1.00$) and amnionitis (**b**) (chorio-deciduitis grade 1: 46.8% (22/47); chorio-deciduitis grade 2: 42.3% (22/52); Fisher's exact test, $p = 0.69$). Of 195 cases which met the entry for this study, 191 patients had an AF culture result; however, 4 patients did not have an AF culture result because of the limited amount of AF.

3. Results

3.1. Clinical Characteristics and Pregnancy Outcomes According to Chorio-Deciduitis Grade in the Context of Inflammation Restricted to Chorio-Decidua (CD) and Amnionitis

Inflammation restricted to CD and amnionitis were present in 47.7% (93/195) and 52.3% (102/195) of study population, respectively, (Tables 1 and 2). Tables 1 and 2 demonstrated there was no significant difference in clinical characteristics and pregnancy outcomes between chorio-deciduitis grade 1 and grade 2 in the context of inflammation restricted to CD (Table 1) and amnionitis (Table 2).

3.2. Amniotic Fluid (AF) MMP-8 Concentrations and AF WBC Counts According to Chorio-Deciduitis Grade in the Context of Inflammation Restricted to Chorio-Decidua (CD) and Amnionitis

AF MMP-8 concentrations (ng/mL) (Figure 1a) and AF WBC counts (cells/mm^3) (Figure 2a) were significantly higher in cases with chorio-deciduitis grade 2 than in those with chorio-deciduitis grade 1 in the context of inflammation restricted to CD. However, there was no significant increase in AF MMP-8 concentrations (Figure 1b) and AF WBC counts (cells/mm^3) (Figure 2b) when chorio-deciduitis progressed from grade 1 to grade 2 in the context of amnionitis.

3.3. Early Onset Neonatal Sepsis According to Chorio-Deciduitis Grade in the Context of Inflammation Restricted to Chorio-Decidua (CD) and Amnionitis

In the context of inflammation restricted to CD, proven early onset neonatal sepsis was more frequent in cases with chorio-deciduitis grade 2 than in those with chorio-deciduitis grade 1 without reaching statistical significance (Table 1, 10.5% vs. 2.9%; $p = 0.199$). However, there was no significant difference in the frequency of proven early onset neonatal sepsis between chorio-deciduitis grade 1 and 2 in the context of amnionitis (Table 2, 6.2% vs. 6.2%; $p = 1.000$). These patterns correspond to those of IAIR (Figures 1 and 2).

3.4. Positive Amniotic Fluid (AF) Culture According to Chorio-Deciduitis Grade in the Context of Inflammation Restricted to Chorio-Decidua (CD) and Amnionitis

Unlike AF MMP-8 concentrations and AF WBC counts, there was no significant difference in the frequency of positive AF culture between chorio-deciduitis grade 1 and grade 2 in the context of both inflammation restricted to CD (Figure 3a) and amnionitis (Figure 3b). We did not find the relationship between the type of specific organisms and chorio-deciduitis grade in the context of either inflammation restricted to CD or amnionitis. However, we consistently found genital mycoplasmas in more than 50% of positive AF culture in each group (data is not shown).

3.5. Histopathology According to Chorio-Deciduitis Grade in the Context of Inflammation Restricted to Chorio-Decidua (CD) and Amnionitis

Figure 4 shows representative images for chorio-deciduitis grade 1 in inflammation restricted to CD (Figure 4a), chorio-deciduitis grade 2 in inflammation restricted to CD (Figure 4b), chorio-deciduitis grade 1 in amnionitis (Figure 4c), and chorio-deciduitis grade 2 in amnionitis (Figure 4d) in H&E-stained histologic sections of EPM.

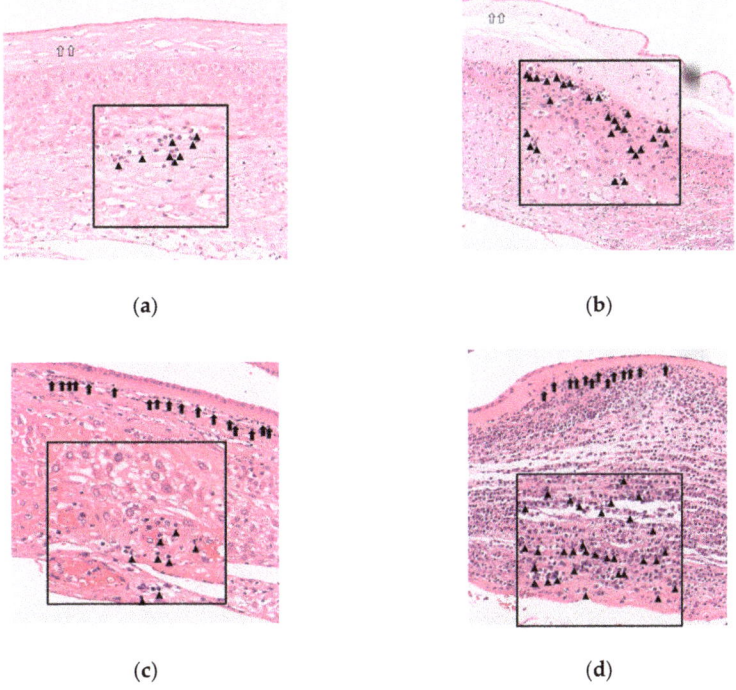

Figure 4. Histopathology according to chorio-deciduitis grade in the context of inflammation restricted to chorio-decidua (CD) and amnionitis. Hematoxylin and eosin-stained histologic sections of extra-placental membrane (EPM) are shown as follows: (**a**) chorio-deciduitis grade 1, inflammation restricted to CD; (**b**) chorio-deciduitis grade 2, inflammation restricted to CD; (**c**) chorio-deciduitis grade 1, amnionitis; and (**d**) chorio-deciduitis grade 2, amnionitis. These images are based on the magnification setting ×200, and the insets of panels are based on the magnification setting ×400. Open arrows indicate inflammation-free amnion (**a**,**b**), and black arrows show amnionitis with infiltrated neutrophils into amnion (**c**,**d**). Arrow heads indicate neutrophils infiltration into chorio-decidua (**a**–**d**).

4. Discussion

Principal finding of this study is that the inflammatory milieu of AF increases with chorio-deciduitis grade in inflammation restricted to CD, but not amnionitis, of EPM. This finding suggests that chorio-deciduitis grade may have little effect on the intensification of IAIR in the context of advanced stage acute-HCA (i.e., amnionitis) (Figure 5). This finding supports our previous assertion that the advanced compartment in the involved anatomical regions is more important than the grade by infiltrated neutrophils for the severity of IAIR in the progression of acute-HCA [33].

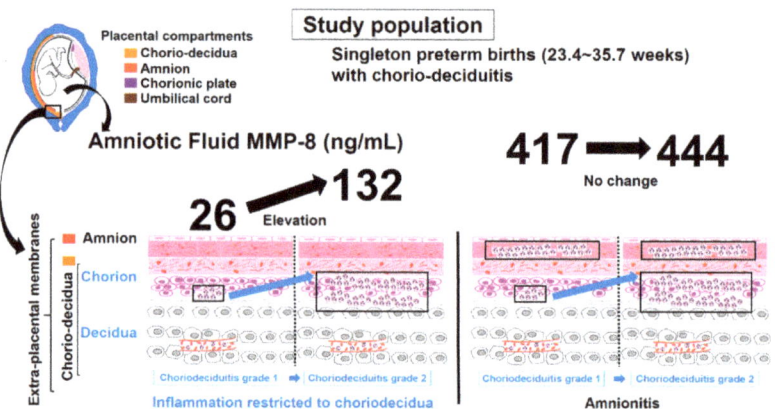

Figure 5. Schema of AF MMP-8 concentrations according to chorio-deciduitis grade in the context of inflammation restricted to chorio-decidua (CD) and amnionitis.

Our previous studies demonstrated IAIR increased according to the progression of inflammation in the detailed subdivisions of each placental compartment [25–31]. However, there is a paucity of data about the relationship between chorio-deciduitis grade and IAIR in the context of early stage and advanced stage acute-HCA in EPM. Moreover, very few previous studies about this issue had a limitation as in the following: (1) although only one previous study analyzed the relationship between positive AF culture and chorio-deciduitis grade in chorio-deciduitis, they did not control the presence of inflammation in other placental compartments (i.e., amnion) failing to exclude a major source of bias leading to a more inclusion of amnionitis in cases of higher chorio-deciduitis grade [38]; and (2) although another previous study examined the relationship between the total grade of acute-HCA and IAIR [32], that study did not examine on the effect of chorio-deciduitis grade on the intensity of IAIR. Indeed, we could not find any study controlling or adjusting for the stage (i.e., the advanced compartment in the involved anatomical regions of acute-HCA) in the analysis about the relationship between chorio-deciduitis grade and IAIR.

The conventional idea of ascending intrauterine infection depicts a model in which the micro-organism of cervical canal enters the decidua, followed by a widespread invasion of the chorion and amnion before crossing the intact membranes into the amniotic cavity [1–9,39–43]. However, one study using fluorescent in situ hybridization with a bacterial 16S rRNA probe demonstrated that focal infection of the CD in the vicinity of the cervical canal leads to intra-amniotic infection before the invasion of amnion and a diffuse inflammation of CD in the context of intact membranes [44,45]. Both mechanisms are plausible but there is insufficient evidence to determine which mechanism represents in vivo pathology of ascending intrauterine infection in humans. Nevertheless, it is well-known that intra-amniotic micro-organisms incite an IAIR resulting in an increase of chemokine level (e.g., CXCL6, IL-8) and chemotactic gradient [3,7,14,15]. Ultimately, this phenomenon causes amniotrophic outside-in neutrophil migration within EPM [7,14]. The extent of migration by neutrophils within EPM is thought to be dependent on the chemotactic gradient developed by chemokines concentration within AF, given that there is a stepwise increase in IAIR according to outside-in neutrophil migration from the decidua via the chorion to the amnion [20–23,25–28]. However, we should explain why the advanced compartment in involved anatomical regions (i.e., amnionitis) is more important than the chorio-deciduitis grade in EPM for the intensity of IAIR, and chorio-deciduitis grade may have little effect on the intensification of IAIR in the context of advanced stage acute-HCA (i.e., amnionitis). Our explanation is as follows (Figure 4). Firstly, neutrophils are likely to begin to gather in the CD (i.e., chorio-deciduitis grade 1 [focal aggregation] in the context of inflammation restricted to CD) in response to initial IAIR, and subsequently accumulate (i.e., chorio-deciduitis grade 2 [diffuse infiltration] in the context of inflammation restricted to CD) but still remain within CD according to a mild and significant increase of IAIR. Secondly, when IAIR surpasses a certain threshold, there is good chance that neutrophils within the CD migrate to the amnion leading to a subsequent decrease in the number of neutrophils in the CD, which means the regression from chorio-deciduitis grade 2 to chorio-deciduitis grade 1 (i.e., chorio-deciduitis grade 1 in the context of amnionitis). Finally, as only a secondary result of IAIR leading to amnionitis, neutrophils in the CD may be replenished from maternal decidual vessels resulting in an increase of chorio-deciduitis grade (i.e., chorio-deciduitis grade 2 in the context of amnionitis). However, all these explanations are only speculation because there is no clear animal or experimental model for the explanation of our current study's results up to now. Therefore, further studies are needed for the elucidation of these issues.

In current study, the frequency of positive AF culture remained unaltered according to chorio-deciduitis grade in the context of both early and advanced stage acute-HCA. Although AF culture is the gold standard for the diagnosis of intra-amniotic infection, it is not a reliable proxy for IAIR as follows: (1) the frequency of positive AF culture remained low in clinical situation at high risk for ascending intrauterine infection such as PTL (10–13%) [46–49] and preterm-PROM (23–32%) [46,47,50–52]; (2) the footprint of micro-organism was identifiable even in the negative AF culture samples via molecular microbiologic techniques [53–61] implying the low sensitivity of culture technique; and (3) intra-amniotic inflammation, but not intra-amniotic infection, may be accompanied by an extra-amniotic infection in the early stage of ascending intrauterine infection, where micro-organisms reside in the CD. Therefore, AF culture results are unlikely to preserve the integrity of the inflammatory milieu of AF (i.e., AF MMP-8 and AF WBC count).

Major strengths of this study are as follows. Firstly, we controlled the involved placental compartments of acute-HCA (i.e., inflammation restricted to chorio-decidua, and amnionitis) for the analysis of the effect of chorio-deciduitis grade on the intensity of IAIR. This allowed us to assess the pure effect of chorio-deciduitis grade on the intensity of IAIR in the context of both early and advanced stage acute-HCA in EPM. Secondly, the intensity of IAIR was gauged with both AF MMP-8 concentration [62–67] and AF WBC count [34,35,68–71], well-known laboratory markers for IAIR in spontaneous PTB. These two markers showed consistent results adding to the credibility in current study. The limitations of this study are as follows. Firstly, this study is retrospective and has a small sample size. Secondly, chorio-deciduitis was not divided into detailed sub-divisions such as inflammation restricted to decidua, inflammation restricted to membranous trophoblast and inflammation in connective tissue of chorion. Thirdly, our study shows a huge variability in AF MMP-8 concentrations even in the same context of chorio-deciduitis grade 1 and grade 2 among patients with inflammation restricted to chorio-deciduitis or amnionitis. It is well-known that IAIR was greatly influenced by the grade and stage of placental inflammation. Moreover, GA at delivery [72] and the cause of PTB [73] have some influence on IAIR. Our previous studies demonstrated the relationship between GA at delivery and IAIR [72] and the relationship between the cause of PTB and IAIR [73] as in the following: (1) The inflammatory milieu of AF decrease in acute-chorioamnionitis with GA [72] and (2) IAIR is more severe in PTL than in preterm-PROM in the context of funisitis, despite less common positive AF culture [73]. Therefore, it is likely that AF MMP-8 concentrations are variable even in the same context of chorio-deciduitis grade 1 and grade 2 among patients with inflammation restricted to chorio-deciduitis or amnionitis, because GA at delivery is not the same and the cause of PTB is either PTL or preterm-PROM even in the same context of placental inflammatory condition. However, we did not adjust GA at delivery and the cause of PTB because GA at delivery and the cause of PTB were not significantly different between chorio-deciduitis grade 1 and grade 2 among patients with inflammation restricted to chorio-deciduitis or amnionitis (Tables 1 and 2).

The classification of acute-HCA usually includes the stage (i.e., the location (compartment) of neutrophil infiltration) and grade (i.e., the degree of neutrophil infiltration in a specific compartment). However, we cannot find any studies examining the interaction between chorio-deciduitis grade and the advanced compartment (i.e., amnionitis) in the involved compartments of acute-HCA for the intensity of IAIR. To our knowledge, this is the first human study reporting that the severity of IAIR is higher in chorio-deciduitis grade 2 than chorio-deciduitis grade 1 in the context of early stage acute-HCA (i.e., inflammation restricted to CD), whereas in advanced stage acute-HCA (i.e., amnionitis), chorio-deciduitis grade 2 is not associated with a more severe IAIR than chorio-deciduitis grade 1. This finding may provide the obstetricians and researchers the information that chorio-deciduitis grade should not be overlooked in the context of early stage acute-HCA (i.e., inflammation restricted to CD) and may have little effect on the intensification of IAIR in the context of advanced stage acute-HCA (i.e., amnionitis).

The CD in itself is a large territory with the detailed sub-divisions composing of the outermost decidua, the membranous trophoblast of chorion as a middle layer, and the innermost connective tissue of chorion [25–28]. Our recent study has suggested that intra-amniotic inflammation is more frequent and intense according to outside-in neutrophil migration in the detailed subdivisions (i.e., the outermost decidua, the membranous trophoblast of chorion as a middle layer, and the innermost connective tissue of chorion) within the same CD [25]. Considering the results of our recent and current studies, neutrophils found in the innermost sub-divisional layer of CD (the connective tissue of chorion) is more likely to be associated with chorio-deciduitis grade 2 than chorio-deciduitis grade 1. Therefore, we should examine whether chorio-deciduitis grade 2 is associated with a more frequent neutrophil infiltration in the innermost connective tissue of chorion than chorio-deciduitis grade 1.

5. Conclusions

The inflammatory milieu of AF increases with chorio-deciduitis grade in early stage, but not advanced stage, acute-HCA in EPM. This finding suggests that chorio-deciduitis grade may have little effect on the intensification of IAIR in the context of advanced stage acute-HCA.

Author Contributions: Conceptualization, C.-W.P. and J.H.L.; methodology, C.-W.P.; software, C.-W.P.; validation, C.-W.P. and J.H.L.; formal analysis, C.-W.P.; investigation, C.-W.P. and J.H.L.; resources, C.-W.P.; data curation, C.-W.P.; writing—original draft preparation, C.-W.P. and J.H.L.; writing—review and editing, all authors; visualization, C.-W.P.; supervision, C.-W.P.; project administration, C.-W.P.; funding acquisition, C.-W.P. All authors have read and agreed to the published version of the manuscript.

Funding: This work was supported by Research Resettlement Fund for the new faculty of Seoul National University (800-20160056).

Institutional Review Board Statement: The study was conducted according to the guidelines of the Declaration of Helsinki, and the Institutional Review Board of Seoul National University Hospital specifically approved this study (IRB-No: 1909-120-106, and 27 September 2019).

Informed Consent Statement: Informed consent was obtained from all subjects involved in the study.

Data Availability Statement: Not applicable.

Conflicts of Interest: The authors declare no conflict of interest.

References

1. Goldenberg, R.L.; Hauth, J.C.; Andrews, W.W. Intrauterine infection and preterm delivery. *N. Engl. J. Med.* **2000**, *342*, 1500–1507. [CrossRef] [PubMed]
2. Helmo, F.R.; Alves, E.A.R.; Moreira, R.A.A.; Severino, V.O.; Rocha, L.P.; Monteiro, M.L.G.D.R.; Reis, M.A.D.; Etchebehere, R.M.; Machado, J.R.; Corrêa, R.R.M. Intrauterine infection, immune system and premature birth. *J. Matern. Fetal Neonatal Med.* **2018**, *31*, 1227–1233. [CrossRef] [PubMed]
3. Agrawal, V.; Hirsch, E. Intrauterine infection and preterm labor. *Semin. Fetal Neonatal Med.* **2012**, *17*, 12–19. [CrossRef] [PubMed]
4. Kemp, M.W. Preterm birth, intrauterine infection, and fetal inflammation. *Front. Immunol.* **2014**, *5*, 574. [CrossRef]
5. Chen, H.J.; Gur, T.L. Intrauterine Microbiota: Missing, or the Missing Link? *Trends Neurosci.* **2019**, *42*, 402–413. [CrossRef]
6. Romero, R.; Mazor, M. Infection and preterm labor. *Clin. Obstet. Gynecol.* **1988**, *31*, 553–584. [CrossRef] [PubMed]
7. Cappelletti, M.; Presicce, P.; Kallapur, S.G. Immunobiology of Acute Chorioamnionitis. *Front. Immunol.* **2020**, *11*, 649. [CrossRef] [PubMed]
8. Petit, E.; Abergel, A.; Dedet, B. The role of infection in preterm birth. *J. Gynecol. Obstet. Biol. Reprod.* **2012**, *41*, 14–25. [CrossRef] [PubMed]
9. Menon, R.; Dunlop, A.L.; Kramer, M.R.; Fortunato, S.J.; Hogue, C.J. An overview of racial disparities in preterm birth rates: Caused by infection or inflammatory response? *Acta Obstet. Gynecol. Scand.* **2011**, *90*, 1325–1331. [CrossRef] [PubMed]
10. Gonçalves, L.F.; Chaiworapongsa, T.; Romero, R. Intrauterine infection and prematurity. *Ment. Retard. Dev. Disabil. Res. Rev.* **2002**, *8*, 3–13. [CrossRef]
11. Stinson, L.F.; Payne, M.S. Infection-mediated preterm birth: Bacterial origins and avenues for intervention. *Aust. N. Z. J. Obstet. Gynaecol.* **2019**, *59*, 781–790. [CrossRef] [PubMed]
12. Pavlidis, I.; Spiller, O.B.; Demarco, G.S.; MacPherson, H.; Howie, S.E.M.; Norman, J.E.; Stock, S.J. Cervical epithelial damage promotes Ureaplasma parvum ascending infection, intrauterine inflammation and preterm birth induction in mice. *Nat. Commun.* **2020**, *11*, 199. [CrossRef] [PubMed]
13. Bayar, E.; Bennett, P.R.; Chan, D.; Sykes, L.; MacIntyre, D.A. The pregnancy microbiome and preterm birth. *Semin. Immunopathol.* **2020**, *42*, 487–499. [CrossRef]
14. Kim, C.J.; Romero, R.; Chaemsaithong, P.; Chaiyasit, N.; Yoon, B.H.; Kim, Y.M. Acute chorioamnionitis and funisitis: Definition, pathologic features, and clinical significance. *Am. J. Obstet. Gynecol.* **2015**, *213*, S29–S52. [CrossRef]
15. Nadeau, H.C.; Subramaniam, A.; Andrews, W.W. Infection and preterm birth. *Semin. Fetal Neonatal Med.* **2016**, *21*, 100–105. [CrossRef]
16. Park, C.W.; Kim, S.M.; Park, J.S.; Jun, J.K.; Yoon, B.H. Fetal, amniotic and maternal inflammatory responses in early stage of ascending intrauterine infection, inflammation restricted to chorio-decidua, in preterm gestation. *J. Matern. Fetal Neonatal Med.* **2014**, *27*, 98–105. [CrossRef] [PubMed]
17. Abehsera, D.; Rodrigues, Y.; Mingorance, J.; Suárez, A.; Magdaleno, F.; Bartha, J.L. Prediction and clinical relevance of pathologic patterns of injury associated with chorioamnionitis. *Placenta* **2014**, *35*, 70–71. [CrossRef]
18. Buhimschi, I.A.; Zambrano, E.; Pettker, C.M.; Bahtiyar, M.O.; Paidas, M.; Rosenberg, V.A.; Thung, S.; Salafia, C.M.; Buhimschi, C.S. Using proteomic analysis of the human amniotic fluid to identify histologic chorioamnionitis. *Obstet. Gynecol.* **2008**, *111*, 403–412. [CrossRef] [PubMed]
19. Hockney, R.; Waring, G.J.; Taylor, G.; Cummings, S.P.; Robson, S.C.; Orr, C.H.; Nelson, A. Fetal membrane bacterial load is increased in histologically confirmed inflammatory chorioamnionitis: A retrospective cohort study. *Placenta* **2020**, *91*, 43–51. [CrossRef]
20. Park, C.W.; Moon, K.C.; Park, J.S.; Jun, J.K.; Romero, R.; Yoon, B.H. The involvement of human amnion in histologic chorioamnionitis is an indicator that a fetal and an intra-amniotic inflammatory response is more likely and severe: Clinical implications. *Placenta* **2009**, *30*, 56–61. [CrossRef]
21. Yoneda, S.; Shiozaki, A.; Ito, M.; Yoneda, N.; Inada, K.; Yonezawa, R.; Kigawa, M.; Saito, S. Accurate Prediction of the Stage of Histological Chorioamnionitis before Delivery by Amniotic Fluid IL-8 Level. *Am. J. Reprod. Immunol.* **2015**, *73*, 568–576. [CrossRef]
22. Kidokoro, K.; Furuhashi, M.; Kuno, N.; Ishikawa, K. Amniotic fluid neutrophil elastase and lactate dehydrogenase: Association with histologic chorioamnionitis. *Acta Obstet. Gynecol. Scand.* **2006**, *85*, 669–674. [CrossRef]
23. Miura, H.; Ogawa, M.; Hirano, H.; Sanada, H.; Sato, A.; Obara, M.; Terada, Y. Neutrophil elastase and interleukin-6 in amniotic fluid as indicators of chorioamnionitis and funisitis. *Eur. J. Obstet. Gynecol. Reprod. Biol.* **2011**, *158*, 209–213. [CrossRef] [PubMed]
24. Park, C.W.; Moon, K.C.; Park, J.S.; Jun, J.K.; Yoon, B.H. The frequency and clinical significance of intra-uterine infection and inflammation in patients with placenta previa and preterm labor and intact membranes. *Placenta* **2009**, *30*, 613–618. [CrossRef] [PubMed]
25. Oh, J.W.; Park, C.W.; Moon, K.C.; Park, J.S.; Jun, J.K. Acute Chorioamnionitis and Intra-amniotic Inflammation are More Severe according to Outside-in Neutrophil Migration within the Same Chorio-decidua. *Taiwan J. Obstet. Gynecol.* accepted.

26. Mauri, A.; Perrini, M.; Mateos, J.M.; Maake, C.; Ochsenbein-Koelble, N.; Zimmermann, R.; Ehrbar, M.; Mazza, E. Second harmonic generation microscopy of fetal membranes under deformation: Normal and altered morphology. *Placenta* **2013**, *34*, 1020–1026. [CrossRef] [PubMed]
27. Gupta, A.; Kedige, S.D.; Jain, K. Amnion and Chorion Membranes: Potential Stem Cell Reservoir with Wide Applications in Periodontics. *Int. J. Biomater.* **2015**, *2015*, 274082. [CrossRef]
28. Avila, C.; Santorelli, J.; Mathai, J.; Ishkin, S.; Jabsky, M.; Willins, J.; Figueroa, R.; Kaplan, C. Anatomy of the fetal membranes using optical coherence tomography: Part 1. *Placenta* **2014**, *35*, 1065–1069. [CrossRef]
29. Park, C.W.; Oh, J.W.; Moon, K.C.; Park, J.S.; Jun, J.K. Amniotic necrosis is associated with severe and advanced acute histologic chorioamnionitis. *Placenta* **2017**, *57*, 285. [CrossRef]
30. Seong, J.S.; Park, C.W.; Moon, K.C.; Park, J.S.; Jun, J.K. Necrotizing funisitis is an indicator that intra-amniotic inflammatory response is more severe and amnionitis is more frequent in the context of the extension of inflammation into Wharton's jelly. *Taiwan J. Obstet. Gynecol..* accepted.
31. Moon, K.C.; Oh, J.W.; Park, C.W.; Park, J.S.; Jun, J.K. The Relationship Among Intra-Amniotic Inflammatory Response, The Progression of Inflammation in Chorionic Plate and Early-Onset Neonatal Sepsis. *Front. Pediatr.* **2021**, *9*, 582472:1–582472:9. [CrossRef]
32. Kim, S.M.; Romero, R.; Park, J.W.; Oh, K.J.; Jun, J.K.; Yoon, B.H. The relationship between the intensity of intraamniotic inflammation and the presence and severity of acute histologic chorioamnionitis in preterm gestation. *J. Matern. Fetal Neonatal Med.* **2015**, *28*, 1500–1509. [CrossRef]
33. Park, C.W.; Yoon, B.H.; Kim, S.M.; Park, J.S.; Jun, J.K. Which is more important for the intensity of intra-amniotic inflammation between total grade or involved anatomical region in preterm gestations with acute histologic chorioamnionitis? *Obstet. Gynecol. Sci.* **2013**, *56*, 227–233. [CrossRef]
34. Yoon, B.H.; Jun, J.K.; Park, K.H.; Syn, H.C.; Gomez, R.; Romero, R. Serum C-reactive protein, white blood cell count, and amniotic fluid white blood cell count in women with preterm premature rupture of membranes. *Obstet. Gynecol.* **1996**, *88*, 1034–1040. [CrossRef]
35. Yoon, B.H.; Yang, S.H.; Jun, J.K.; Park, K.H.; Kim, C.J.; Romero, R. Maternal blood C-reactive protein, white blood cell count, and temperature in preterm labor: A comparison with amniotic fluid white blood cell count. *Obstet. Gynecol.* **1996**, *87*, 231–237. [CrossRef]
36. Yoon, B.H.; Romero, R.; Kim, C.J.; Jun, J.K.; Gomez, R.; Choi, J.H.; Syn, H.C. Amniotic fluid interleukin-6: A sensitive test for antenatal diagnosis of acute inflammatory lesions of preterm placenta and prediction of perinatal morbidity. *Am. J. Obstet. Gynecol.* **1995**, *172*, 960–970. [CrossRef]
37. Park, J.S.; Romero, R.; Yoon, B.H.; Moon, J.B.; Oh, S.Y.; Han, S.Y.; Ko, E.M. The relationship between amniotic fluid matrix metalloproteinase-8 and funisitis. *Am. J. Obstet. Gynecol.* **2001**, *185*, 1156–1161. [CrossRef]
38. Romero, R.; Salafia, C.M.; Athanassiadis, A.P.; Hanaoka, S.; Mazor, M.; Sepulveda, W.; Bracken, M.B. The relationship between acute inflammatory lesions of the preterm placenta and amniotic fluid microbiology. *Am. J. Obstet. Gynecol.* **1992**, *166*, 1382–1388. [CrossRef]
39. Goldenberg, R.L.; Andrews, W.W.; Hauth, J.C. Choriodecidual infection and preterm birth. *Nutr. Rev.* **2002**, *60*, S19–S25. [CrossRef] [PubMed]
40. Grigsby, P.L.; Novy, M.J.; Waldorf, K.M.A.; Sadowsky, D.W.; Gravett, M.G. Choriodecidual inflammation: A harbinger of the preterm labor syndrome. *Reprod. Sci.* **2010**, *17*, 85–94. [CrossRef] [PubMed]
41. Suff, N.; Karda, R.; Diaz, J.A.; Ng, J.; Baruteau, J.; Perocheau, D.; Tangney, M.; Taylor, P.W.; Peebles, D.; Buckley, S.M.K.; et al. Ascending Vaginal Infection Using Bioluminescent Bacteria Evokes Intrauterine Inflammation, Preterm Birth, and Neonatal Brain Injury in Pregnant Mice. *Am. J. Pathol.* **2018**, *188*, 2164–2176. [CrossRef] [PubMed]
42. Waldorf, K.M.A.; Rubens, C.E.; Gravett, M.G. Use of nonhuman primate models to investigate mechanisms of infection-associated preterm birth. *BJOG Int. J. Obstet. Gynaecol.* **2011**, *118*, 136–144. [CrossRef] [PubMed]
43. Fortner, K.B.; Grotegut, C.A.; Ransom, C.E.; Bentley, R.C.; Feng, L.; Lan, L.; Heine, R.P.; Seed, P.C.; Murtha, A.P. Bacteria localization and chorion thinning among preterm premature rupture of membranes. *PLoS ONE* **2014**, *9*, e83338. [CrossRef] [PubMed]
44. Kim, M.J.; Romero, R.; Gervasi, M.T.; Kim, J.S.; Yoo, W.; Lee, D.C.; Mittal, P.; Erez, O.; Kusanovic, J.P.; Hassan, S.S.; et al. Widespread microbial invasion of the chorioamniotic membranes is a consequence and not a cause of intra-amniotic infection. *Lab. Investig.* **2009**, *89*, 924–936. [CrossRef]
45. Jefferson, K.K. The bacterial etiology of preterm birth. *Adv. Appl. Microbiol.* **2012**, *80*, 1–22. [CrossRef]
46. Romero, R.; Gómez, R.; Chaiworapongsa, T.; Conoscenti, G.; Kim, J.C.; Kim, Y.M. The role of infection in preterm labour and delivery. *Paediatr. Perinat. Epidemiol.* **2001**, *15* (Suppl. S2), 41–56. [CrossRef]
47. Stranik, J.; Kacerovsky, M.; Andrys, C.; Soucek, O.; Bolehovska, R.; Holeckova, M.; Matulova, J.; Jacobsson, B.; Musilova, I. Intra-amniotic infection and sterile intra-amniotic inflammation are associated with elevated concentrations of cervical fluid interleukin-6 in women with spontaneous preterm labor with intact membranes. *J. Matern. Fetal Neonatal Med.* **2021**. [CrossRef]
48. Yoon, B.H.; Romero, R.; Moon, J.B.; Shim, S.S.; Kim, M.; Kim, G.; Jun, J.K. Clinical significance of intra-amniotic inflammation in patients with preterm labor and intact membranes. *Am. J. Obstet. Gynecol.* **2001**, *185*, 1130–1136. [CrossRef]

49. Combs, C.A.; Gravett, M.; Garite, T.J.; Hickok, D.E.; Lapidus, J.; Porreco, R.; Rael, J.; Grove, T.; Morgan, T.K.; Clewell, W.; et al. Amniotic fluid infection, inflammation, and colonization in preterm labor with intact membranes. *Am. J. Obstet. Gynecol.* **2014**, *210*, 125.e1–125.e15. [CrossRef]
50. Shim, S.S.; Romero, R.; Hong, J.S.; Park, C.W.; Jun, J.K.; Kim, B.I.; Yoon, B.H. Clinical significance of intra-amniotic inflammation in patients with preterm premature rupture of membranes. *Am. J. Obstet. Gynecol.* **2004**, *191*, 1339–1345. [CrossRef]
51. Cobo, T.; Kacerovsky, M.; Palacio, M.; Hornychova, H.; Hougaard, D.M.; Skogstrand, K.; Jacobsson, B. Intra-amniotic inflammatory response in subgroups of women with preterm prelabor rupture of the membranes. *PLoS ONE* **2012**, *7*, e43677. [CrossRef]
52. Cobo, T.; Kacerovsky, M.; Holst, R.M.; Hougaard, D.M.; Skogstrand, K.; Wennerholm, U.B.; Hagberg, H.; Jacobsson, B. Intra-amniotic inflammation predicts microbial invasion of the amniotic cavity but not spontaneous preterm delivery in preterm prelabor membrane rupture. *Acta Obstet. Gynecol. Scand.* **2012**, *91*, 930–935. [CrossRef] [PubMed]
53. Han, Y.W.; Shen, T.; Chung, P.; Buhimschi, I.A.; Buhimschi, C.S. Uncultivated bacteria as etiologic agents of intra-amniotic inflammation leading to preterm birth. *J. Clin. Microbiol.* **2009**, *47*, 38–47. [CrossRef]
54. Yoon, B.H.; Romero, R.; Kim, M.; Kim, E.C.; Kim, T.; Park, J.S.; Jun, J.K. Clinical implications of detection of Ureaplasma urealyticum in the amniotic cavity with the polymerase chain reaction. *Am. J. Obstet. Gynecol.* **2000**, *183*, 1130–1137. [CrossRef] [PubMed]
55. Stinson, L.; Hallingström, M.; Barman, M.; Viklund, F.; Keelan, J.; Kacerovsky, M.; Payne, M.; Jacobsson, B. Comparison of Bacterial DNA Profiles in Mid-Trimester Amniotic Fluid Samples from Preterm and Term Deliveries. *Front. Microbiol.* **2020**, *11*, 415. [CrossRef] [PubMed]
56. Keskin, F.; Ciftci, S.; Keceli, S.A.; Koksal, M.O.; Caliskan, E.; Cakiroglu, Y.; Agacfidan, A. Comparison of culture and real-time polymerase chain reaction methods for detection of Mycoplasma hominis in amniotic fluids samples. *Niger. J. Clin. Pract.* **2018**, *21*, 1127–1131. [CrossRef] [PubMed]
57. Rodríguez, N.; Fernandez, C.; Zamora, Y.; Berdasquera, D.; Rivera, J.A. Detection of Ureaplasma urealyticum and Ureaplasma parvum in amniotic fluid: Association with pregnancy outcomes. *J. Matern. Fetal Neonatal Med.* **2011**, *24*, 47–50. [CrossRef]
58. Yoon, B.H.; Romero, R.; Lim, J.H.; Shim, S.S.; Hong, J.S.; Shim, J.Y.; Jun, J.K. The clinical significance of detecting Ureaplasma urealyticum by the polymerase chain reaction in the amniotic fluid of patients with preterm labor. *Am. J. Obstet. Gynecol.* **2003**, *189*, 919–924. [CrossRef]
59. Morimoto, S.; Usui, H.; Kobayashi, T.; Katou, E.; Goto, S.; Tanaka, H.; Shozu, M. Bacterial-Culture-Negative Subclinical Intra-Amniotic Infection Can Be Detected by Bacterial 16S Ribosomal-DNA-Amplifying Polymerase Chain Reaction. *Jpn. J. Infect. Dis.* **2018**, *71*, 274–280. [CrossRef]
60. Marconi, C.; de Andrade Ramos, B.R.; Peraçoli, J.C.; Donders, G.G.; da Silva, M.G. Amniotic fluid interleukin-1 beta and interleukin-6, but not interleukin-8 correlate with microbial invasion of the amniotic cavity in preterm labor. *Am. J. Reprod. Immunol.* **2011**, *65*, 549–556. [CrossRef] [PubMed]
61. DiGiulio, D.B. Diversity of microbes in amniotic fluid. *Semin. Fetal Neonatal Med.* **2012**, *17*, 2–11. [CrossRef] [PubMed]
62. Park, C.W.; Yoon, B.H.; Kim, S.M.; Park, J.S.; Jun, J.K. The frequency and clinical significance of intra-amniotic inflammation defined as an elevated amniotic fluid matrix metalloproteinase-8 in patients with preterm labor and low amniotic fluid white blood cell counts. *Obstet. Gynecol. Sci.* **2013**, *56*, 167–175. [CrossRef] [PubMed]
63. Revello, R.; Alcaide, M.J.; Dudzik, D.; Abehsera, D.; Bartha, J.L. Differential amniotic fluid cytokine profile in women with chorioamnionitis with and without funisitis. *J. Matern. Fetal Neonatal Med.* **2016**, *29*, 2161–2165. [CrossRef]
64. Angus, S.R.; Segel, S.Y.; Hsu, C.D.; Locksmith, G.J.; Clark, P.; Sammel, M.D.; Macones, G.A.; Strauss, J.F., 3rd; Parry, S. Amniotic fluid matrix metalloproteinase-8 indicates intra-amniotic infection. *Am. J. Obstet. Gynecol.* **2001**, *185*, 1232–1238. [CrossRef]
65. Kim, A.; Lee, E.S.; Shin, J.C.; Kim, H.Y. Identification of biomarkers for preterm delivery in mid-trimester amniotic fluid. *Placenta* **2013**, *34*, 873–878. [CrossRef] [PubMed]
66. Myntti, T.; Rahkonen, L.; Nupponen, I.; Pätäri-Sampo, A.; Tikkanen, M.; Sorsa, T.; Juhila, J.; Andersson, S.; Paavonen, J.; Stefanovic, V. Amniotic Fluid Infection in Preterm Pregnancies with Intact Membranes. *Dis. Markers* **2017**, *2017*, 8167276. [CrossRef]
67. Myntti, T.; Rahkonen, L.; Pätäri-Sampo, A.; Tikkanen, M.; Sorsa, T.; Juhila, J.; Helve, O.; Andersson, S.; Paavonen, J.; Stefanovic, V. Comparison of amniotic fluid matrix metalloproteinase-8 and cathelicidin in the diagnosis of intra-amniotic infection. *J. Perinatol.* **2016**, *36*, 1049–1054. [CrossRef] [PubMed]
68. Romero, R.; Quintero, R.; Nores, J.; Avila, C.; Mazor, M.; Hanaoka, S.; Hagay, Z.; Merchant, L.; Hobbins, J.C. Amniotic fluid white blood cell count: A rapid and simple test to diagnose microbial invasion of the amniotic cavity and predict preterm delivery. *Am. J. Obstet. Gynecol.* **1991**, *165*, 821–830. [CrossRef]
69. Fan, S.R.; Liu, P.; Yan, S.M.; Peng, J.Y.; Liu, X.P. Diagnosis and Management of Intraamniotic Infection. *Matern. Fetal Med.* **2020**, *2*, 223–230. [CrossRef]
70. Romero, R.; Yoon, B.H.; Mazor, M.; Gomez, R.; Diamond, R.X.; Kenney, J.S.; Ramirez, M.; Fidel, P.L.; Sorokin, Y.; Cotton, D.; et al. The diagnostic and prognostic value of amniotic fluid white blood cell count, glucose, interleukin-6, and gram stain in patients with preterm labor and intact membranes. *Am. J. Obstet. Gynecol.* **1993**, *169*, 805–816. [CrossRef]
71. Abdel-Razeq, S.S.; Buhimschi, I.A.; Bahtiyar, M.O.; Rosenberg, V.A.; Dulay, A.T.; Han, C.S.; Werner, E.F.; Thung, S.; Buhimschi, C.S. Interpretation of amniotic fluid white blood cell count in "bloody tap" amniocenteses in women with symptoms of preterm labor. *Obstet. Gynecol.* **2010**, *116*, 344–354. [CrossRef] [PubMed]

72. Park, C.W.; Park, J.S.; Jun, J.K.; Yoon, B.H. The inflammatory milieu of amniotic fluid in acute-chorioamnionitis decreases with increasing gestational age. *Placenta* **2015**, *36*, 1283–1290. [CrossRef] [PubMed]
73. Park, C.W.; Yoon, B.H.; Park, J.S.; Jun, J.K. A fetal and an intra-amniotic inflammatory response is more severe in preterm labor than in preterm PROM in the context of funisitis: Unexpected observation in human gestations. *PLoS ONE* **2013**, *8*, e62521. [CrossRef] [PubMed]

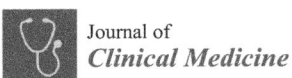

Journal of
Clinical Medicine

Article

MMP-2 and MMP-9 Polymorphisms and Preeclampsia Risk in Tunisian Arabs: A Case-Control Study

Marwa Ben Ali Gannoun [1,2,†], Nozha Raguema [1,3,4,†], Hedia Zitouni [1], Meriem Mehdi [5], Ondrej Seda [6], Touhami Mahjoub [1] and Julie L. Lavoie [3,4,*]

1. Laboratory of Human Genome and Multifactorial Diseases, Faculty of Pharmacy of Monastir, University of Monastir, Monastir 5000, Tunisia; marwabenali24@yahoo.fr (M.B.A.G.); nozharakam@gmail.com (N.R.); hediaztn@gmail.com (H.Z.); touhamimahjoub@gmail.com (T.M.)
2. Laboratory of Histology Embryology and Cytogenetics, Faculty of Medicine, University of Monastir, Monastir 5000, Tunisia
3. Centre de Recherche du Centre Hospitalier de l'Université de Montréal (CRCHUM), Montréal, QC H2X 0A9, Canada
4. School of Kinesiology and Physical Activity Sciences, Université de Montréal, Montréal, QC H3T 1J4, Canada
5. Laboratory of Cytogenetics and Reproductive Biology, Center of Maternity and Neonatology Monastir, Fattouma Bourguiba University Teaching Hospital, Monastir 5000, Tunisia; hbsmahdi@yahoo.fr
6. The First Faculty of Medicine and General University Hospital, Institute of Biology and Medical Genetics, Charles University, 12800 Prague, Czech Republic; oseda@lf1.cuni.cz
* Correspondence: julie.lavoie.3@umontreal.ca; Tel.: +1-(514)-890-8000 (ext. 23612)
† The first and second author have equal contribution.

Abstract: The abnormal production of matrix metalloproteinases (MMPs), especially MMP-9 and MMP-2, plays a pivotal role in hypertensive disorders of pregnancy, and as such, can influence the development of preeclampsia. These alterations may result from functional genetic polymorphisms in the promoter region of MMP-9 and MMP-2 genes, which modify MMP-9 and MMP-2 expression. We investigated the association of MMP-9 polymorphism rs3918242 (-1562 C>T) and MMP-2 polymorphism rs2285053 (-735 C>T) with the risk of preeclampsia. This case–control study was conducted on 345 women with preeclampsia and 281 age-matched women with normal pregnancies from Tunisian hospitals. Genomic DNA was extracted from whole blood collected at delivery. Genotypes for -1562 C>T and -735 C>T polymorphisms were performed using polymerase chain reaction-restriction fragment length polymorphism (PCR-RFLP). An increased frequency of heterozygous MMP-9 -1562 C/T genotype carriers was observed in women with preeclampsia compared to healthy controls (p = 0.03). In contrast, the MMP-2 -735 C>T polymorphism was not significantly different regarding frequency distribution of the allele and genotype between healthy pregnant women and women with preeclampsia. Our study suggests that the MMP-9 -1562 C/T variant, associated with high MMP-9 production, could be a genetic risk factor for preeclampsia in Tunisian women.

Keywords: genotyping; preeclampsia; MMP-9; MMP-2; SNPs

Citation: Gannoun, M.B.A.; Raguema, N.; Zitouni, H.; Mehdi, M.; Seda, O.; Mahjoub, T.; Lavoie, J.L. MMP-2 and MMP-9 Polymorphisms and Preeclampsia Risk in Tunisian Arabs: A Case-Control Study. *J. Clin. Med.* **2021**, *10*, 2647. https://doi.org/10.3390/jcm10122647

Academic Editors: Alex Heazell and Eyal Sheiner

Received: 11 May 2021
Accepted: 10 June 2021
Published: 16 June 2021

Publisher's Note: MDPI stays neutral with regard to jurisdictional claims in published maps and institutional affiliations.

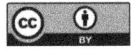

Copyright: © 2021 by the authors. Licensee MDPI, Basel, Switzerland. This article is an open access article distributed under the terms and conditions of the Creative Commons Attribution (CC BY) license (https://creativecommons.org/licenses/by/4.0/).

1. Introduction

Preeclampsia (PE) is a multi-system pregnancy-specific disorder classically characterized by elevated maternal blood pressure and proteinuria after 20 weeks of pregnancy. This syndrome complicates 5–7% of pregnancies worldwide and is responsible for 60,000 maternal deaths annually, and a far greater number of fetal and neonatal deaths [1]. Indeed, it is one of the leading causes of maternal and fetal mortality and morbidity [2,3].

PE has been proposed to result from multiple factors, such as angiogenic, inflammatory, and immune response, potentially due to genetic and external environmental factors [4]. However, the role of genetic predisposition is still not well understood, although there is clear evidence of the contribution of family history supported by several segregation and linkage analysis studies, as well as genome-wide association studies [5]. One of the most proposed mechanisms for PE relates to inadequate maternal blood flow to the placenta, caused by impaired spiral artery remodeling, vascular endothelial injury, altered trophoblast cell activity and an exacerbated inflammatory response [6].

Of interest, MMPs are zinc-dependent endopeptidases that degrade different extracellular matrix components and play a role in the remodeling of various tissues [7]. Consequently, MMP activity dysregulation has been reported in clinical conditions affecting the cardiovascular system [8,9], including gestational hypertensive disorders, such as PE [10].

More specifically, MMPs, such as MMP-2 (gelatinase A) and MMP-9 (gelatinase B), have been implicated in endometrial tissue remodeling during estrous cycles and pregnancy [11]. Indeed, MMP-9 and MMP-2 efficiently degrade type IV collagen, a main component of the basement membrane, and are associated with active neovascularization [12–15]. Of interest, elevated levels of MMP-9 and lower levels of MMP-2 are observed in the serum of women with PE, and similar observations are reported in the umbilical cord plasma of newborns born from women with PE [9,16,17].

MMP-2 and MMP-9 genes contain SNPs, some of which are in the promoter region, that play an essential role in disease development [18,19]. Notably, the MMP-9 -1562 C>T polymorphic substitution, present in this gene's promoter, is associated with higher transcriptional activity of the gene and higher protein levels of MMP-9 [20]. Interestingly, this T allele has been associated with higher MMP-9 plasma levels in men and women with cardiovascular diseases, such as atherosclerosis and restenosis [21,22], as well as with pregnancy complications [23,24]. More specifically, a few groups have reported an association between this polymorphism and PE risk [23–25]. Indeed, six studies have found an association between the -1562 T allele and PE in Brazilian, United Kingdom, Dutch, Polish, and Iranian populations, although in small cohorts (less than 180 cases and 200 controls) [25–30]. Hence, it is important to repeat these studies in different populations and large cohorts, as the size of the cohort, ethnic variation and geographical location can contribute to the differences in -1562 T allele distribution.

Concerning MMP-2, its gene is located on chromosome 16. Interestingly, the -735 C>T polymorphism is present in the promoter region and abolishes a Sp1-binding site, leading to decreased promoter activity and reduced MMP-2 expression. The 'C' to 'T' substitution at the -735 position of the MMP-2 gene may predispose to different conditions, such as increased inflammatory status, tumour metastasis and respiratory diseases [31,32]. However, very few studies have investigated the association between MMP-2 polymorphisms and gestational hypertension and PE [20]. Indeed, only one Iranian study has reported that the maternal -735 T allele is associated with an increased risk of PE in a small cohort (150 cases and 150 controls) [33], while two studies found no association in Brazilian and Polish populations [29,34].

Hence, to date, none of the mentioned MMP polymorphisms have been investigated in the African continent. As genetic variations may differ, depending on ethnicity [35,36], the present study aimed to evaluate the association of MMP-2 -735 C>T (rs2285053) and MMP-9 -1562 C>T (rs3918242) polymorphisms with the risk of PE in a large Tunisian cohort (281 controls and 345 cases).

2. Materials and Methods

2.1. Subjects

This retrospective case–control study, which we previously described in detail [37,38], involved 345 unrelated Tunisian women with PE, who were recruited between May 2012 and June 2013 from the gynecology service (hospitalized and outpatient) of Farhat Hached University Hospital (Sousse, Central Tunisia), Fattouma Bourguiba University Hospital (Monastir, Central Tunisia), Taher Sfar University Hospital (Mahdia, Eastern Tunisia), and Gafsa Hospital (Southern Tunisia). The inclusion criteria were PE during a natural pregnancy, defined as gravid hypertension, assessed as systolic blood pressure (SBP) > 140 mmHg, diastolic blood pressure (DBP) > 90 mmHg, a rise in SBP > 30 mmHg, or DBP > 15 mmHg on at least two measurements, 6 h apart, and significant proteinuria $\geq$ 300 mg/24 h after 20 weeks of gestation [2]. Severe PE was defined as SBP $\geq$ 160 mmHg or DBP $\geq$ 110 mmHg and proteinuria $\geq$ 500 mg/24 h [2]. As subject recruitment was conducted in 2012, we used the definition and classification of PE determined by the American College of Obstetricians and Gynecologists (ACOG), which was active at the time [2]. This is in contrast with the actual ACOG guidelines, where PE is diagnosed by the presence of de novo hypertension after 20 weeks of gestation, accompanied by proteinuria and/or evidence of maternal acute kidney injury (AKI), liver dysfunction, neurological features, hemolysis or thrombocytopenia, or intra-uterine growth restriction [39]. Women who met the criteria for PE, but not severe PE, were defined as moderate PE. Our study included women with previously diagnosed chronic hypertension and a history of PE.

We recruited women with normal pregnancies from the same geographical area and without any obstetrical complications for the control group. Exclusion criteria for this group were known personal or family history of hypertension and PE. The pairing of women with normal pregnancy was done on the basis of the age of preeclampsia cases (+/− 1 year of age). Hence, certain women with normal pregnancies were not chosen based on their age. Local ethics committees approved the study protocol, and both PE cases and control women gave written informed consent for participation in the study. The study participants' demographic and clinical data were collected from a designed questionnaire and medical records, as done previously [40].

2.2. MMPs Genotyping

Genotyping of MMP-2 -735 C>T and MMP-9 -1562 C>T SNPs was performed on DNA extracted from blood samples by the proteinase K/salting-out method [41], using PCR-restriction fragment-length polymorphism (PCR-RFLP) method [42]. The target fragments containing these two polymorphisms were amplified using the following primers: for the -735 C>T: 5′-GGATTCTTGGCTTGGCGCAGGA-3′ (forward) and 5′-GGGGGCTGGGTAAAATGAGGCTG-3′ (reverse); for the -1562 C>T polymorphism: (forward) 5′-GCCTGGCACATAGTAGGCCC-3′ (forward) and 5′-CTTCCTAGCCAGCCGGC-ATC-3′ (reverse). For PCR amplification, the reaction mixture consisted of 2.5 µL of DNA sample, 0.5 µM of each primer, 10× PCR buffer, 1.5 mM of MgCl2, 0.5 U of Taq DNA polymerase (Invitrogen), 0.2 mM of each dNTP and water was added to obtain a final volume of 20 µL. To detect polymorphisms, the samples were denatured at 95 °C for 5 min, followed by 35 cycles of denaturation at 94 °C for 30 s, annealing at 59 °C for 30 s and extension at 72 °C for 30 s. The samples were incubated at 72 °C for an additional 5 min for the final extension. Amplicons were 436 and 391 bp for -1562 C>T and -735 C>T, respectively. The SphI and HinfI restriction enzymes produced 242 and 194 bp fragments for the -1562 T allele and 338 and 53 bp fragments for the -735 T allele. The fragments were analyzed on a 2% agarose gel.

2.3. Statistical Analysis

Continuous data are expressed as mean ± standard deviation (SD) and were compared using the Mann–Whitney U-test. Categorical variables are presented as numbers (percentages of total) and were compared using the Chi-square test (χ^2). Allele frequencies were calculated by the gene-counting method, and each polymorphism was tested for Hardy–Weinberg equilibrium using χ^2 goodness-of-fit test using HPlus 2.5 software. The putative predictors of PE, the clinical factors of study participants, and the two polymorphisms studied were initially evaluated by univariate analysis and then by multivariate logistic regression analysis. We calculated the corresponding crude odds ratio (cOR) and its 95% confidence interval (95% CI) and then the adjusted odds ratio (aOR) and its 95% CI; the main covariates that we adjusted for were gestational age, BMI, delivery method and baby weight. Statistical significance was set at $p < 0.05$.

3. Results

3.1. Study Subjects

Demographic and clinical features of PE cases and control women are shown in Table 1. According to the defined criteria, 162 of the 345 women had severe PE. Among them, 87 (25.2%) developed a severe early onset form (before 34 weeks of gestation); there were 15 cases of eclampsia, but no cases of HELLP (hemolysis, elevated liver enzymes, low platelets) syndrome. As expected, women with PE had significantly elevated SBP and DBP, higher BMI, and gave birth at a lower gestational age. Not surprisingly, women with PE had a significantly higher incidence of primiparous pregnancies, as this is a known risk factor for this disease. In addition, we found that babies born from women with PE had significantly lower weights. Accordingly, gestational age, BMI, delivery method and baby weight were selected as covariates controlled for in the subsequent analysis.

Table 1. Demographic and clinical characteristics of controls and patients.

Characteristic		Controls (n = 289)	Cases (n = 345)	p [1]
Age (years) [2]		30.5 ± 5.8	31.3 ± 7.0	0.121
BMI (kg/m^2) [2]		28.6 ± 4.2	32.2 ± 5.0	<0.001
Newborn weight (g) [2]		3253.3 ± 405.2	2888.0 ± 755.7	<0.001
GA at blood sampling [2]		38.2 ± 3.0	35.8 ± 3.6	<0.001
Region [3]	Sahel region Central Tunisia Southern Tunisia	199 (66.3) 7 (2.3) 94 (31.3)	234 (78.0) 33 (11.0) 33 (11.0)	<0.001
Blood pressure (mmHg) [2]	Systolic Diastolic	112.3 ± 9.3 68.8 ± 7.9	155.4 ± 14.9 95.0 ± 8.7	<0.001
Delivery method [3]	Vaginal delivery Caesarian sections	188 (62.7) 112 (37.3)	165 (55.0) 135 (45.0)	0.068
Pregnancy status [3]	Multiparous Primiparous Nulliparous	164 (54.7) 131 (43.7) 5 (1.7)	75 (25.0) 222 (74.0) 3 (1.00)	<0.001
Chronic hypertension		0 (0.0)	155 (39.1)	<0.001

[1] Student t-test for continuous variables, and Pearson's chi-square for categorical variables. [2] Mean ± SD. [3] Number (percent total). BMI, body mass index; GA, gestational age.

3.2. Association Studies

Minor allele frequencies of MMP-9 -1562 T and MMP-2 -735 T were not significantly different among PE cases and control women (Table 2). Setting the major homozygous genotype C/C as a reference (OR = 1.00), significantly higher frequencies of heterozygous MMP-9 -1562 C/T genotype carriers were observed in PE cases compared to control women (p = 0.03; OR (95% CI) = 1.62 (1.03–2.56)) (Table 3). We found no significant differences in the distribution of the remaining genotypes between PE cases and control women.

Table 2. Distribution of MMP-9 and MMP-2 alleles in PE cases and control women.

Gene (SNP)	Position [1]	MAF	Patients	Controls	χ^2	p Value	OR (95% CI)
MMP-9 (-1562 C>T)	chr8:81279768	T	64 (18.6) [2]	38 (13.5)	2.87	0.09	0.72 (0.50–1.05)
MMP-2 (-735 C>T)	chr16:55478465	T	78 (23.5)	53 (18.9)	1.94	0.16	0.80 (0.58–1.09)

[1] Location on the chromosome. [2] Number of alleles (frequency). MMP: Matrix Metalloproteinases; PE: preeclampsia; SNP: single-nucleotide polymorphism; MAF: minor allele frequency; T: threonine; chr: chromosome.

Table 3. Genotypic frequencies of the studied polymorphisms.

Gene (SNP)	Genotype	Controls [a]	Cases [a]	p	p [c]	OR (95% CI)
MMP-9 (-1562 C>T)	C/C	243 (86.7) [b]	281 (81.4)	0.03	0.14	1
	C/T	33 (11.7)	62 (17.9)			1.62 (1.03–2.56)
	T/T	5 (1.7)	2 (0.5)			0.35 (0.07–1.80)
MMP-2 (-735 C>T)	C/C	228 (81.1)	254 (76.5)	0.26	0.33	1
	C/T	41 (14.6)	65 (19.6)			1.42 (0.93–2.19)
	T/T	12 (4.3)	13 (3.9)			0.97 (0.43–2.17)

[a] Study subjects included 345 PE cases and 281 control women. [b] Number of genotypes/subjects (percent total). [c] p-values adjusted for age, gender, diabetes, smoking, hypertension.

3.3. Association Analysis

Our results showed a lack of association between the tested MMP-9 and MMP-2 polymorphisms and the severity of PE, irrespective of the genetic model used (co-dominant, dominant, or recessive) (Table 4). These associations remained not significant, even after adjustment for gestational age, BMI, delivery method and baby weight.

Table 4. Association of MMP-9 and MMP-2 genotypes with the severity of PE.

Model	Genotype	Genotype Distribution MMP-9				Genotype Distribution MMP-2			
		Moderate PE n = 183	Severe PE n = 162	p	p [b]	Moderate PE n = 178	Severe PE n = 154	p	p [b]
Co-dominant model	C/C	150 (82) [a]	131 (80.9)	0.22	0.29	132 (74.2)	122 (79.2)	0.39	0.65
	C/T	33 (18)	29 (17.9)			37 (20.8)	28 (18.2)		
	T/T	0 (0)	2 (1.2)			9 (5.1)	4 (2.6)		
Dominant model	C/C	150 (82)	131 (80.9)	0.79	0.17	132 (74.2)	122 (79.2)	0.28	0.39
	C/T-T/T	33 (18)	31 (19.1)			46 (25.8)	32 (20.8)		
Recessive model	T/T	0 (0)	2 (1.2)	0.08	0.6	9 (5.1)	4 (2.6)	0.24	0.97
	C/C-C/T	183 (100)	160 (98.8)			169 (94.9)	150 (97.4)		

[a] Number of genotypes/subjects (percent total). [b] p-values adjusted for gestational age, BMI, delivery method and baby weight.

4. Discussion

To our knowledge, in the African continent, this is the first case–control study that investigated the association of polymorphisms in the promoter region of MMP-2 (-735 C>T) and MMP-9 (-1562 C>T) with the risk of PE. More specifically, these polymorphisms were investigated in a large Tunisian Arab cohort (281 controls and 345 cases), compared to most studies, which studied small cohorts. As such, in our study, we may have higher statistical power for the genetic analysis. Notably, the CT genotype of MMP-9 -1562 C>T was associated with an increased risk of PE in our Tunisian cohort. However, the frequency distribution of MMP-2 -735 C>T allele and genotype polymorphism was not associated with PE.

In contrast to our results, most studies have reported no association between the -1562 C/T polymorphism and the risk of PE in the Netherlands [30], Brazilian [25,29], United Kingdom [27], Poland [26] and Iranian [28] populations. However, PE cases with chronic hypertension and a history of PE were excluded in these reports, in contrast to our study. Only one study, conducted by Rahimi et al., found an association with the MMP-9 -1562 C>T polymorphism but only found in women with severe PE. Hence, these differences may result from the cohort size of most of these studies as our cohort is almost twice the size of these other studies. As such, they may have been underpowered to find any MMP-2 and MMP-9 polymorphism association with PE. Importantly, they investigated a heterogeneous population. As such, ethnic variations and geographical location could have contributed to the lack of association.

With regard to the lack of association of the polymorphism MMP-2 -735 C>T with PE, these are in agreement with two previous studies which looked at this SNP in Brazilian [34] and Polish [26] populations. However, another investigation conducted on 144 women with PE and 103 healthy control subjects in Iran found an association between the MMP-2 -735 T polymorphism and PE risk [33]. Interestingly, in this Iranian study, all women had a Kurdish ethnic background and women with chronic hypertension were excluded from their cohort. As such, this may have contributed to a more homogenous cohort and allowed them to uncover this association. As such, the inclusion of women with chronic hypertension in our study and our unique geographical location and ethnicity may have contributed to the lack of association in our study.

Mechanistically, changes in MMP expression and activity may lead to increased oxidative stress and inflammatory mediators, which are associated with endothelial dysfunction and, in turn, contribute to the pathogenesis of PE [43,44]. More specifically, in healthy pregnancies, MMPs, such as MMP-9 and MMP-2, play a crucial role in the process of trophoblast cell invasion, remodelling spiral arteries as well as in angiogenesis [7]. In contrast, in women with PE, high MMP-9 activity has been implicated in the pathological remodelling of the extracellular matrix of the arterial wall by causing an accumulation of collagen [45]. MMP-2 and MMP-9 dysregulation could lead to altered endometrial matrix degradation and impaired trophoblastic invasion and placentation, thus, inducing PE symptoms [15,16]. As the MMP-9 -1562 C/T and MMP-2 -735 C/T polymorphisms are located in the promoter region, they may regulate the protein production of these MMPs [26]. Interestingly, the presence of the T allele of the MMP-9 -1562 C>T polymorphism is associated with higher transcriptional activity of the gene and elevated MMP-9 protein levels in biological fluids and tissues [46]. Additionally, it has been reported that MMP-9 protein levels in the umbilical cord arterial wall and the plasma of newborns from preeclamptic pregnancies are increased compared to those from women with normal pregnancies [10].

In contrast to the study by Rahimi et al., we found a lack of association between the tested MMP-9 and MMP-2 variants and PE severity. Indeed, they found a significantly higher frequency of the MMP-9 CT + TT genotypes among women with severe PE [45]. This discordance may be due to the small number of cases of women with severe PE in our cohort or may relate to differences in PE subtypes and other ethnic/racial factors in the study population. Moreover, this result was irrespective of the genetic model used (co-dominant, dominant, or recessive) and remained insignificant, even after adjustment for clinical parameters (gestational age, BMI, delivery method and baby weight).

Finally, the differences observed between our results and those previously published may stem from ethnic and racial variations in the distribution of MMP variants. Additional studies in large cohorts from other ethnic groups will be required to confirm this speculation. One of the strengths of our study is the homogeneity of the population. This minimized the differences in genetic background, inherent to gene association studies and the possibility of ethnic stratification on the distribution of the MMPs allele and genotype, as well as the potential covariates to control. A limitation of the present case–control study was that we did not correlate genotypic data with MMP plasma levels. Follow-up studies are needed to analyze other variants in these genes and assess if altered MMP activity in PE pathogenesis.

5. Conclusions

In conclusion, MMP-9 promoter polymorphism could influence the risk of PE development through increased production of MMP-9 protein in the maternal circulation and at the maternal–fetal interface. Our results indicate, for the first time, that such an association is present in a Tunisian population where we found that the carriage of the heterozygous MMP-9 -1562 C/T genotype, which is associated with higher MMP-9 production, was associated with PE risk.

Author Contributions: M.B.A.G. and N.R.: patient recruitment, sample collection, all experimental procedures and interpretation of data and draft of the manuscript. H.Z.: patient recruitment, sample collection and DNA extraction. M.M.: patient recruitment. O.S.: statistical analysis. T.M.: project experimental design and management of laboratory experiments and revision of the manuscript. J.L.L.: interpretation of the data, revision and correction of the manuscript. All authors have read and agreed to the published version of the manuscript.

Funding: This work was supported by the Ministry of Higher Education and Scientific Research Tunisia, Faculty of Pharmacy of Monastir, University of Monastir (Tunisia) and by a CIHR operating grant (PJT-169020) for Julie L. Lavoie.

Institutional Review Board Statement: The study was conducted according to the guidelines of the Declaration of Helsinki, and approved by the ethics committee of Hospital Farhat Hached Sousse, chaired by Tasnim Masmoudi (project number: PI-15-91, approved in 2012).

Informed Consent Statement: Informed consent was obtained from all subjects involved in the study.

Conflicts of Interest: The authors declare no conflict of interest.

References

1. Kallela, J.; Jaaskelainen, T.; Kortelainen, E.; Heinonen, S.; Kajantie, E.; Kere, J.; Kivinen, K.; Pouta, A.; Laivuori, H. The diagnosis of pre-eclampsia using two revised classifications in the Finnish Pre-eclampsia Consortium (FINNPEC) cohort. *BMC Pregnancy Childbirth* **2016**, *16*, 221. [CrossRef] [PubMed]
2. American College of Obstetricians and Gynecologists. Hypertension in pregnancy. Report of the American College of Obstetricians and Gynecologists' Task Force on Hypertension in Pregnancy. *Obs. Gynecol* **2013**, *122*, 1122–1131.
3. Gathiram, P.; Moodley, J. Pre-eclampsia: Its pathogenesis and pathophysiolgy. *Cardiovasc. J. Afr.* **2016**, *27*, 71–78. [CrossRef] [PubMed]
4. Cerdeira, A.S.; Karumanchi, S.A. Angiogenic factors in preeclampsia and related disorders. *Cold Spring Harb. Perspect. Med.* **2012**, *2*, a006585. [CrossRef]
5. Abou, E.L.; Hassan, M.; Diamandis, E.P.; Karumanchi, S.A.; Shennan, A.H.; Taylor, R.N. Preeclampsia: An old disease with new tools for better diagnosis and risk management. *Clin. Chem.* **2015**, *61*, 694–698. [CrossRef]
6. De Vivo, A.; Baviera, G.; Giordano, D.; Todarello, G.; Corrado, F.; D'Anna, R. Endoglin, PlGF and sFlt-1 as markers for predicting pre-eclampsia. *Acta Obstet. Gynecol. Scand.* **2008**, *87*, 837–842. [CrossRef]
7. Su, M.T.; Tsai, P.Y.; Tsai, H.L.; Chen, Y.C.; Kuo, P.L. miR-346 and miR-582-3p-regulated EG-VEGF expression and trophoblast invasion via matrix metalloproteinases 2 and 9. *Biofactors* **2017**, *43*, 210–219. [CrossRef]
8. Goncalves, F.M.; Jacob-Ferreira, A.L.; Gomes, V.A.; Casella-Filho, A.; Chagas, A.C.; Marcaccini, A.M.; Gealach, R.F.; Tanus-Santos, J.E. Increased circulating levels of matrix metalloproteinase (MMP)-8, MMP-9, and pro-inflammatory markers in patients with metabolic syndrome. *Clin. Chim. Acta* **2009**, *403*, 173–177. [CrossRef]
9. Narumiya, H.; Zhang, Y.; Fernandez-Patron, C.; Guilbert, L.J.; Davidge, S.T. Matrix metalloproteinase-2 is elevated in the plasma of women with preeclampsia. *Hypertens. Pregnancy* **2001**, *20*, 185–194. [CrossRef] [PubMed]
10. Montagnana, M.; Lippi, G.; Albiero, A.; Scevarolli, S.; Salvagno, G.L.; Franchi, M.; Guidi, G.C. Evaluation of metalloproteinases 2 and 9 and their inhibitors in physiologic and pre-eclamptic pregnancy. *J. Clin. Lab. Anal.* **2009**, *23*, 88–92. [CrossRef]
11. Ulbrich, S.E.; Meyer, S.U.; Zitta, K.; Hiendleder, S.; Sinowatz, F.; Bauersachs, S.; Büttner, M.; Fröhlich, T.; Arnold, G.J.; Reichenbach, H.-D. Bovine endometrial metallopeptidases MMP14 and MMP2 and the metallopeptidase inhibitor TIMP2 participate in maternal preparation of pregnancy. *Mol. Cell. Endocrinol.* **2011**, *332*, 48–57. [CrossRef]
12. Gai, X.; Zhang, Z.; Liang, Y.; Chen, Z.; Yang, X.; Hou, J.; Lan, X.; Zheng, W.; Hou, J.; Huang, M. MMP-2 and TIMP-2 gene polymorphisms and susceptibility to atrial fibrillation in Chinese Han patients with hypertensive heart disease. *Clin. Chim. Acta* **2010**, *411*, 719–724. [CrossRef] [PubMed]
13. Lacchini, R.; Jacob-Ferreira, A.L.; Luizon, M.R.; Gasparini, S.; Ferreira-Sae, M.C.; Schreiber, R.; Nadruz, W.J.; Tanus-Santos, J.E. Common matrix metalloproteinase 2 gene haplotypes may modulate left ventricular remodelling in hypertensive patients. *J. Hum. Hypertens.* **2012**, *26*, 171–177. [CrossRef] [PubMed]
14. Yu, Y.; Wang, L.; Liu, T.; Guan, H. MicroRNA-204 suppresses trophoblast-like cell invasion by targeting matrix metalloproteinase-9. *Biochem. Biophys. Res. Commun.* **2015**, *463*, 285–291. [CrossRef] [PubMed]
15. Love, C.; Dave, S. MicroRNA expression profiling using microarrays. *Methods Mol. Biol.* **2013**, *999*, 285–296. [PubMed]
16. Eleuterio, N.M.; Palei, A.C.; Rangel Machado, J.S.; Tanus-Santos, J.E.; Cavalli, R.C.; Sandrim, V.C. Positive correlations between circulating adiponectin and MMP2 in preeclampsia pregnant. *Pregnancy Hypertens.* **2015**, *5*, 205–208. [CrossRef] [PubMed]
17. Yeh, C.C.; Chao, K.C.; Huang, S.J. Innate immunity, decidual cells, and preeclampsia. *Reprod. Sci.* **2013**, *20*, 339–353. [CrossRef] [PubMed]
18. Lou, X.Y.; Chen, G.B.; Yan, L.; Ma, J.Z.; Zhu, J.; Elston, R.C.; Li, M.D. A generalized combinatorial approach for detecting gene-by-gene and gene-by-environment interactions with application to nicotine dependence. *Am. J. Hum. Genet.* **2007**, *80*, 1125–1137. [CrossRef]

19. Lyall, F. Mechanisms regulating cytotrophoblast invasion in normal pregnancy and pre-eclampsia. *Aust. N. Z. J. Obstet. Gynaecol.* **2006**, *46*, 266–273. [CrossRef]
20. Blankenberg, S.; Rupprecht, H.J.; Poirier, O.; Bickel, C.; Smieja, M.; Hafner, G.; Meyer, J.; Cambie, F.; Tiret, L. Plasma concentrations and genetic variation of matrix metalloproteinase 9 and prognosis of patients with cardiovascular disease. *Circulation* **2003**, *107*, 1579–1585. [CrossRef]
21. Apple, F.S.; Wu, A.H.; Mair, J.; Ravkilde, J.; Panteghini, M.; Tate, J.; Pagani, F.; Christenson, R.H.; Mockel, M.; Danne, O.; et al. Future biomarkers for detection of ischemia and risk stratification in acute coronary syndrome. *Clin. Chem.* **2005**, *51*, 810–824. [CrossRef]
22. Thompson, M.M.; Squire, I.B. Matrix metalloproteinase-9 expression after myocardial infarction: Physiological or pathological? *Cardiovasc. Res.* **2002**, *54*, 495–498. [CrossRef]
23. Lockwood, C.J.; Oner, C.; Uz, Y.H.; Kayisli, U.A.; Huang, S.J.; Buchwalder, L.F.; Murk, W.; Funai, E.F.; Schatz, F. Matrix metalloproteinase 9 (MMP9) expression in preeclamptic decidua and MMP9 induction by tumor necrosis factor alpha and interleukin 1 beta in human first trimester decidual cells. *Biol. Reprod.* **2008**, *78*, 1064–1072. [CrossRef] [PubMed]
24. Poon, L.C.; Nekrasova, E.; Anastassopoulos, P.; Livanos, P.; Nicolaides, K.H. First-trimester maternal serum matrix metalloproteinase-9 (MMP-9) and adverse pregnancy outcome. *Prenat. Diagn.* **2009**, *29*, 553–559. [CrossRef]
25. Palei, A.C.; Sandrim, V.C.; Amaral, L.M.; Machado, J.S.; Cavalli, R.C.; Lacchini, R.; Duarte, G.; Tanus-Santos, J.E. Matrix metalloproteinase-9 polymorphisms affect plasma MMP-9 levels and antihypertensive therapy responsiveness in hypertensive disorders of pregnancy. *Pharm. J.* **2012**, *12*, 489–498. [CrossRef] [PubMed]
26. Sakowicz, A.; Lisowska, M.; Biesiada, L.; Rybak-Krzyszkowska, M.; Gach, A.; Sakowicz, B.; Grzesiak, M.; Huras, H.; Pietrucha, T. Association of Maternal and Fetal Single-Nucleotide Polymorphisms in Metalloproteinase (MMP1, MMP2, MMP3, and MMP9) Genes with Preeclampsia. *Dis. Markers* **2018**, *2018*, 1371425. [CrossRef] [PubMed]
27. Fraser, R.; Walker, J.J.; Ekbote, U.V.; Martin, K.L.; McShane, P.; Orsi, N.M. Interleukin-4 -590 (C>T), toll-like receptor-2 +2258 (G>A) and matrix metalloproteinase-9 -1562 (C>T) polymorphisms in pre-eclampsia. *BJOG* **2008**, *115*, 1052–1056. [CrossRef]
28. Rahimi, Z.; Rahimi, Z.; Aghaei, A.; Vaisi-Raygani, A. AT2R -1332 G:A polymorphism and its interaction with AT1R 1166 A:C, ACE I/D and MMP-9 -1562 C:T polymorphisms: Risk factors for susceptibility to preeclampsia. *Gene* **2014**, *538*, 176–181. [CrossRef]
29. Leonardo, D.P.; Albuquerque, D.M.; Lanaro, C.; Baptista, L.C.; Cecatti, J.G.; Surita, F.G.; Parpinelli, M.A.; Costa, F.F.; Franco-Penteado, C.F.; Fertrin, K.B.; et al. Association of Nitric Oxide Synthase and Matrix Metalloprotease Single Nucleotide Polymorphisms with Preeclampsia and Its Complications. *PLoS ONE* **2015**, *10*, e0136693.
30. Coolman, M.; De Maat, M.; Van Heerde, W.; Felida, L.; Schoormans, S.; Steegers, E.; Bertina, R.; De Groot, C. Matrix Metalloproteinase-9 Gene -1562C/T Polymorphism Mitigates Preeclampsia. *Placenta* **2007**, *28*, 709–713. [CrossRef]
31. Goncalves, F.M.; Martins-Oliveira, A.; Lacchini, R.; Belo, V.A.; Speciali, J.G.; Dach, F.; Tanus-Santos, J. E Matrix metalloproteinase (MMP)-2 gene polymorphisms affect circulating MMP-2 levels in patients with migraine with aura. *Gene* **2013**, *512*, 35–40. [CrossRef]
32. Yu, C.; Zhou, Y.; Miao, X.; Xiong, P.; Tan, W.; Lin, D. Functional haplotypes in the promoter of matrix metalloproteinase-2 predict risk of the occurrence and metastasis of esophageal cancer. *Cancer Res.* **2004**, *64*, 7622–7628. [CrossRef] [PubMed]
33. Rahimi, Z.; Lotfi, S.; Ahmadi, A.; Jalilian, N.; Shakiba, E.; Vaisi-Raygani, A.; Rahimi, Z. Matrix metalloproteinase-2 C-735T and its interaction with matrix metalloproteinase-7 A-181G polymorphism are associated with the risk of preeclampsia: Influence on total antioxidant capacity and blood pressure. *J. Obs. Gynaecol* **2018**, *38*, 327–332. [CrossRef] [PubMed]
34. Palei, A.C.; Sandrim, V.C.; Amaral, L.M.; Machado, J.S.; Cavalli, R.C.; Duarte, G.; Tanus-Santos, J.E. Association between matrix metalloproteinase (MMP)-2 polymorphisms and MMP-2 levels in hypertensive disorders of pregnancy. *Exp. Mol. Pathol.* **2012**, *92*, 217–221. [CrossRef] [PubMed]
35. Johnson, J.D.; Louis, J.M. Does race or ethnicity play a role in the origin, pathophysiology, and outcomes of preeclampsia? An expert review of the literature. *Am. J. Obstet. Gynecol.* **2020**. [CrossRef]
36. Ghosh, G.; Grewal, J.; Männistö, T.; Mendola, P.; Chen, Z.; Xie, Y.; Laughon, S.K. Racial/ethnic differences in pregnancy-related hypertensive disease in nulliparous women. *Ethn. Dis.* **2014**, *24*, 283–289.
37. Ben Ali Gannoun, M.; Bourrelly, S.; Raguema, N.; Zitouni, H.; Nouvellon, E.; Maleh, W.; Chemilia, A.B.; Elfeleh, R.; Almawi, W.; Mahjoub, T.; et al. Placental growth factor and vascular endothelial growth factor serum levels in Tunisian Arab women with suspected preeclampsia. *Cytokine* **2016**, *79*, 1–6. [CrossRef]
38. Ben Ali, M.; Messaoudi, S.; Ezzine, H.; Mahjoub, T. Contribution of eNOS variants to the genetic susceptibility of coronary artery disease in a Tunisian population. *Genet. Test. Mol. Biomark.* **2015**, *19*, 203–208. [CrossRef]
39. American College of Obstetricians and Gynecologists. Gestational Hypertension and Preeclampsia: ACOG Practice Bulletin, Number 222. *Obs. Gynecol.* **2020**, *135*, e237–e260. [CrossRef]
40. Raguema, N.; Zitouni, H.; Ben Ali Gannoun, M.; Benletaifa, D.; Almawi, W.Y.; Mahjoub, T.; Lavoie, J.L. FAS A-670G and Fas ligand IVS2nt A 124G polymorphisms are significantly increased in women with pre-eclampsia and may contribute to HELLP syndrome: A case-controlled study. *BJOG* **2018**, *125*, 1758–1764. [CrossRef]
41. Miller, S.A.; Dykes, D.D.; Polesky, H.F. A simple salting out procedure for extracting DNA from human nucleated cells. *Nucleic Acids Res.* **1988**, *16*, 1215. [CrossRef] [PubMed]
42. Wolf, C.; Rentsch, J.; Hubner, P. PCR-RFLP analysis of mitochondrial DNA: A reliable method for species identification. *J. Agric. Food Chem.* **1999**, *47*, 1350–1355. [CrossRef]

43. Demir-Weusten, A.Y.; Seval, Y.; Kaufmann, P.; Demir, R.; Yucel, G.; Huppertz, B. Matrix metalloproteinases-2, -3 and -9 in human term placenta. *Acta Histochem.* **2007**, *109*, 403–412. [CrossRef] [PubMed]
44. Chen, J.; Khalil, R.A. Matrix Metalloproteinases in Normal Pregnancy and Preeclampsia. *Prog. Mol. Biol. Transl. Sci.* **2017**, *148*, 87–165. [PubMed]
45. Rahimi, Z.; Rahimi, Z.; Shahsavandi, M.O.; Bidoki, K.; Rezaei, M. MMP-9 (-1562 C:T) polymorphism as a biomarker of susceptibility to severe pre-eclampsia. *Biomark. Med.* **2013**, *7*, 93–98. [CrossRef] [PubMed]
46. Medley, T.L.; Cole, T.J.; Dart, A.M.; Gatzka, C.D.; Kingwell, B.A. Matrix metalloproteinase-9 genotype influences large artery stiffness through effects on aortic gene and protein expression. *Artern. Thromb. Vasc. Biol.* **2004**, *24*, 1479–1484. [CrossRef] [PubMed]

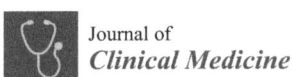

Article

Uterine Cervical Change at Term Examined Using Ultrasound Elastography: A Longitudinal Study

Hyun Soo Park [1],*, Hayan Kwon [2], Ja-Young Kwon [2], Yun Ji Jung [2], Hyun-Joo Seol [3], Won Joon Seong [4], Hyun Mi Kim [4], Han-Sung Hwang [5], Ji-Hee Sung [6] and Soo-young Oh [6] on behalf of the Korean Consortium for the Study of Cervical Elastography in the Prediction of Preterm Delivery

[1] Department of Obstetrics and Gynecology, Dongguk University Ilsan Hospital, Dongguk University, Goyang 10326, Korea
[2] Division of Maternal-Fetal Medicine, Department of Obstetrics and Gynecology, Institute of Women's Medical Life Science, Yonsei University College of Medicine, Yonsei University Health System, Seoul 03722, Korea; whitekwonmd@gmail.com (H.K.); jaykwon@yuhs.ac (J.-Y.K.); ccstty@yuhs.ac (Y.J.J.)
[3] Department of Obstetrics and Gynecology, Kyung Hee University Hospital at Gangdong, Seoul 05278, Korea; seolhj@khu.ac.kr
[4] Department of Obstetrics and Gynecology, Kyungpook National University Hospital, Daegu 41944, Korea; wjseong@knu.ac.kr (W.J.S.); hyunmik@gmail.com (H.M.K.)
[5] Department of Obstetrics and Gynecology, Konkuk University Medical Center, Konkuk University School of Medicine, Seoul 05030, Korea; hwanghs@kuh.ac.kr
[6] Samsung Medical Center, Department of Obstetrics and Gynecology, Sungkyunkwan University School of Medicine, Seoul 06351, Korea; obgysung@gmail.com (J.-H.S.); ohsymd@skku.edu (S.-y.O.)
* Correspondence: hsparkmd@gmail.com; Tel.: +82-31-961-7367

Abstract: The aim of the study was to investigate if there are changes in elastographic parameters in the cervix at term around the time of delivery and if there are differences in the parameters between women with spontaneous labor and those without labor (labor induction). Nulliparous women at 36 weeks of gestation eligible for vaginal delivery were enrolled. Cervical elastography was performed and cervical length were measured using the E-Cervix^{TM} system (WS80A Ultrasound System, Samsung Medison, Seoul, Korea) at each weekly antenatal visit until admission for spontaneous labor or labor induction. E-Cervix parameters of interest included elasticity contrast index (ECI), internal os strain mean level (IOS), external os strain mean level (EOS), IOS/EOS strain mean ratio, strain mean level, and hardness ratio. Regression analysis was performed using days from elastographic measurement at each visit to admission for delivery and the presence or absence of labor against cervical length, and each E-Cervix parameter fitted to a linear model for longitudinal data measured repeatedly. A total of 96 women were included in the analysis, (spontaneous labor, $n = 39$; labor induction, $n = 57$). Baseline characteristics were not different between the two groups except for cesarean delivery rate. Cervical length decreased with advancing gestation and was different between the two groups. Most elastographic parameters including ECI, IOS, EOS, strain mean, and hardness ratio were significantly different between the two groups. In addition, ECI, IOS, and strain mean values significantly increased with advancing gestation. Our longitudinal study using ultrasound elastography indicated that E-cervix parameters tended to change linearly at term near the time of admission for delivery and that there were differences in E-Cervix parameters according to the presence or absence of labor.

Keywords: ultrasonography; elastography; uterine cervix; term pregnancy; parturition

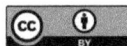

1. Introduction

Human parturition begins with structural and biochemical changes in the uterus, including the uterine body and cervix. The pregnant cervix becomes soft from early pregnancy and ripens shortly before labor through the biochemical changes [1]. Such biochemical change during cervical ripening include decreased collagen concentration, increased hydrophilic glycosaminoglycans, hyaluronic acid, and water [2]. Extensive remodeling before labor subsequently leads to uterine cervical effacement and dilatation from forceful uterine contractions.

Since the report of association between short cervical length and increased risk of preterm delivery, cervical length measurement has been used to predict spontaneous preterm delivery [3]. However, as the prevalence of high-risk population is low, and cervical length measurement has low sensitivity to predict preterm birth, the utility of cervical length measurements has been limited. In addition, some researchers reported considerable inter-observer variability [4,5] and inadequate measurement of cervical length, especially when using transabdominal ultrasound, which limits the utility of cervical length measurement as a screening tool [6]. Therefore, researchers are investigating various methods to detect biomechanical or biochemical changes of the cervix to improve the ability to predict spontaneous preterm delivery using ultrasonography, which includes quantitative cervical texture analysis (mean gray level histogram) and elastography.

Quantitative cervical texture analysis uses a histogram with different indices such as mean gray level [7], mean gray-scale values [8] or cervical texture-based score [9] from gray-scale ultrasound image of the uterine cervix. Some of them report promising results in predicting spontaneous preterm birth [8,9]. Recently, ultrasound elastography has been introduced to assess the elasticity or compressibility of tissues for the diagnosis of breast cancer and liver fibrosis [10]. In the obstetrical field, elastography has been studied in the uterine cervix, and the diagnostic performance has been validated in predicting successful induction of labor and preterm delivery in low and high-risk pregnancies [11]. All these efforts to predict labor focus on the changes in the elastic or biomechanical properties of the cervix, and that is based on the premise that elastic changes reflect the biochemical changes inside the cervix. The traditional way to evaluate cervical change is to measure the cervical length, which has been used for the prediction of preterm birth and successful labor induction [12,13]. However, cervical length measurements only detect changes in the physical dimension of the cervix. Detecting biomechanical and biochemical changes before labor could help us understand and predict the common labor processes in preterm or term pregnancy. There are many studies looking into preterm delivery prediction using elastography, and there is a recent report regarding elastographic changes in each trimester [14]. On the other hand, there is a paucity of information regarding immediate changes in the cervix near term parturition.

E-Cervix^{TM} elastography is one of the strain elastographic ultrasound applications that gets compression signals using internal or in vivo compression forces such as adjacent arterial pulsation and breathing. As it uses internal compression, E-Cervix elastography is less operator-dependent than other ultrasound elastography machines that employ external compression. We have reported its reproducibility and utility in predicting preterm delivery in pregnancies with a moderately short cervix [15–17]. We found that there were changes in E-Cervix parameters antedating preterm delivery. However, our understanding of the temporal cervical change is poor, especially in term cervix around the time of labor. Therefore, we planned a longitudinal study to investigate if we could detect cervical changes in the strain as well as the length using E-Cervix elastography. We also wanted to look at the differences in the elastographic parameters in the cervix between spontaneous labor and no labor (labor induction) groups. The aim of the study was to investigate if there were changes in elastographic parameters in the cervix at term around the time of delivery and if there were differences in the parameters between women with spontaneous labor and those without labor (labor induction).

2. Materials and Methods

2.1. Subjects

Between July 2019 and April 2020, nulliparous women eligible for vaginal delivery were invited to participate in this study. They were enrolled at 36 weeks of gestation from three institutions (Dongguk University Ilsan Hospital, Konkuk University Medical

Center, and Kyung Hee University Hospital at Gangdong). Four investigators (H.-J.S., H.K., H.-S.H., H.S.P.) who had experience in the use of E-Cervix elastography for more than three years performed cervical elastography. Ultrasound elastography was carried out by one operator in each patient. Cervical elastography and cervical length were measured at each weekly antenatal visit until admission for spontaneous labor or labor induction. Labor was induced according to the managing clinician's discretion. Multiple pregnancies or pregnancies with cerclage were excluded from this study. Pregnancy outcomes, demographic data, and obstetric data were collected. The study protocol was reviewed and approved by the Institutional Review Board of each participating hospital. Written informed consent was collected from all women.

2.2. Cervical Length and Elastographic Measurements

We performed cervical elastography with a vaginal ultrasound (WS80A Ultrasound System, Samsung Medison, Seoul, Korea) using a 6-MHz transvaginal probe. After measuring cervical length, elastography was performed three times in the same plane with the same transvaginal probe using an E-Cervix^{TM} system. The median values of the three measurements were used for the analysis. The cervical length measurement and E-Cervix elastography were performed according to previously described protocol [17]. E-Cervix uses in vivo compression by internally generating fine vibration through organ motion, such as adjacent arterial pulsation and breathing without manual compression. The E-Cervix parameters included in the analysis were elasticity contrast index (ECI), internal (IOS) and external os (EOS) of cervix strain mean level, IOS/EOS strain mean ratio, strain mean level, and hardness ratio (Table 1).

Table 1. Selected E-Cervix parameters.

Measurement Parameter	Description
ECI	ECI score within the ROI, value range: 0 (homogeneity)–81 (heterogeneity)
IOS strain mean level	Standardized strain mean level in 1 cm circle of IOS, value range: 0 (hard)–1 (soft)
EOS strain mean level	Standardized strain mean level in 1 cm circle of EOS, value range: 0 (hard)–1 (soft)
Ratio (IOS/EOS)	IOS strain level/EOS strain level
Strain mean level	Strain mean level within the ROI, value range: 0 (hard)–1 (soft)
Hardness ratio	30-percentile hardness area ratio within the ROI, value range: 0% (soft)–100% (hard)

IOS, internal os of the cervix; EOS, external os of the cervix; ROI, a region of interest; ECI, elasticity contrast index.

2.3. Plots and Regression Analysis

Spaghetti plots were depicted to visualize the serial changes of the cervical length and E-Cervix parameters. Each measurement from an individual was connected and plotted against days from measurements to admission. Fitted lines from linear regression were drawn to represent serial changes in the parameters. We also made the lasagna plot, which is a heatmap for longitudinal data where each subject's trajectory over time is a horizontal layer, with the simultaneous plotting of trajectories resulting in the stacking of layers, as in lasagna [18].

As we were interested in the elastographic changes of the cervix near the time of the delivery, subjects whose last measurement before delivery was within seven days and measurements within three weeks from the admission were included in the analysis. We hypothesized that E-Cervix parameters would change over time, and there would be differences in the elastographic parameters between the spontaneous labor and labor induction groups. To test the hypothesis, we performed regression analysis using days from elastographic measurement at each visit to the admission for the delivery (Days, Figure 1) and the presence or absence of the labor (Labor) against cervical length and each E-Cervix parameter (y) using the following equation: y = ß0+ ß1* Days + ß2* Labor group. To evaluate the changes of the parameters with time only, we also performed regression analysis using the equation: y= α0 + α1*Days. We used a linear model for longitudinal data by employing mixed procedure in SAS statistical analysis packages, which enables us to handle covariances [19].

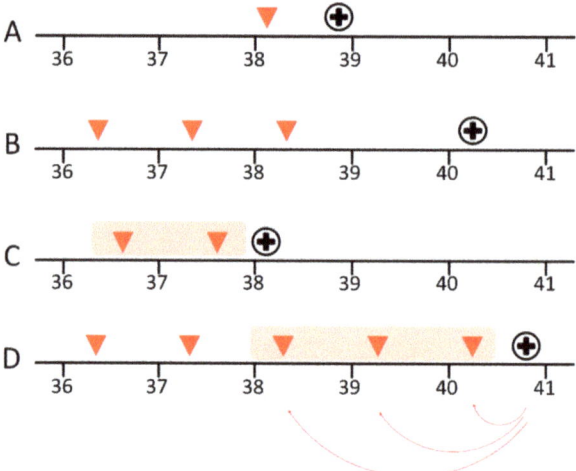

Figure 1. Scheme of measurements. From 36 weeks of gestation, E-Cervix was measured at each weekly visit until admission for spontaneous labor or labor induction. Days from admission to measurements were counted and used for analysis. Subjects whose last measurement before delivery was within seven days and measurements within three weeks were included in the analysis (data in the shaded area in cases of C and D). As elastography was measured only once in case A, and the last measurement was more than seven days from the admission in case B, data were not included in the analysis. Numbers, weeks of gestation; Red arrowhead, time of each measurement; Black cross in a circle, admission for delivery; Red curved arrow, calculation of days from measurement to admission (e.g., −4. −11, and −18); Shades, data used in the analysis.

2.4. Other Statistical Analysis

Maternal baseline characteristics and obstetric outcomes were collected and compared between the spontaneous labor and labor induction groups. Continuous variables were compared using Mann–Whitney U tests. Categorical variables were compared using Fisher's exact tests. A p-value of less than 0.05 was considered significant. STATA 14.0 (StataCorp LLC, College Station, TX, USA) and SAS 9.3 (SAS Institute Inc., Cary, NC, USA) were used for statistical analyses.

3. Results

During the study period, a total of 122 women were enrolled. Of those, elastography was performed only once in 12 patients. The last measurement was more than seven days before the day of admission in 13 patients. One was not followed up. Finally, 96 women were included in the analysis (spontaneous labor, $n = 39$; labor induction, $n = 57$) (Figure 2). The elastography was performed 2, 3, and 4 times in 27 (28.1%), 64 (66.7%), and 5 (5.2%) patients, respectively. Indications for labor induction were as follows: post-term pregnancy (31.6%, 18/57), pre-labor rupture of membranes (24.6%, 14/57), maternal request (14.0%, 8/57), large for gestational age (7.0%, 4/57), hypertensive disorders (5.3%, 3/57), oligohydramnios (5.3%, 3/57), fetal growth restriction (5.3%, 3/57), and others (7.2%, 4/57).

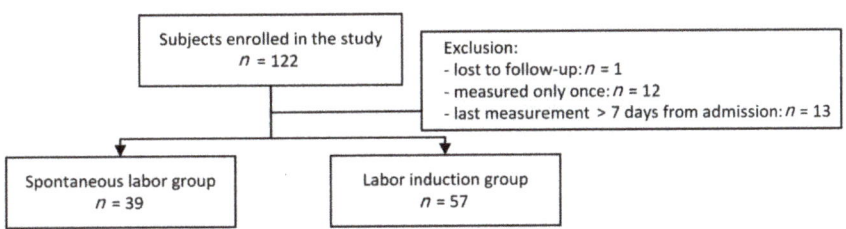

Figure 2. Flow diagram showing the number of subjects enrolled in this study.

The baseline characteristics of the participants and pregnancy outcomes are shown in Table 2. The mean maternal age in spontaneous labor and labor induction group was 31.9 (range, 24–39) and 33.4 (range, 24–41), respectively. The cesarean delivery rate was higher in the labor induction group than in the spontaneous labor group. Hypertensive diseases were found in 5.26% of the labor induction group only but were not statistically different. The frequency of pregnancies with in vitro fertilization-embryo transfer (IVF-ET) was 20.8% (20/96). Gestational diabetes consisted of 13.5% (13/96) of the study population. Other variables did not show a statistically significant difference between the two groups.

Table 2. Characteristics and pregnancy outcomes of the participants.

	Spontaneous Labor $n = 39$	Labor Induction $n = 57$	p-Value
Maternal age	32.00 (29.00–35.00)	33.00 (31.00–36.00)	0.067
History of abortion	6 (15.38%)	15 (26.32%)	0.220
History of CIN	2 (5.13%)	2 (3.51%)	1.000
History of LEEP	1 (2.56%)	1 (1.75%)	1.000
IVF-ET	7 (17.95%)	13 (22.81%)	0.620
pre-pregnancy BMI	21.77 (20.32–23.50)	21.30 (19.71–23.44)	0.480
Smoking	1 (2.56%)	2 (3.51%)	1.000
Hypertensive diseases	0 (0.00%)	3 (5.26%)	0.270
GDM	6 (15.38%)	7 (12.28%)	0.760
Progesterone use	2 (5.13%)	1 (1.75%)	0.560
Maternal weight at delivery	71.90 (64.70–76.50)	70.30 (65.00–79.90)	0.880
GA at admission	39.57 (39.14–40.29)	39.71 (39.00–40.29)	0.960
GA at delivery	39.57 (39.14–40.43)	39.86 (39.14–40.43)	0.630
Cesarean delivery	3 (7.69%)	21 (36.84%)	0.001
Birthweight	3244 (3000–3404)	3340 (3110–3498)	0.120
NICU admission	2 (5.13%)	1 (1.79%)	0.570

Data are presented as median (interquartile range) or n (%). CIN, cervical intraepithelial neoplasia; LEEP, loop electrosurgical excision procedure; IVF-ET, in vitro fertilization and embryo transfer; BMI, body mass index; GDM, gestational diabetes mellitus; GA, gestational age; NICU, neonatal intensive care unit.

Table 3 shows the regression results against cervical length and the E-Cervix parameters using days from the measurement to admission with or without spontaneous labor (labor induction and spontaneous labor). When only days from the measurements to admission were put in the regression analysis, ECI, IOS strain mean level, and strain mean significantly increased with advancing gestation along with cervical length. In the model including both days from the measurements to admission and labor groups, ECI, IOS strain mean level, and strain mean again significantly increased with advancing gestation, and they also were significantly different between the two groups. ECI, IOS strain, and strain mean increased by 0.122 and 0.011 and 0.008 per week three weeks from the admission, respectively. EOS and hardness ratio were different between the two groups. Although the hardness ratio decreased with time, such a decrease did not reach statistical significance. With this table, we can explain the change of the cervix according to time and labor group. If we take the example with cervical length, we can say that "Cervical length of the singleton pregnancy at term will decrease by 0.02468 cm everyday within 3 weeks before the admission for delivery in both spontaneous labor and labor induction group. In addition, the cervical length of the spontaneous labor group is 0.481 cm shorter than that of labor induction group throughout the period." Other parameters can be interpreted in the same manner.

Figure 3 shows the combination of the spaghetti plots that connect cervical length and E-Cervix parameter measurements at each visit for each individual. In the middle and right columns, the measured values were fitted in a regression equation to generate red lines illustrating the overall levels of the values in the labor induction and spontaneous labor groups and the change of the parameters with time. For example, the parameter of ECI tended to increase with time, and the levels of the parameter were different between spontaneous labor and labor induction groups, reflecting the regression results.

Figure 4 is the lasagna plots of the cervical length and the selected E-Cervix parameters against each visit. The horizontal axis of each plot represents a visit counted from the admission for delivery (e.g., -1 being the last visit before admission). The color bar located right to each plot represents each parameter's value range, red being the highest and yellow being the lowest. The color change from left to right in each picture can be interpreted as change of each parameter's value at each visit. For example, middle panel in row A shows the change of the cervical length at each visit in the labor induction group. From the visit -3 to visit -1, the color tends to change from red to yellow which indicates shortening of the cervix toward the admission for delivery.

Table 3. The results of the regression analyses.

	Days from the Measurement to Admission ($α_1$) in Equation (1)	SEM	p-Value	Days from the Measurement to Admission ($ß_1$) in Equation (2)	SEM	p-Value	Labor Group ($ß_2$) in Equation (2)	SEM	p-Value
Cervical length	−0.02459	0.00483	<0.001	−0.02468	0.00483	<0.001	−0.4810	0.1692	0.0055
ECI	0.0175	0.00824	0.0363	0.01756	0.00824	0.0357	0.2872	0.1386	0.0442
IOS strain mean level	0.00159	0.00072	0.0284	0.001605	0.00072	0.0272	0.0318	0.0122	0.0105
EOS strain mean level	0.001	0.00074	0.1788	0.001033	0.00074	0.1673	0.03131	0.0133	0.0209
IOS/EOS ratio	−0.0004	0.00279	0.8799	−0.00041	0.0028	0.8831	0.02319	0.0418	0.5805
Strain mean	0.00113	0.00053	0.0353	0.001140	0.00053	0.0323	0.03204	0.0103	0.0025
Hardness ratio	−0.2049	0.1142	0.0759	−0.2084	0.1137	0.0699	−6.3078	2.1683	0.0045

SEM, standard error of mean; ECI, elasticity contrast index; IOS, internal os of the cervix; EOS, external os of the cervix; The Equation (1): $y = α_0 + α_1*$(days from the measurement to admission); The Equation (2): $y = ß_0 + ß_1*$(days from the measurement to admission) + $ß_2*$ (labor group), Labor group = 0 in labor induction group, labor group = 1 in spontaneous labor group (i.e., the Equation (2) will be $y = ß_0 + ß_1*$(days from the measurement to admission) in labor induction group, and it will be $y = (ß_0 + ß_2) + ß_1*$(days from the measurement to admission) in spontaneous labor group). Both $α_0$ and $ß_0$ are constants and not listed.

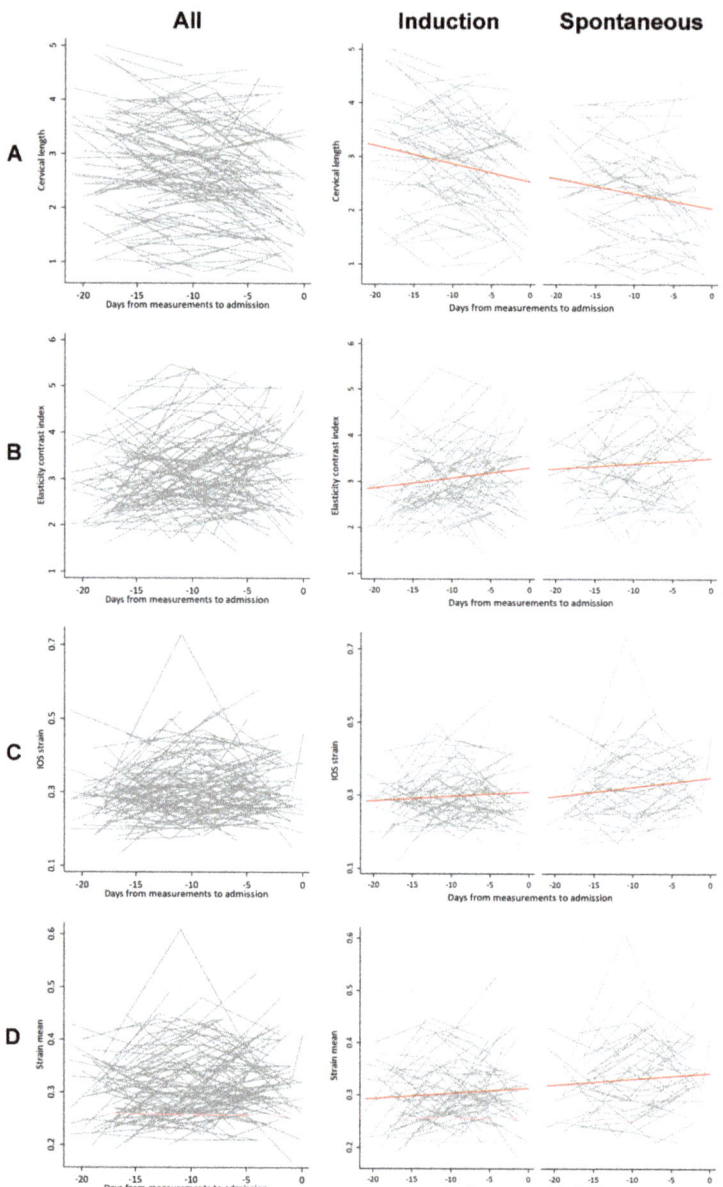

Figure 3. Spaghetti plots of the cervical length and the selected E-Cervix parameters against days from measurement to admission. The number on the *x*-axis represents days from admission (indicated as 0), and the number on the *y*-axis represents the value of cervical length and each E-Cervix parameter. Red lines in the middle and right column indicate line fitted by linear regression. (**A**): Cervical length; (**B**): Elasticity contrast index; (**C**): Strain mean of the internal os of the cervix; (**D**): Strain mean level; **Left** column, plots including all subjects; **Middle** column, plots of the labor induction group; **Right** column, plots of the spontaneous labor group.

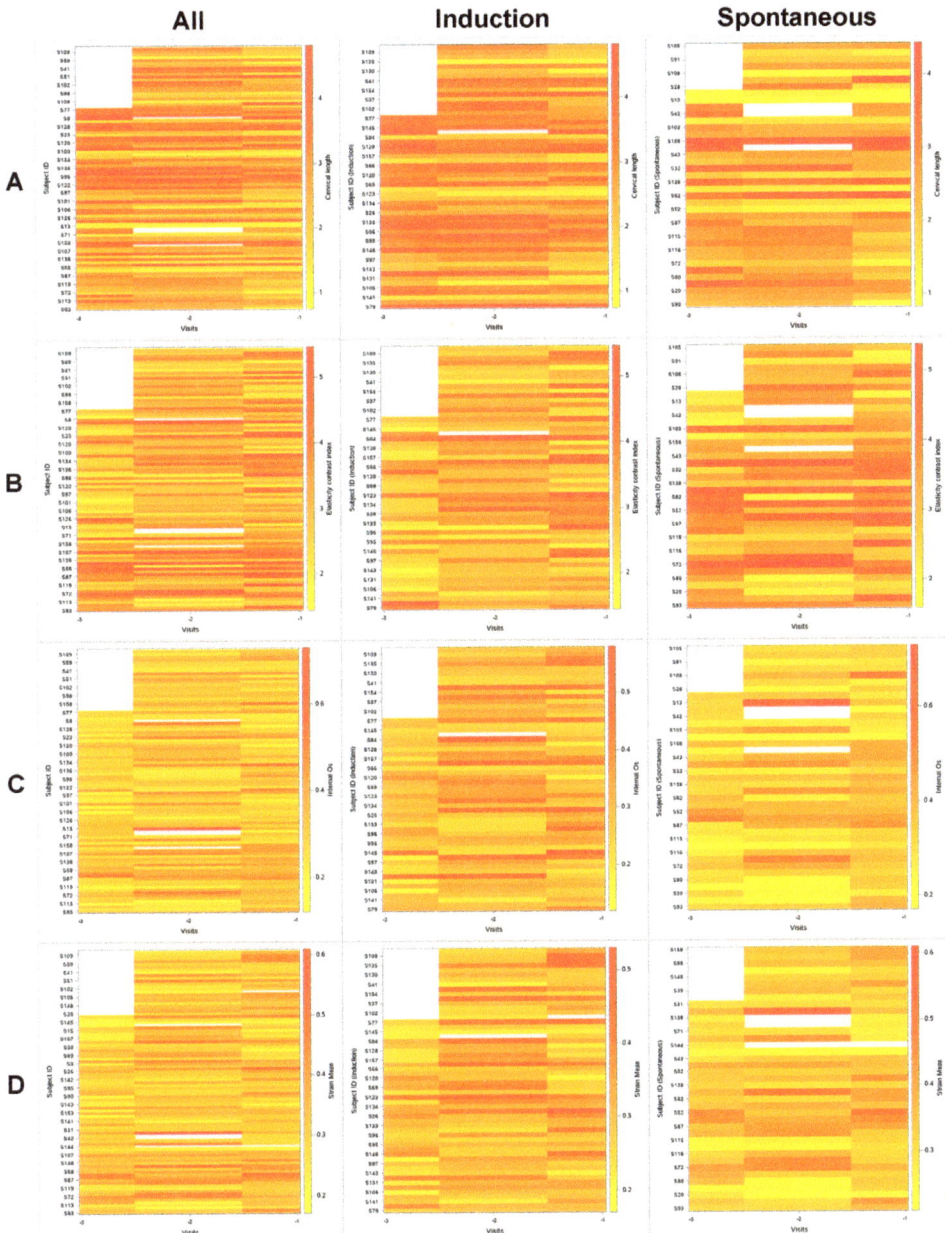

Figure 4. Lasagna plots of the cervical length and the selected E-Cervix parameters against each visit. A lasagna plot is a heatmap for longitudinal data where each subject's trajectory over time is a horizontal layer, with the simultaneous plotting of trajectories resulting in the stacking of layers, as in lasagna [18]. The horizontal axis of each plot represents a visit counted from the admission for delivery (e.g., −1 being the last visit before admission). The color bar located right to each plot represents each parameter's value range, red being the highest value, and yellow being the lowest value. The color change from left to right in each picture can be interpreted as change of each parameter's value at each visit. (**A**): Cervical length; (**B**): Elasticity contrast index; (**C**): Strain mean of the internal os of the cervix; (**D**): Strain mean level; **Left** column, plots including all subjects; **Middle** column, plots of the labor induction group; **Right** column, plots of the spontaneous labor group.

4. Discussion

This longitudinal study showed that the E-Cervix parameters tended to change during the three weeks before the admission for the delivery in women with singleton pregnancies at term. Our results also revealed that there were significant differences in E-Cervix parameters according to the presence or absence of spontaneous labor in these women.

The changes in most E-Cervix parameters, including ECI, IOS, EOS, strain mean, and hardness ratio were in agreement with previous reports. For example, it was previously reported that ECI was significantly higher in patients with a moderately short cervix and who ultimately deliver preterm [16]. In the report, we suggested that ECI values increase with increasing heterogeneity as the uterine cervix ripens. The current data support our suggestion regarding ECI, as ECI increased with advancing gestation irrespective of the development of spontaneous labor. The finding that ECI value was higher in women with spontaneous labor also indicated that there would be more biochemical change and heterogeneity in the cervix of patients with spontaneous labor. Elastographic measurement around the internal os of the cervix has been extensively studied to determine whether it can predict preterm delivery in high- and low-risk pregnancies [20–22]. These early reports have all indicated that soft cervix or higher strain values were related to spontaneous preterm delivery. In addition, those values were increased in the spontaneous labor group, as in the case of ECI. All these findings demonstrate that E-Cervix elastography can differentiate the cervical changes according to the time and labor group in term pregnancy. However, there are differences in significance observed among E-Cervix parameters. There may be some difference in sensitivity among E-Cervix parameters in detecting changes of the cervix. For example, in all the E-Cervix parameters except IOS/EOS ratio, there were significant differences between the two labor groups. However, the change according to the days might have been enough to be detected only in several parameters such as ECI, IOS strain, and strain mean. Reproducibility should also be taken into consideration. We previously reported reproducibility in terms of intra- and inter-observer intraclass correlation coefficient (ICC), which ranged between 0.838 and 0.887 for intra-observer ICC and between 0.901 and 0.988 for inter-observer ICC [17]. Although the results showed good to excellent reproducibility, it would be reasonable, and customary to present mean or median values from multiple measurements.

This research is unique in that it is a longitudinal study in which serial measurements were performed so that we can learn the changes of the cervix with regard to the time and the presence or absence of labor around the time of delivery at term. However, there was no abrupt change in any E-Cervix elastographic parameters or cervical length near the onset of labor. The changes seemed to be constant throughout three weeks before admission in both spontaneous labor and labor induction groups (Figure 3). One study has investigated cervical length changes from 17 to 34 weeks and found that the cervical length was predicted to decrease by 0.6 mm per week of advancing gestation, and the changes were linear in singleton pregnancies [23]. According to our data (Table 3), the cervical length is expected to decrease by 1.7 mm per week for three weeks before the admission, and those changes seem to be linear. Although the rate of change was higher than the cervical length change between 17 to 34 weeks, we could not detect accelerated changes in cervical length near the time of admission. Our data provide an insight into the cervical change at term around delivery. The cervix probably continues to change constantly without any further accelerated ripening around the time of birth at least within three weeks from spontaneous labor. We included the labor induction (no labor) group in this study to contrast the cervical changes of the spontaneous labor group with an assumption that there may be "additional" differences in the spontaneous labor group near the time of spontaneous labor. Cervical ripening of the women who are destined to have spontaneous labor is more advanced than that in women who would not.

In a textbook of obstetrics, the process of parturition is divided into four phases, with cervical ripening occurring in phase two of the parturition. The cervix must undergo "extensive remodeling". The transition from the softening to the ripening phase begins "weeks or days before labor" [24]. However, our data did not support such an argument. The transition from the softening to ripening might have started even earlier.

We enrolled the patients from 36 weeks of gestation because the cervical ripening may ensue before term, and the labor may begin at any time near term. In addition, as the patients should visit every week from 36 weeks of gestation, we thought that it would be best to enroll patients from 36 weeks. Our study implies that cervical ripening near term parturition could be detected by cervical elastographic measurement. Further studies are needed to confirm this. For example, considering that cervical ripening is one of the most important parameters affecting induction failure, cervical elastography could be used to predict successful induction of labor in women with term pregnancies.

There are things to consider when interpreting our results. First, although we assumed a linear relationship between time and variables, it might have been curvilinear if we had performed elastography more frequently. Second, while we presented statistically significant changes in E-Cervix elastography parameters near term pregnancies, the actual differences were relatively small in values to be useful in clinical settings. Finally, as the participating institutions are referral hospitals where patients with high-risk pregnancies are taken care of, this feature is reflected in the subject population. Gestational diabetes mellitus (GDM) comprised 13.6% (13/96), which is quite high, and 5% of patients with hypertensive diseases were included in the labor induction group. When those findings are taken into consideration, the readers should be reminded that the study population in this study was from high-risk patients and showed much heterogeneity.

Author Contributions: Conceptualization: H.S.P.; data curation: H.-S.H., H.K., H.S.P., and H.-J.S.; formal analysis: H.S.P. and S.-y.O.; funding acquisition: J.-Y.K. and S.-y.O.; investigation: H.-S.H., H.S.P., and H.-J.S.; methodology: H.S.P.; project administration: H.K. and J.-H.S.; resources: all authors; software: H.S.P.; supervision: W.J.S., H.M.K., and Y.J.J.; validation: H.-J.S. and H.-S.H.; visualization: H.S.P.; writing-original draft: H.S.P., J.-H.S., and H.K.; writing—review and editing: H.S.P., W.J.S., H.M.K., J.-Y.K., S.-y.O., H.-S.H., and Y.J.J. All authors have read and agreed to the published version of the manuscript.

Funding: This research was supported by Korea Health Technology R&D Project through the Korea Health Industry Development Institute (KHIDI), funded by the Ministry of Health & Welfare, Republic of Korea (grant number: HI18C1696).

Institutional Review Board Statement: The study was conducted according to the guidelines of the Declaration of Helsinki, and approved by the Institutional Review Board of Dongguk University Ilsan Hospital (IRB file No.: DUIH 2019-06-013-001, and date of approval: 24 July 2019), Kyung Hee University Hospital at Gangdong (IRB file No.: KHNMC 2019-07-005 and date of approval: 14 August 2019), and Konkuk University Medical Center (IRB file No.: KUMC 2019-07-008 and date of approval: 11 July 2019).

Informed Consent Statement: Informed consent was obtained from all subjects involved in the study.

Data Availability Statement: The data presented in this study are available on request from the corresponding author. The data are not publicly available due to privacy policy.

Acknowledgments: Part of the data in this article was presented at the 29th World Congress on Ultrasound in Obstetrics and Gynecology, which was held in Berlin, Germany, on 12–16 October 2019.

Conflicts of Interest: The authors declare no conflict of interest. The funders had no role in the design of the study; in the collection, analyses, or interpretation of data; in the writing of the manuscript, or in the decision to publish the results.

References

1. Yellon, S.M. Immunobiology of Cervix Ripening. *Front. Immunol.* **2019**, *10*, 3156. [CrossRef] [PubMed]
2. Word, R.A.; Li, X.H.; Hnat, M.; Carrick, K. Dynamics of cervical remodeling during pregnancy and parturition: Mechanisms and current concepts. *Semin. Reprod. Med.* **2007**, *25*, 69–79. [CrossRef] [PubMed]
3. Iams, J.D.; Goldenberg, R.L.; Meis, P.J.; Mercer, B.M.; Moawad, A.; Das, A.; Thom, E.; McNellis, D.; Copper, R.L.; Johnson, F.; et al. The length of the cervix and the risk of spontaneous premature delivery. National Institute of Child Health and Human Development Maternal Fetal Medicine Unit Network. *N. Engl. J. Med.* **1996**, *334*, 567–572. [CrossRef] [PubMed]

4. Kuusela, P.; Wennerholm, U.B.; Fadl, H.; Wesstrom, J.; Lindgren, P.; Hagberg, H.; Jacobsson, B.; Valentin, L. Second trimester cervical length measurements with transvaginal ultrasound: A prospective observational agreement and reliability study. *Acta Obstet. Gynecol. Scand.* **2020**, *99*, 1476–1485. [CrossRef]
5. Valentin, L.; Bergelin, I. Intra- and interobserver reproducibility of ultrasound measurements of cervical length and width in the second and third trimesters of pregnancy. *Ultrasound Obstet. Gynecol.* **2002**, *20*, 256–262. [CrossRef]
6. Hernandez-Andrade, E.; Romero, R.; Ahn, H.; Hussein, Y.; Yeo, L.; Korzeniewski, S.J.; Chaiworapongsa, T.; Hassan, S.S. Transabdominal evaluation of uterine cervical length during pregnancy fails to identify a substantial number of women with a short cervix. *J. Matern. Fetal Neonatal Med.* **2012**, *25*, 1682–1689. [CrossRef]
7. Kuwata, T.; Matsubara, S.; Taniguchi, N.; Ohkuchi, A.; Ohkusa, T.; Suzuki, M. A novel method for evaluating uterine cervical consistency using vaginal ultrasound gray-level histogram. *J. Perinat. Med.* **2010**, *38*, 491–494. [CrossRef]
8. Tekesin, I.; Hellmeyer, L.; Heller, G.; Romer, A.; Kuhnert, M.; Schmidt, S. Evaluation of quantitative ultrasound tissue characterization of the cervix and cervical length in the prediction of premature delivery for patients with spontaneous preterm labor. *Am. J. Obstet. Gynecol.* **2003**, *189*, 532–539. [CrossRef]
9. Banos, N.; Perez-Moreno, A.; Julia, C.; Murillo-Bravo, C.; Coronado, D.; Gratacos, E.; Deprest, J.; Palacio, M. Quantitative analysis of cervical texture by ultrasound in mid-pregnancy and association with spontaneous preterm birth. *Ultrasound Obstet. Gynecol.* **2018**, *51*, 637–643. [CrossRef]
10. Sigrist, R.M.S.; Liau, J.; Kaffas, A.E.; Chammas, M.C.; Willmann, J.K. Ultrasound Elastography: Review of Techniques and Clinical Applications. *Theranostics* **2017**, *7*, 1303–1329. [CrossRef]
11. Swiatkowska-Freund, M.; Preis, K. Cervical elastography during pregnancy: Clinical perspectives. *Int. J. Womens Health* **2017**, *9*, 245–254. [CrossRef] [PubMed]
12. Papillon-Smith, J.; Abenhaim, H.A. The role of sonographic cervical length in labor induction at term. *J. Clin. Ultrasound* **2015**, *43*, 7–16. [CrossRef] [PubMed]
13. Glover, A.V.; Manuck, T.A. Screening for spontaneous preterm birth and resultant therapies to reduce neonatal morbidity and mortality: A review. *Semin. Fetal Neonatal Med.* **2018**, *23*, 126–132. [CrossRef] [PubMed]
14. Du, L.; Lin, M.F.; Wu, L.H.; Zhang, L.H.; Zheng, Q.; Gu, Y.J.; Xie, H.N. Quantitative elastography of cervical stiffness during the three trimesters of pregnancy with a semiautomatic measurement program: A longitudinal prospective pilot study. *J. Obstet. Gynaecol. Res.* **2020**, *46*, 237–248. [CrossRef] [PubMed]
15. Kwak, D.W.; Kim, M.; Oh, S.Y.; Park, H.S.; Kim, S.J.; Kim, M.Y.; Hwang, H.S. Reliability of strain elastography using in vivo compression in the assessment of the uterine cervix during pregnancy. *J. Perinat. Med.* **2020**, *48*, 256–265. [CrossRef]
16. Park, H.S.; Kwon, H.; Kwak, D.W.; Kim, M.Y.; Seol, H.J.; Hong, J.S.; Shim, J.Y.; Choi, S.K.; Hwang, H.S.; Oh, M.J.; et al. Addition of Cervical Elastography May Increase Preterm Delivery Prediction Performance in Pregnant Women with Short Cervix: A Prospective Study. *J. Korean Med. Sci.* **2019**, *34*, e68. [CrossRef]
17. Seol, H.J.; Sung, J.H.; Seong, W.J.; Kim, H.M.; Park, H.S.; Kwon, H.; Hwang, H.S.; Jung, Y.J.; Kwon, J.Y.; Oh, S.Y. Standardization of measurement of cervical elastography, its reproducibility, and analysis of baseline clinical factors affecting elastographic parameters. *Obstet. Gynecol. Sci.* **2020**, *63*, 42–54. [CrossRef]
18. Swihart, B.J.; Caffo, B.; James, B.D.; Strand, M.; Schwartz, B.S.; Punjabi, N.M. Lasagna plots: A saucy alternative to spaghetti plots. *Epidemiology* **2010**, *21*, 621–625. [CrossRef]
19. Fitzmaurice, G.M.; Laird, N.M.; Ware, J.H. *Applied Longitudinal Analysis*, 2nd ed.; Wiley: Hoboken, NJ, USA, 2011; pp. 144–145.
20. Hernandez-Andrade, E.; Garcia, M.; Ahn, H.; Korzeniewski, S.J.; Saker, H.; Yeo, L.; Chaiworapongsa, T.; Hassan, S.S.; Romero, R. Strain at the internal cervical os assessed with quasi-static elastography is associated with the risk of spontaneous preterm delivery at ≤34 weeks of gestation. *J. Perinat. Med.* **2015**, *43*, 657–666. [CrossRef]
21. Wozniak, S.; Czuczwar, P.; Szkodziak, P.; Milart, P.; Wozniakowska, E.; Paszkowski, T. Elastography in predicting preterm delivery in asymptomatic, low-risk women: A prospective observational study. *BMC Pregnancy Childbirth* **2014**, *14*, 238. [CrossRef]
22. Wozniak, S.; Czuczwar, P.; Szkodziak, P.; Wrona, W.; Paszkowski, T. Elastography for predicting preterm delivery in patients with short cervical length at 18–22 weeks of gestation: A prospective observational study. *Ginekol. Pol.* **2015**, *86*, 442–447. [CrossRef] [PubMed]
23. Meath, A.J.; Ramsey, P.S.; Mulholland, T.A.; Rosenquist, R.G.; Lesnick, T.; Ramin, K.D. Comparative longitudinal study of cervical length and induced shortening changes among singleton, twin, and triplet pregnancies. *Am. J. Obstet. Gynecol.* **2005**, *192*, 1410–1415. [CrossRef] [PubMed]
24. Cunningham, F.G. *Williams Obstetrics*, 25th ed.; McGraw-Hill: New York, NY, USA, 2018; pp. 400–420.

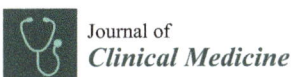

Review

Sex Differences Are Here to Stay: Relevance to Prenatal Care

Amy M. Inkster [1,2,†], Icíar Fernández-Boyano [1,2,†] and Wendy P. Robinson [1,2,*]

1. BC Children's Hospital Research Institute, Vancouver, BC V5Z 4H4, Canada; ainkster@bcchr.ca (A.M.I.); iciar.fernandez@bcchr.ca (I.F.-B.)
2. Department of Medical Genetics, University of British Columbia, Vancouver, BC V6H 3N1, Canada
* Correspondence: wrobinson@bcchr.ca; Tel.: +1-(604)-875-3229
† Considered co-first authors.

Abstract: Sex differences exist in the incidence and presentation of many pregnancy complications, including but not limited to pregnancy loss, spontaneous preterm birth, and fetal growth restriction. Sex differences arise very early in development due to differential gene expression from the X and Y chromosomes, and later may also be influenced by the action of gonadal steroid hormones. Though offspring sex is not considered in most prenatal diagnostic or therapeutic strategies currently in use, it may be beneficial to consider sex differences and the associated mechanisms underlying pregnancy complications. This review will cover (i) the prevalence and presentation of sex differences that occur in perinatal complications, particularly with a focus on the placenta; (ii) possible mechanisms underlying the development of sex differences in placental function and pregnancy phenotypes; and (iii) knowledge gaps that should be addressed in the development of diagnostic or risk prediction tools for such complications, with an emphasis on those for which it would be important to consider sex.

Keywords: sex as a biological variable; sex differences; pregnancy complications; placenta; prenatal diagnosis; preeclampsia; preterm birth; fetal growth restriction; miscarriage

Citation: Inkster, A.M.; Fernández-Boyano, I.; Robinson, W.P. Sex Differences Are Here to Stay: Relevance to Prenatal Care. *J. Clin. Med.* **2021**, *10*, 3000. https://doi.org/10.3390/jcm10133000

Academic Editor: Alex Heazell

Received: 22 June 2021
Accepted: 2 July 2021
Published: 5 July 2021

Publisher's Note: MDPI stays neutral with regard to jurisdictional claims in published maps and institutional affiliations.

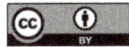

Copyright: © 2021 by the authors. Licensee MDPI, Basel, Switzerland. This article is an open access article distributed under the terms and conditions of the Creative Commons Attribution (CC BY) license (https://creativecommons.org/licenses/by/4.0/).

1. Introduction

Sex differences exist throughout the life course, with the earliest differences evident well before birth and spanning gestation. Pregnancies carrying male and female fetuses may differ in their risks of early pregnancy loss, preterm birth, and placental insufficiency associated with preeclampsia and/or fetal growth restriction. However, establishing the influence of sex on these outcomes is complicated by the different diagnostic criteria and genetic and environmental risk factors in the populations studied. As the placenta mediates fetal growth and underlies many pregnancy complications, sex differences arising in gestation are likely due to effects of sex on placental development and function. Compared to females (XX), male (XY) fetuses are larger by the second trimester of pregnancy (based on ultrasound data) [1,2], show a more pro-inflammatory immune response across gestation, and are at a higher risk of infection leading to preterm birth and other pregnancy complications [3–5]. This in turn may contribute to sex differences in early susceptibility to childhood conditions including neurodevelopmental disorders [6–8]. Throughout life, females remain at lower risk of infection, but are more likely than males to develop adult-onset autoimmune diseases [9]. Sex differences extend well beyond steroid hormones, reproductive organs, and body size; sex differences also affect factors such as disease incidence, and are of value to consider with respect to diagnostic criteria and therapeutic efficacy [10].

Characterizing the mechanisms that underlie sex differences observed in pre- and perinatal complications may contribute to our understanding of why these sex differences are observed, including the key pathways involved, and has the potential to lead to more effective sex-informed diagnostic and therapeutic practices. Fetal sex steroid hormone production begins partway through the first trimester [11], and therefore sex differences arising earlier in gestation are likely to be due to differential expression of genes on the sex chromosomes, or other sex chromosome effects. Later in development, sex differences may be influenced by transient higher testosterone levels produced by the male fetal testes between 12 and 16 weeks of gestation [12–14]. Importantly, sex differences are generally not discrete: for example, testosterone levels and fetal size measurements show considerable variation within each sex, and measurements can overlap between the sexes. In this review, we discuss the sex differences observed in common pregnancy complications, discuss the underlying mechanisms that may be involved, and emphasize the need for collection of fetal sex-specific data when assessing diagnostic and screening tools aimed at promoting healthy birth outcomes (Figure 1).

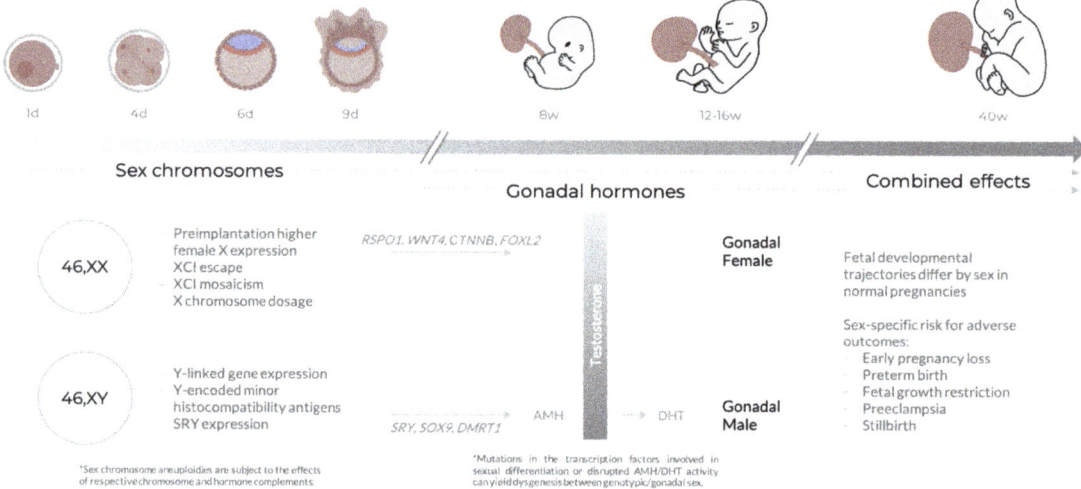

Figure 1. Typical sex differences across gestational age. Throughout pregnancy, sex differences may arise as a consequence of both sex chromosome and sex hormone (testosterone) biology. The combined effects of sex chromosomes and hormones on placental function may contribute to sex differences in healthy development and risk for adverse pregnancy outcomes. Section 3 contains more detailed descriptions of the processes mentioned in this figure, in particular those relating to the X chromosome.

Sex differences arise as consequences of the processes of sex determination and differentiation; for more information on these processes, see [15,16]. In XY embryos, gonadal upregulation of sex-determining *SRY* initiates a gene expression cascade, leading to sexual differentiation. *SRY* activates *SOX9*, which triggers testis differentiation pathways including the upregulation of *AMH* (anti-Mullerian hormone), leading to regression of the Mullerian ducts. In males, expression of *DMRT1* is also required to antagonize female differentiation pathways. Testosterone, produced by the Leydig cells of the male testes after internal differentiation, is oxidized to the more potent dihydroxytestosterone (DHT), which induces differentiation of the male external genitalia. In the female, lack of *SRY* expression enables upregulation of *RSPO1* and *WNT4*, which cooperatively upregulate *CTNNB* (coding for β-catenin) and accordingly inhibit *SOX9* expression; this allows for the differentiation of the Mullerian ducts into the female reproductive tract. β-catenin also activates *FOXL2* to further repress male differentiation factors including *SOX9*. Mutations in these important transcription factors, or in several other transcription factors involved in downstream gene regulatory networks leading to sexual differentiation, have the potential to lead to gonadal dysgenesis, a spectrum of conditions in which the gonads develop out of accord with genetic sex.

2. Sex Differences in Prenatal and Perinatal Complications

Although an increased male vulnerability to several adverse pregnancy outcomes and complications is well recognized [17], the so-called "male disadvantage" is not consistent across pregnancy complications or throughout gestation. Recent work suggests that although male mortality is elevated in later pregnancy, the opposite is true in early gestation [18]. The notion of a "fragile sex", whether male or female, is likely an oversimplification, as pregnancy complications differ in their multifactorial etiologies and underlying mechanisms. Furthermore, variation exists in diagnostic criteria for pregnancy complication across institutions. As many adverse pregnancy outcomes have been associated with abnormal placentation, this review will focus on sex differences in perinatal complications associated with placental insufficiency.

2.1. Early Pregnancy Loss

Worldwide, sex ratio at birth is consistently biased toward males [19]. The sex ratio at conception appears to be balanced [18], which suggests preferential loss of female conceptuses during implantation or early development. Approximately 10% of clinically recognized pregnancies [20–23] and ~30% of all pregnancies [21–23] are spontaneously lost in the first trimester, referred to as early pregnancy loss (EPL), thought to arise from placentation failure secondary to other factors. Studies on sex biases in pregnancy loss have been conflicting. An excess of females has been observed among karyotypically normal spontaneous losses during the first two trimesters [18,24–26]; however, such bias can also result from maternal contamination confounding cytogenetic analysis of products of conception [27]. Indeed, other studies have reported that male conceptuses are more susceptible to both early and late pregnancy loss [28–31], suggesting that female embryos may be preferentially lost during implantation, prior to the detection of pregnancy.

Most sporadic pregnancy losses occur prior to the identification of fetal sex during the routine second trimester anatomy ultrasound [32,33], so early fetoplacental sex data are largely limited to referral for prenatal genetic testing [34,35] or karyotyping of products of conception after miscarriage. Karyotyping after miscarriage is not routine practice, and as such is often limited to cases of recurrent miscarriage (RM), defined as the loss of three of more consecutive pregnancies [36]. Chromosomal abnormalities are associated with approximately 50% of all pregnancy losses [37,38], and with most cases of EPL [39]. In some cases, the fetus carries normal diploid cells while the chromosomal abnormality is confined to the placenta (confined placental mosaicism, CPM), which may allow progression of a pregnancy to term that might otherwise result in early loss [40].

Intriguingly, it appears that mosaic trisomy may be more likely to persist to term in females. CPM for trisomy 16, typically originating from trisomy rescue and diagnosed at 10–12 weeks gestational age by chorionic villus sampling (CVS), shows a strong female bias [41]. This could indicate that CPM16 female pregnancies are more resistant to EPL or that mosaicism arises more often in female embryos, though the underlying mechanism is unknown. Similarly, a female preponderance is observed in trisomy 18 cases surviving to term [42,43], which is also associated with placental mosaicism [44], as well as in mosaic trisomy 21 [45,46]. Thus, the susceptibility of either sex to pregnancy loss may be dependent on both the underlying cause and gestational age. Given the importance of chromosomal abnormalities in pregnancy loss, the apparent female bias for prolonged survival of mosaic trisomy pregnancies deserves further study.

2.2. Preterm Birth

Preterm birth (PTB), defined as a live birth prior to 37 weeks of gestation, is a major cause of neonatal morbidity and mortality, and of life-long health complications [47,48]. As with many other pregnancy complications, PTB disproportionately affects individuals of lower socioeconomic status and/or living in lower-average-income countries. Spontaneous PTB is the result of preterm labor with either intact membranes or following preterm premature rupture of membranes (PPROM) [49]. This can arise from a myriad of pathologic processes including infection and decidual senescence. In contrast, iatrogenic PTB is usually indicated by maternal and fetal complications such as preeclampsia and/or fetal growth restriction [49].

Pregnancies carrying a male fetus have a higher incidence of spontaneous PTB independent of other risk factors [5,50–57] (Table 1). Stratification of analyses by gestational age has revealed that male prevalence in spontaneous PTB is greater at earlier gestational ages [5,54,56,58,59]. The trophoblast in male-bearing pregnancies shows a greater pro-inflammatory response to infection, which may contribute to an increase in early spontaneous PTB. Higher rates of spontaneous PTB in male-bearing pregnancies may also indicate a mechanistic link between fetal sex and labor-inducing processes [60]. As opposed to spontaneous PTB, a male excess is not observed for iatrogenic PTB [5,54,56]. This may be explained by the lack of male excess in pregnancy complications that commonly lead to iatrogenic PTB. Either no sex bias or an underrepresentation of males is observed in early iatrogenic PTB (<28 weeks) [59,61,62], most often indicated for preterm preeclampsia [58,59], although this effect may depend on statistical methods used [62]. Therefore, sex differences observed in PTB may differ according to the clinical etiology, and sex differences observed in iatrogenic PTB may further depend on the underlying cause. In addition, preterm males and females also differ in their postnatal clinical course. Morbidities associated with PTB such as bronchopulmonary dysplasia, intraventricular haemorrhage, and infection consistently occur at higher rates in PTB males compared to their female counterparts in various populations [63–65]. Moreover, even significant improvements in neonatal care have not narrowed the gap between males and females for neonatal morbidity [66].

It is important to note that many studies of sex biases in PTB have been limited to predominantly white populations, and both genetic risk variants and predisposing environmental risk factors may vary in other populations. As such, these findings may not generalize to all pregnancies; for instance, male excess in spontaneous PTB is insignificant in high-risk pregnancies, where competing risk factors of larger effect may mask the predisposing risk of carrying a male [67]. In addition, while several studies have reported the absence of a male excess among spontaneous PTB in Black and Australian Indigenous populations [51,54,68], other studies disagree [69,70]. It is vital to consider ancestry, ethnicity, and socioeconomic factors when studying the impact of fetoplacental sex on pregnancy complications.

Table 1. Summary of findings from preterm birth (PTB) studies. An asterisk (*) indicates $n_{PTB} < 1000$.

M/F Ratio > 1 (Male Predominance)	Population(s)	Reference
• High in spontaneous PTB (not in induced PTB or with any antenatal pathology) • Low at/after term	Aberdeen, UK	[50]
• High in PTB among white singleton births • Balanced in Black singleton births	New England, US	[51]
• High in PTB compared to term births up to 37 w	Italy	[52]
• High in PTB; particularly in early and spontaneous PTB • Balanced in two cohorts of PTB Black singleton births, induced PTB, and spontaneous PTB after IVF	Europe	[54]
• High in PTB; males account for 55% of all newborns at 23–32 w • High in neonatal mortality, particularly at early GA	Sweden	[71]
• High in spontaneous PTB • Balanced in induced PTB • Low in early PTB with hypertension	France	[60]
• High in spontaneous PTB • High in perinatal mortality throughout pregnancy • Low in PTB with preeclampsia	Norway	[58]

Table 1. Cont.

M/F Ratio > 1 (Male Predominance)	Population(s)	Reference
• High in spontaneous PTB • Low in induced PTB	Oxford, UK	[59]
• High in spontaneous PTB between 34 and 36 w but not <34 w, and after adjustment for confounding factors	Southern China	[72]
• High in PTB and PPROM, even after adjusting for fetal weight	Spain	[57]
• High in PTB even after controlling for birth weight	Libya	[69]
• High in PTB even after adjustment for cofounders including hospital grade, maternal age, bad obstetric history, and other medical disorders	Mainland China	[73]
• High in spontaneous PTB with intact membranes and with PPROM, with a more pronounced effect in PTB at <32 w	Netherlands	[56]
• High in preterm labor and PTB • Balanced in preterm labor and PTB in non-Caucasian women	Netherlands	[74] *
• High in spontaneous and iatrogenic PTB, although iatrogenic PTB shows a bias for either sex depending on the statistical method used	South Australia	[62]
• High in PTB in an African, Asian and Mediterranean population, although the population-attributable risk of male fetal sex on spontaneous PTB was lowest in African women and highest in Mediterranean women	African, Asian and Mediterranean	[70]
M/F Ratio < 1 (Female Predominance)	**Population (s)**	**Reference**
• Low in PTB	Indigenous Australian	[68]
• Low in spontaneous and iatrogenic PTB in a cohort of high-risk women for PTB	White, Black, South Asian, and Other	[67]
• Low in iatrogenic PTB	Belgium	[61] *

2.3. Fetal Growth Restriction

Fetal growth restriction (FGR) is the condition in which a fetus does not reach its potential for intrauterine growth and development, and is typically caused by poor placental function [75,76]. Fetuses with FGR are at an increased risk of poor perinatal and neonatal outcomes, and they have higher rates of morbidity and mortality. In the absence of a diagnostic standard, a variety of metrics including fetal biometry, Doppler ultrasound, and small for gestational age (SGA), are used across studies to define FGR SGA describes fetal size at a given gestational age (e.g., below the 10th percentile) without considering the cause for small size or the growth trajectory in utero, and is commonly used as a surrogate for FGR [75,76]. However, most SGA infants do not show signs of placental dysfunction, nor are they at increased risk of adverse outcomes [77]. Therefore, discrepancies in reports of sex differences in FGR and SGA could be partly due to varying criteria, and using SGA as a surrogate for FGR could inflate the reported female risk of FGR. The threshold used to define SGA should be carefully considered.

For decades, female fetuses have been reported to be at an increased risk of FGR in several populations [55,57,73,78–80] (Table 2). Females also appear to be at higher risk of FGR in association with maternal hypertension [79], smoking [79,81], or asthma [82]. However, it is important to note that many of these studies use FGR interchangeably with SGA; only a few consider the presence of additional obstetric factors, or other metrics of serial ultrasonography. In a study using the head-to-abdominal circumference ratio, male fetal sex was identified as a risk factor for FGR only in women with a low pre-pregnancy weight and BMI [79]. Conversely, one study reported no sex differences in the incidence of preterm FGR [60]. It is possible that the risk of FGR in either sex may depend on additional factors, with males appearing more vulnerable to maternal anthropometric factors that limit fetal growth [79]. In addition, gestational age must also be considered, as early FGR (diagnosed < 32 weeks) is more often associated with abnormal Doppler studies and severe outcomes than late FGR (diagnosed > 32 weeks) [75].

While females can be over-diagnosed with SGA if using growth curves that are undifferentiated for sex, in studies using sex-specific growth curves, SGA females appear to be at a lower risk of experiencing adverse outcomes than SGA males [81]. SGA defined with sex-agnostic growth curves is less likely to reflect FGR or increased risk for other adverse outcomes [83,84], and may thus lead to unnecessary obstetric interventions, inadvertently increasing neonatal morbidity [83,85]. In addition, SGA defined with a fully customized fetal growth standard (adjusting for sex, parity, height, weight, and ethnicity) is associated with increased risk of poor outcomes [86].

Table 2. Summary of findings from fetal growth restriction (FGR) and small for gestational age (SGA) studies, PTB indicates pre-term birth. An asterisk (*) indicates $n_{FGR} < 1000$ or $n_{SGA} < 1000$.

Criteria Used to Define FGR/SGA	Main Findings	Population(s)	Reference
Female Predominance			
BW < 10th percentile for GA, included some studies with <2500 g birth weight plus GA > 37 w.	• Male fetuses have a higher BW and lower risk of SGA across all populations studied. • Female fetal sex is more significantly associated with SGA in developed countries.	North America, Western Europe, Africa, Latin America, Southeast Asia, India	[78]
BW < 10th percentile for GA.	• Female fetuses at higher risk of SGA.	Lebanon	[80]
BW and GA < 10th percentile.	• Higher female risk for SGA with maternal smoking.	Germany	[81]
Unspecified.	• Greater incidence of SGA among female fetuses, independent of other SGA risk factors such as preeclampsia.	Israel	[55]
Echographic diagnosis (criteria unspecified).	• FGR more frequent among female fetuses.	Spain	[57]
BW < 10th percentile.	• SGA more frequent among female fetuses.	Mainland China	[73]
Suspicion of FGR based on poor fetal growth for BW percentile, and presence of obstetric risk factors.	• Females more often suspected of FGR according to risk factors for SGA infants with a birthweight <10th and <3rd percentile.	France	[85]
Serial ultrasonography (SU); increase in the head-to-abdominal circumference ratio up to >2 SDs above the mean, or failure of either abdominal or head circumference to grow on 2 consecutive examinations 2 w apart.	• FGR more frequent among females according to SU and SGA curves. • Female risk higher with maternal hypertension and smoking. • Male risk higher with low maternal pre-pregnancy weight and BMI.	Italy	[79] *
No Effect or Male Predominance			
Ethnicity- and sex-specific BW < 10th percentile for GA.	• FGR slightly more frequent in males • FGR males at higher risk of all adverse outcomes studied, including neonatal death, necrotizing enterocolitis, and respiratory distress syndrome.	Vermont (white and African American)	[87]
Unspecified.	• No male excess among PTB associated with FGR.	France	[60]
BW < 10th percentile for GA.	• No differences in SGA outcomes by sex. • Fetal sex not an independent risk factor for adverse outcomes in SGA.	Pennsylvania, US	[88] *

2.4. Preeclampsia

Preeclampsia (PE) is commonly defined as maternal hypertension arising de novo after 20 weeks' gestation accompanied by one or more adverse conditions, including proteinuria and/or maternal organ dysfunction [89,90]. The two most common clinical subtypes of PE are early-onset (EOPE) and late-onset (LOPE), depending on timing of diagnosis (prior to or at/after 34 weeks) [91,92]. While EOPE is more commonly associated with abnormal placentation, both forms are now thought to result from placental malperfusion, leading to syncytiotrophoblast damage [91,92]. Dividing PE into EOPE and LOPE at 34 weeks does not fully capture the spectrum of clinical, molecular, and pathophysiological features that vary across patients. This heterogeneity is important to consider when studying how sex affects PE, as illustrated by the conflicting results found in the literature.

Considering PE as a single entity irrespective of factors such as gestational age often reveals no differential incidence by sex [57,93,94], although sex differences have been reported in a few studies [95,96] (Table 3). More consistent sex differences are observed when stratifying PE by gestational age, with a female predominance in preterm PE (<37 weeks) [58,94]. A female excess is also observed in very preterm PE (<34 weeks) in several populations [69,94,97,98]. In contrast, either an equal sex ratio or slight male bias is reported for PE with term delivery (>37 weeks) [58,93]. The diversity of findings across studies highlights the importance of considering the heterogeneity of PE and gestational age when considering sex differences. Based on our current understanding, categorizing PE with variables such as gestational age, severity, or co-morbidities provides a more complete picture of sex differences in this disorder.

Table 3. Summary of findings from preeclampsia (PE) studies. An asterisk indicates n_{PE} < 1000.

Main Findings	Population(s)	Reference
Male Predominance		
• Slightly more male pregnancies with PE (not stratified for gestational age).	Denmark	[96]
• Male preponderance in PE, • No significant sex differences in any of the studied obstetric complications usually secondary to PE, including placental abruption, placenta previa, and stillbirth.	Missouri, US	[95]
Female Predominance in Preterm PE		
• Preterm PE (<37 weeks) more frequent among females. • Sex ratio reversed >37 weeks, male fetal sex associated with PE. • 40–42 weeks, equal proportion of males and females with PE.	Norway	[58]
• Compared to all infants born <32 weeks, those with PE <32 weeks more often female. • At term, the M/F ratio is increased in PE.	Sweden	[93]
• Female singleton pregnancies had increased incidence of PE. • Female–female monochorionic diamniotic (MD) and dichorionic diamniotic (DD) pregnancies had a higher incidence of PE than their male counterparts in both MD and DD pregnancies, respectively.	Japan	[98]
• Overall incidence of PE not associated with fetal sex. • Preterm PE more common in pregnancies carrying a female fetus, even after adjustment for confounders.	Northern China	[97]
• No sex difference in incidence of PE (not stratified for GA). • Female fetal sex associated with preterm PE. • Post-term PE more frequent among male fetuses. • Male fetuses of primigravid women had a greater likelihood of developing PE than female-bearing primigravid women.	Libya	[69] *
• No sex differences in all PE, term PE (>37 w), and PE 34–37 w. • Female predominance in very preterm (<34 w) PE.	Europe, US, New Zealand, Australia	[94]
No Sex Differences		
• No sex differences in incidence of PE (not stratified for GA).	Spain	[57]

2.5. Stillbirth

Stillbirth is most commonly defined as fetal death at or beyond 20 weeks of gestation or weight >500 g [99]. Some of the leading causes of stillbirth are asphyxia during labor, maternal factors, and placental dysfunction, which accounts for more than 50% of cases [100,101]. Unfortunately, most stillbirths occurring after 28 weeks of gestation are unexplained [101]. Male fetal sex has been recognized as one of the most prevalent risk factors for stillbirth [102]. A heightened male risk of perinatal morbidity and mortality is well reported in the literature [71,103–106], and a higher frequency of stillbirth among males has also been described [106–108]. However, nuances exist regarding male risk of stillbirth; for instance, one study noted that while male fetuses were at an increased risk of stillbirth, the association diminished with increasing birth weight quintile [103]. A few studies report no sex differences in the rates of stillbirth [71,104], while one study found female excess in stillbirths without any observed demographic or obstetric differences by sex at diagnosis [109]. In addition, a study of infant mortality in India and Pakistan, where the probable causes for stillbirth were similar in both male and female groups, revealed a significantly higher rate of male stillbirths and an increased risk for early perinatal mortality among male infants [107].

Findings are more variable for stillbirth coincident with other complications. There is an excess of males in stillbirths co-occurring with placental abruption [109,110], whereas an excess of females is observed for stillbirths associated with placental insufficiency or hypertension [109]. Sex differences in stillbirth risk are likely dependent on the underlying cause, and further research is needed to elucidate the role of fetoplacental sex as a risk factor for stillbirth.

3. Mechanisms for Sex Differences across Gestation

The cascade leading to phenotypic sex differences in both healthy and complicated pregnancies begins with the basic actions of sex chromosomes and steroid hormones (Table 4), which yield molecular consequences such as autosomal gene expression sex differences, and culminate in observable sex-specific phenotypes. Except in rare cases, the placenta harbours the same sex chromosome complement as the fetus and is subject to the effects of X and Y chromosome dosage disparities. Additionally, the fetoplacental unit produces hormones throughout gestation including estrogen, progesterone, and testosterone. Notable molecular consequences of prenatal sex differences include sex-specific patterns of gene expression, sex differences in key pregnancy hormones such as human chorionic gonadotropin, and sex differences in the fetoplacental response to maternal inflammation and infection.

Table 4. Mechanisms underlying sex differences across gestation, XCI indicates X-chromosome inactivation.

Mechanism	Description
Escape from XCI	• Genes that escape XCI may be more highly expressed in females. • Proportion of XCI escape in placenta may be greater than other somatic tissues.
Mosaicism for XCI	• Patterns of XCI across placenta (mosaicism for parental inactive X) may enable females to better tolerate deleterious alleles.
X chromosome dosage	• Before implantation, females have two active X chromosomes. During this period, X-linked genes are biallelically and more highly expressed in female cells. • Coincident autosomal gene expression sex differences observed. • Single X chromosome associated with larger placentas at term (in humans; in mice this holds true and is independent of gonadal steroids).
Y chromosome	• Preimplantation expression of Y-linked genes in XY embryos. • Y chromosome minor histocompatibility antigens in placenta may interact with maternal immune system to mediate perinatal complications including secondary RM.
Estrogen and progesterone	• Amniotic fluid levels not reported to differ by sex, likely do not have strong influence on sex-biased phenotypes.
Testosterone	• Initially synthesized mid-late first trimester, peak concentration in male amniotic fluid 12–16 weeks' gestation and is 2–5-fold higher than observed in females. • Has the potential to contribute to sex-biased phenotypes

3.1. Sex Chromosome Effects

3.1.1. Peri-Implantation X Chromosome Dynamics

Female-biased expression of X chromosome genes is one mechanism by which sex chromosomes may underlie phenotypic differences. In female (XX) mammals, one of the two X chromosomes is epigenetically silenced early in development by X-chromosome inactivation (XCI). XCI in humans occurs between implantation and tissue differentiation, and is completed approximately between 12 days and 1 month post-fertilization [111,112]. Prior to XCI, female X-linked genes are biallelically expressed as early as embryonic day three [112], and by embryonic day four, more than 25% of X-linked transcripts are expressed 2-fold higher in females [113]. It has been suggested that preimplantation growth differences are attributable to X chromosome effects, as male preimplantation embryos of several species exhibit faster metabolism and growth rates [114–117]. However, it is not yet clear whether sex-specific growth rates are also observed in vivo, and these observations may be artefacts of in vitro culture conditions [118,119]

3.1.2. Escape from X-Chromosome Inactivation

Following the establishment of XCI, cells of the female conceptus have one active and one inactive X chromosome. Though XCI dramatically reduces inactive X chromosome gene expression, up to 12% of genes escape XCI, and another 15% are reported to variably escape between tissues, individuals, or studies [120,121]. Genes that escape XCI are generally more highly expressed in females, though not always [120,122].

XCI escape genes in the placenta and fetus may contribute to phenotypic sex differences. DNA methylation is an epigenetic mark that assists with silencing gene expression on the inactive X [123,124]. Overall, DNA methylation levels are lower in the placental genome as compared to other tissues [125], and are specifically depleted on the placental inactive X chromosome [126]. Low placental inactive X DNA methylation may suggest that the placenta has a higher load of XCI escape genes than other tissues [126], which could widen the transcriptional gap between male and female placentae and contribute to phenotypic sex differences across gestation.

3.1.3. Mosaic X-Chromosome Inactivation

In human embryonic and extraembryonic tissue, XCI is random and not imprinted via parent-of-origin; this in contrast to rodent extraembryonic lineages with paternally imprinted XCI. The human female placenta is thus a mosaic tissue often harbouring cell populations with a paternally active X chromosome and cell populations with a maternally active X chromosome [127,128]. Skewed XCI is the phenomenon by which >90% of cells within a tissue or individual inactivate the same parentally inherited X chromosome; skewed XCI in females can occur by chance, particularly if tissues are derived from a small pool of precursor cells or can occur if inactivation of one parental allele leads to a selective survival or proliferation advantage [129]. In placenta, such selection appears weak; instead due to clonal villous tree development there is a patchiness to XCI [130].

Aside from XY homologs in the pseudoautosomal regions, males have only a single copy of X chromosome genes and thus each X-linked variant in males has the potential to exert a greater phenotypic impact than in females [131]. Expression of mildly deleterious variants would have stronger effects in males [131] because they are constitutively expressed across the placenta, while the female placenta in theory could better moderate the effects of deleterious variants by the presence of some cell populations across the placenta inactivating the deleterious allele and limiting its impact.

3.1.4. X Chromosome Dosage

A more general effect of X chromosome biology on prenatal development is X chromosome dosage disparity by sex. Male (XY) and female (XX) cells differ in their typical X and Y chromosome complements. Several effects of X and Y chromosome dosage on prenatal development have been reported, though the precise mechanisms by which they act have not yet been elucidated. For example, presence of a single X chromosome has been associated with larger placentae in male compared to female pregnancies [3]. This effect replicates in mouse models where X chromosome dosage can be manipulated independently of phenotypic sex [132]; larger murine placentae were associated with offspring bearing a single X chromosome, independent of gonadal sex (male or female) and parental origin of the single X chromosome [133]. The precise mechanism by which X chromosome dosage affects placental size is not known but could involve any of the specific mechanisms described above.

3.1.5. The Forgotten Y

In addition to X chromosomal effects, the Y chromosome in male conceptuses may also drive sex differences. In the preimplantation period, 13 Y-linked genes are expressed at detectable levels [113], including four that lack X-linked homologs with similar function and are thus candidates for underlying phenotypic sex differences. Later in gestation, the mammalian sex-determining gene *SRY* is transcribed, and is critical for phenotypic masculinization [15]. Lack of *SRY* in males due to mutational events can in some cases result in gonadal dysgenesis or a disconnect between typical genotype and gonadal sex, as can *SRY* expression in females [134].

In other tissues, Y-linked genes have been found to contribute to autoimmune disease [135,136], likely owing to Y chromosome-encoded minor histocompatibility antigens (mHAgs) [137]. Y-linked mHAgs may also play a role in maternal immune tolerance of the male conceptus; at least six mHAgs are expressed in the human placenta, derived from the DDX3Y, KDM5D, and RPS4Y1 proteins [138]. Dysfunctional maternal immune tolerance of the fetus may therefore be sex specific, as women affected by RM secondary to one or more successful live births appear to be overrepresented for having a live born male preceding their recurrent losses [139,140]. This pattern has been independently confirmed [141], though a third study found no significant difference in the sex of the live birth preceding RM [142]. These women are also more likely to possess class II major histocompatibility antigens against Y-linked mHAgs, presumably arising from a maternal immune response to the preceding live born male [139]. A lower male/female birth ratio in subsequent live births has also been observed [139,143,144]. Together, these results suggest a Y-chromosomal contribution to sex biased pregnancy outcomes.

3.2. Steroid Hormone Effects

3.2.1. Estrogens and Progesterone

Both male and female fetuses are exposed to high levels of estrogens throughout pregnancy, primarily in the form of estriol, with smaller contributions from estrone and estradiol [145]. Prenatally, estrone and estradiol are synthesized in the placenta from the fetal adrenal cortex-derived precursors dehydroepiandrosterone (DHEA) and dehydroepiandrosterone sulfate (DHEA-S), while estriol is placentally synthesized from 16-α-hydroxyl DHEA-S arising in the fetal liver [146]. Prenatal levels of estriol and estradiol do not appear to differ by fetal sex [12,147], it is likely that estrone levels also do not differ by fetal sex, though studies are limited. DHEA levels also do not appear to differ by fetal sex [13,148], while the association of fetal sex and DHEA-S concentration has not been widely investigated. Estrogen is not be expected to be a major driver of prenatal sex differences, corroborated by evidence for normal fetal and placental growth in estrogen-deficient pregnancies [149]. However, a link exists between estrogen biology and prenatal complications. Estradiol promotes angiogenesis, vasodilation, and trophoblast proliferation/differentiation, processes which are compromised in PE [150]. A decrease in maternal blood estradiol, produced by the placenta, is also observed in pregnant women that subsequently develop PE [150,151]. Several genetic variants that decrease aromatase activity are associated with higher incidence of PE in a Japanese population, supporting an indirect mechanistic link between decreased estradiol production and PE [152].

Similar to estrogen, circulating fetal and maternal progesterone primarily derives from the placental syncytiotrophoblast [12]. Generally, progesterone is required for the maintenance of pregnancy and suppresses uterine contractility by direct inhibition of contraction-associated proteins in the myometrial tissue [153]. Amniotic fluid progesterone does not appear to differ by fetal sex in early or mid-gestation [12,13,154]. Though placental progesterone does not differ by sex, fetal response to maternal progesterone may: when progesterone is given to ovine mothers during early gestation, only male fetal progesterone concentration increases, apparently mediated by lower rates of progesterone metabolism in the male liver [155].

3.2.2. Testosterone

In uncomplicated gestations, prenatal androgens function to masculinize the male external genitalia approximately between the 8th and 16th weeks of gestation [12,13,156,157]. Masculinization is driven by fetal testosterone, mainly synthesized in the fetal adrenal cortex, testis, and the fetal ovary [12,158]. Androgen signalling occurs via the X-linked androgen receptor (AR) protein, loss of which leads to reduced male intrauterine growth in both mice and humans; variation in *AR* expression may also contribute to sex differences in fetal growth [159]. Fetal testosterone facilitates masculinization through its conversion to the more bioactive 5a-dihydroxytestosterone (DHT) upon reaching target organs [160]. However, a second and equally essential route to DHT relies on placental progesterone as an intermediate [13]. Placental insufficiency and FGR are frequently associated with abnormal external genital development in affected male offspring, possibly attributable to insufficient placental progesterone production [13].

Males experience maximum amniotic fluid testosterone concentrations between the 12th and 16th weeks of gestation [12–14]. At its peak, testosterone concentration is 2–5-fold higher in male amniotic fluid than in females [161–164], though there is overlap between the ranges observed in both sexes [13]. During this period of maximal sex difference in testosterone concentration, testosterone may establish the basis for sex-biased phenotypes. Beyond approximately 24 weeks of gestation until term, there are no significant sex differences in serum or amniotic fluid testosterone levels [12,13].

3.3. Molecular Consequences of Prenatal Sex Differences

Though the effects of sex chromosomes and gonadal hormones are the basis of mammalian phenotypic sex differences, over the course of gestation there are notable downstream molecular consequences that are very sex divergent and likely have widespread impacts on development. Among the more immediate molecular consequences of either sex chromosome or sex hormone effects are widespread autosomal gene expression sex differences: up to 60% of sex-differentially expressed genes in the human placenta are autosomal [165,166]. Even during the preimplantation period, alongside X-linked expression differences, multiple autosomal genes (n = 58) are differentially expressed by sex [113]. Before the onset of fetal steroid hormone production, autosomal sex differences imply a relationship between sex chromosome dosage and autosomal gene expression. Though precise mechanisms of sex chromosome–autosome crosstalk in general are not yet clear, X chromosome effects have been somewhat explored and may be related to factors including X chromosome-encoded transcription factors, correlated networks of gene expression, or participation of autosomal genes in the process of XCI [167,168]. The epigenetically inactive X chromosome in each female nucleus also may impact autosomal gene regulation by acting as either a sink or source of epigenetic silencing factors [169].

While the levels of placentally synthesized steroid hormones do not tend to show sex biases, female-carrying pregnancies are associated with average higher maternal serum human chorionic gonadotropin (hCG) after the 3rd week of gestation, though precise male/female ratios vary across populations [170,171]. hCG is produced by the placenta, and the genes encoding the four hCG β subunits are among the most sex-differentially expressed placental autosomal genes [166]. hCG supports growth and invasion of the placenta, and regulates placental vascular endothelial growth factor (VEGF) and its receptors [172]. Though higher levels of hCG are observed in female-bearing pregnancies, females do not have larger placentas than males. This contradicts what one may expect if hCG promotes placental growth, and the reason for this apparent controversy is not yet understood. Additionally, while both the male fetus and placenta are larger than their female counterparts, there is a higher fetal/placental weight ratio in males, indicating that the male placenta is more efficient at promoting fetal growth [3].

Male and female placentae also exhibit marked differences in response to maternal glucocorticoid signalling, either endogenously derived or synthetically administered as antenatal betamethasone for expected preterm delivery [173,174]. In response to maternal glucocorticoid signalling, female fetal growth trajectories adaptively decrease due to alterations in placental glucocorticoid metabolism mediated by the 11β-hydroxysteroid dehydrogenase type 2 (11β-HSD2) enzyme, while male growth trajectories remain unchanged [173]. Higher levels of anti-inflammatory testosterone may protect males from the inflammatory effects of maternal glucocorticoid signaling elicit reduced growth [173], but also the lack of male adrenal adaptation to increased maternal glucocorticoid stimulation may leave males at a disadvantage in the face of preterm delivery [174].

Prenatal sex differences may also arise from sex differences in immunological function and response to inflammation. A higher rate of inflammation and infection is observed in male fetuses during intrauterine life, which may contribute to higher male perinatal mortality [4,175]. Chronic inflammation is more common in the decidua and basal plates of women carrying male offspring, suggesting greater maternal immune response to a male fetus [4]. Conversely, mothers carrying females exhibit greater stimulated cytokine production: across all trimesters, maternal serum levels of IL-6, IL-8, and TNF-a proinflammatory cytokines were significantly higher in association with a female fetus after PBMC lipopolysaccharide stimulation [176]. The cause of these differences is unknown, though, as discussed earlier, it is possible that some portion of the maternal immune response to the male fetus is mediated by Y chromosome antigens.

4. Sex Differences in Diagnostic and Screening Approaches

Given the well-established sex differences in prenatal development, it is important that diagnostic and screening methods for pregnancy complications consider fetal sex and potentially optimize approaches separately for each sex. Sex-specific growth charts are a routinely-used tool, but other diagnostic approaches may similarly benefit from explicit consideration of sex.

There has been growing interest in the development of maternal serum screening tools for early diagnosis of pregnancy complication. However, the concentrations of many trophoblast-derived molecules assessed by such approaches may vary both by pathology and fetoplacental sex. For example, higher levels of two angiogenic factors involved in PE, soluble fms-like tyrosine kinase protein 1 (sFlt1) and placental growth factor (PLGF), are observed in maternal serum in association with a female fetus [177]. In terms of serum proteins evaluated prenatally, hCG and AFP are among several that differ by sex: the presence of a female fetus is associated with higher average maternal serum chorionic gonadotropin (hCG) after the 3rd week of gestation [170,171], and lower average second-trimester maternal serum alpha-fetoprotein (AFP) [178–180]. Female-carrying pregnancies are also associated with higher levels of maternal serum cell-free fetal DNA (cffDNA) [181], which is used for non-invasive prenatal testing (NIPT) of chromosomal abnormalities and fetal sex determination [181]. This cffDNA originates from trophoblast cells and represents 3–6% of the total cell-free circulating DNA in maternal circulation during gestation. Of note, cffDNA levels may correlate with the levels of serum proteins including hCG [182]. Maternal cervical fluid is also a source of trophoblast-derived nucleic acids; cervical fluid has valuable diagnostic potential and can be used to accurately assess fetal sex [183]. It is possible that the interactions of sex and trophoblast-derived markers in cervical fluid may differ from those measured in maternal serum. These examples illustrate the interdependence of biomarker species with fetoplacental sex.

Sex should especially be considered when phenotypes, etiologies, or prognostic markers are a priori known to interact with sex. For example, elevated hCG and low AFP are both observed in association with female offspring, and separately, are indicative of elevated risk of aneuploidy [184]. Though there does not appear to be a bias for higher hCG positive screen rates in females [178,185], an excess in female positive screens is observed for AFP [186]. As AFP and hCG in combination with other factors may also be prognostic for PTB, FGR, and/or PE, sex should be of special consideration given its association with both the markers of interest and the disorders themselves [177,187]. Maternal serum sFlt1/PlGF ratios have been proposed for predicting PE and FGR [188–191]. However, higher levels of maternal serum sFlt1 in female-bearing pregnancies should elevate sFlt1/PlGF ratios [191], while conflicting reports suggest PlGF may also vary with fetal sex [177,192]. The effect of fetal sex on sFlt1/PlGF ratios should be carefully elucidated in both healthy gestations and in the context of PE, to understand the interaction of sex and pathology on this ratio prior to effective clinical implementation [177]. An increase in maternal plasma leptin was observed in EOPE pregnancies carrying a male fetus, suggesting an interaction between sex and PE [193]. More research is needed to evaluate how sex affects the diagnostic utility of such biomarkers.

During pregnancy, fetal sex can be assigned genetically (by NIPT, chorionic villus sampling, or amniotic fluid sampling) or anatomically via ultrasound. Depending on the driver of particular sex differences (sex chromosomes or gonadal hormones), as well as their timing and persistence, different sex assessment methods may prove differentially valuable. Additionally, while sex is typically considered a binary trait, research has illustrated high degrees of variability and overlap in many sex-related phenotypes. Specifically, neuropsychiatric research has begun to adopt a model of sex differences that range from defining male–female differences as sexually dimorphic (categorically distinct and not overlapping) to sex differences with continuous endpoints, to differences with the same endpoint achieved by distinct mechanisms in each sex [194]. The state of this field is reviewed in [195–197].

Prenatal diagnostics should also consider ethnicity or ancestry, as healthy phenotypes in one population could be labelled pathogenic if measured with standards developed in another. When considering genomic screening methods, one must consider the frequency at which "risk" variants exist in certain populations. For example, it has been reported that an *IL6* variant associated with acute chorioamnionitis risk is only present in East Asian populations [198], and that selection in the progesterone receptor gene may have led to specific polymorphisms that underlie differential rates of progesterone-associated pregnancy complications by population [199]. Other maternal factors associated with risk of adverse pregnancy outcomes include socioeconomic status, comorbid health conditions, and smoking status. Some of these factors are well known to interact with sex and are therefore of particular importance to consider; for example, both socioeconomic status and maternal asthma influence maternal glucocorticoid signaling, known to elicit different fetal responses based on sex [82,200].

5. Conclusions

Epidemiological studies have revealed sex differences associated with the incidence and outcomes of several obstetric complications, with the widespread claim of a "male disadvantage" being more nuanced than initially thought, and dependent on additional variables such as gestational age. These findings have warranted further study into the biological mechanisms underlying prenatal sex differences, which we must continue to elucidate if fetal sex is to be incorporated into clinical consideration in the context of diagnostic tests and interventions. As clinical practice is steadily evolving towards precision medicine initiatives, prenatal care will follow suit, and it is clear that the evidence suggests it will be of value for researchers and clinicians to consider how proper integration of sex considerations can improve current or future diagnostic methods for pregnancy complications. Lastly, incorporating fetoplacental sex in diagnosis and screening should not obscure the equal importance of other variables such as genetic ancestry, which are also extremely relevant to perinatal health and may in fact interact with sex in many contexts.

Author Contributions: Conceptualization, writing, and editing A.M.I., I.F.-B. and W.P.R. All authors have read and agreed to the published version of the manuscript.

Funding: This work was supported by a Canadian Institutes of Health Research (CIHR) grant to WPR [SVB-158613 and F19-04091]. WPR holds a CIHR Research Chair in Sex and Gender Science [GSK-171375] and receives salary support through an investigatorship award from the BC Children's Hospital Research Institute. AMI receives support from a CIHR Doctoral Fellowship.

Institutional Review Board Statement: Not applicable.

Informed Consent Statement: Not applicable.

Data Availability Statement: Not applicable.

Acknowledgments: We thank the scientific community for their commitment to the study and inclusion of sex as a variable in biomedical research. We acknowledge members of the Robinson lab for thoughtful discussion and feedback on the analysis and manuscript, especially Giulia F. Del Gobbo and Maria S. Peñaherrera A.

Conflicts of Interest: The authors declare no conflict of interest. The funders had no role in conceptualization or writing of the manuscript.

References

1. Bukowski, R.; Smith, G.C.S.; Malone, F.D.; Ball, R.H.; Nyberg, D.A.; Comstock, C.H.; Hankins, G.D.V.; Berkowitz, R.L.; Gross, S.J.; Dugoff, L.; et al. Human Sexual Size Dimorphism in Early Pregnancy. *Am. J. Epidemiol.* **2007**, *165*, 1216–1218. [CrossRef] [PubMed]
2. Galjaard, S.; Ameye, L.; Lees, C.C.; Pexsters, A.; Bourne, T.; Timmerman, D.; Devlieger, R. Sex Differences in Fetal Growth and Immediate Birth Outcomes in a Low-Risk Caucasian Population. *Biol. Sex Differ.* **2019**, *10*, 48. [CrossRef] [PubMed]
3. Eriksson, J.G.; Kajantie, E.; Osmond, C.; Thornburg, K.; Barker, D.J.P. Boys Live Dangerously in the Womb. *Am. J. Hum. Biol.* **2010**, *22*, 330–335. [CrossRef] [PubMed]
4. Goldenberg, R.L.; Andrews, W.W.; Faye-Petersen, O.M.; Goepfert, A.R.; Cliver, S.P.; Hauth, J.C. The Alabama Preterm Birth Study: Intrauterine Infection and Placental Histologic Findings in Preterm Births of Males and Females Less than 32 Weeks. *Am. J. Obstet. Gynecol.* **2006**, *195*, 1533–1537. [CrossRef] [PubMed]
5. Challis, J.; Newnham, J.; Petraglia, F.; Yeganegi, M.; Bocking, A. Fetal Sex and Preterm Birth. *Placenta* **2013**, *34*, 95–99. [CrossRef]
6. Bale, T.L. The Placenta and Neurodevelopment: Sex Differences in Prenatal Vulnerability. *Dialogues Clin. Neurosci.* **2016**, *18*, 459–464. [PubMed]
7. Grether, J.K.; Nelson, K.B.; Walsh, E.; Willoughby, R.E.; Redline, R.W. Intrauterine Exposure to Infection and Risk of Cerebral Palsy in Very Preterm Infants. *Arch. Pediatr. Adolesc. Med.* **2003**, *157*, 26. [CrossRef] [PubMed]
8. Gardener, H.; Spiegelman, D.; Buka, S.L. Prenatal Risk Factors for Autism: A Comprehensive Meta-Analysis. *Br. J. Psychiatry J. Ment. Sci.* **2009**, *195*, 7–14. [CrossRef]
9. Jaillon, S.; Berthenet, K.; Garlanda, C. Sexual Dimorphism in Innate Immunity. *Clin. Rev. Allergy Immunol.* **2019**, *56*, 308–321. [CrossRef] [PubMed]
10. Mauvais-Jarvis, F.; Merz, N.B.; Barnes, P.J.; Brinton, R.D.; Carrero, J.-J.; DeMeo, D.L.; Vries, G.J.D.; Epperson, C.N.; Govindan, R.; Klein, S.L.; et al. Sex and Gender: Modifiers of Health, Disease, and Medicine. *Lancet* **2020**, *396*, 565–582. [CrossRef]
11. Makieva, S.; Saunders, P.T.K.; Norman, J.E. Androgens in Pregnancy: Roles in Parturition. *Hum. Reprod. Update* **2014**, *20*, 542–559. [CrossRef] [PubMed]
12. Kogan, S.J.; Hafez, E.S.E. (Eds.) *Pediatric Andrology*; Springer: Dordrecht, The Netherlands, 1981; ISBN 978-94-010-3721-1.
13. O'Shaughnessy, P.J.; Antignac, J.P.; Le Bizec, B.; Morvan, M.-L.; Svechnikov, K.; Söder, O.; Savchuk, I.; Monteiro, A.; Soffientini, U.; Johnston, Z.C.; et al. Alternative (Backdoor) Androgen Production and Masculinization in the Human Fetus. *PLoS Biol.* **2019**, *17*, e3000002. [CrossRef] [PubMed]
14. Künzig, H.J.; Meyer, U.; Schmitz-Roeckerath, B.; Broer, K.H. Influence of Fetal Sex on the Concentration of Amniotic Fluid Testosterone: Antenatal Sex Determination? *Arch. Gynakol.* **1977**, *223*, 75–84. [CrossRef]
15. Rey, R.; Josso, N.; Racine, C. Sexual Differentiation. In *Endotext*; Feingold, K.R., Anawalt, B., Boyce, A., Chrousos, G., de Herder, W.W., Dhatariya, K., Dungan, K., Grossman, A., Hershman, J.M., Hofland, J., et al., Eds.; MDText.com, Inc.: South Dartmouth, MA, USA, 2000.

16. Pannetier, M.; Chassot, A.-A.; Chaboissier, M.-C.; Pailhoux, E. Involvement of FOXL2 and RSPO1 in Ovarian Determination, Development, and Maintenance in Mammals. *Sex. Dev.* **2016**, *10*, 167–184. [CrossRef]
17. Stevenson, D.K.; Verter, J.; Fanaro, A.A.; Oh, W.; Ehrenkranz, R.A.; Shankaran, S.; Donovan, E.F.; Wright, L.L.; Lemons, J.A.; Tyson, J.E.; et al. Sex Differences in Outcomes of Very Low Birthweight Infants: The Newborn Male Disadvantage. *Arch. Dis. Child. Fetal Neonatal* **2000**, *83*, F182–F185. [CrossRef]
18. Orzack, S.H.; Stubblefield, J.W.; Akmaev, V.R.; Colls, P.; Munné, S.; Scholl, T.; Steinsaltz, D.; Zuckerman, J.E. The Human Sex Ratio from Conception to Birth. *Proc. Natl. Acad. Sci. USA* **2015**, *112*, E2102–E2111. [CrossRef]
19. Chao, F.; Gerland, P.; Cook, A.R.; Alkema, L. Systematic Assessment of the Sex Ratio at Birth for All Countries and Estimation of National Imbalances and Regional Reference Levels. *Proc. Natl. Acad. Sci. USA* **2019**, *116*, 9303–9311. [CrossRef]
20. American College of Obstetricians and Gynecologists' Committee on Practice Bulletins—Gynecology. ACOG Practice Bulletin No. 200: Early Pregnancy Loss. *Obstet. Gynecol.* **2018**, *132*, e197. [CrossRef]
21. Wilcox, A.J.; Weinberg, C.R.; O'Connor, J.F.; Baird, D.D.; Schlatterer, J.P.; Canfield, R.E.; Armstrong, E.G.; Nisula, B.C. Incidence of Early Loss of Pregnancy. *N. Engl. J. Med.* **1988**, *319*, 189–194. [CrossRef]
22. Wang, X.; Chen, C.; Wang, L.; Chen, D.; Guang, W.; French, J. Conception, Early Pregnancy Loss, and Time to Clinical Pregnancy: A Population-Based Prospective Study. *Fertil. Steril.* **2003**, *79*, 577–584. [CrossRef]
23. Griebel, C.P.; Halvorsen, J.; Golemon, T.B.; Day, A.A. Management of Spontaneous Abortion. *Am. Fam. Physician* **2005**, *72*, 1243–1250.
24. Eiben, B.; Bartels, I.; Bähr-Porsch, S.; Borgmann, S.; Gatz, G.; Gellert, G.; Goebel, R.; Hammans, W.; Hentemann, M.; Osmers, R. Cytogenetic Analysis of 750 Spontaneous Abortions with the Direct-Preparation Method of Chorionic Villi and Its Implications for Studying Genetic Causes of Pregnancy Wastage. *Am. J. Hum. Genet.* **1990**, *47*, 656–663.
25. Cheng, H.-H.; Ou, C.-Y.; Tsai, C.-C.; Chang, S.-D.; Hsiao, P.-Y.; Lan, K.-C.; Hsu, T.-Y. Chromosome Distribution of Early Miscarriages with Present or Absent Embryos: Female Predominance. *J. Assist. Reprod. Genet.* **2014**, *31*, 1059–1064. [CrossRef]
26. Del Fabro, A.; Driul, L.; Anis, O.; Londero, A.P.; Bertozzi, S.; Bortotto, L.; Marchesoni, D. Fetal Gender Ratio in Recurrent Miscarriages. *Int. J. Womens Health* **2011**, *3*, 213–217. [CrossRef]
27. Lathi, R.B.; Gustin, S.L.F.; Keller, J.; Maisenbacher, M.K.; Sigurjonsson, S.; Tao, R.; Demko, Z. Reliability of 46,XX Results on Miscarriage Specimens: A Review of 1222 First-Trimester Miscarriage Specimens. *Fertil. Steril.* **2014**, *101*, 178–182. [CrossRef]
28. Tricomi, V.; Serr, D.; Solish, G. The Ratio of Male to Female Embryos as Determined by the Sex Chromatin. *Am. J. Obstet. Gynecol.* **1960**, *79*, 504–509. [CrossRef]
29. Byrne, J.; Warburton, D.; Opitz, J.M.; Reynolds, J.F. Male Excess among Anatomically Normal Fetuses in Spontaneous Abortions. *Am. J. Med. Genet.* **1987**, *26*, 605–611. [CrossRef]
30. Mizuno, R. The Male/Female Ratio of Fetal Deaths and Births in Japan. *Lancet* **2000**, *356*, 738–739. [CrossRef]
31. Jakobovits, Á.A. Sex Ratio of Spontaneously Aborted Fetuses and Delivered Neonates in Second Trimester. *Eur. J. Obstet. Gynecol. Reprod. Biol.* **1991**, *40*, 211–213. [CrossRef]
32. Van den Hof, M.C.; Demanczuk, N. No. 192-Fetal Sex Determination and Disclosure Policy Statement. *J. Obstet. Gynaecol. Can.* **2017**, *39*, e65–e66. [CrossRef]
33. Practice Bulletin No. 175: Ultrasound in Pregnancy. *Obstet. Gynecol.* **2016**, *128*, e241. [CrossRef] [PubMed]
34. Acog Practice Bulletin: No 24, Feb 2001, Management of Recurrent Early Pregnancy Loss. *Int. J. Gynecol. Obstet.* **2002**, *78*, 179–190. [CrossRef]
35. Maithripala, S.; Durland, U.; Havelock, J.; Kashyap, S.; Hitkari, J.; Tan, J.; Iews, M.; Lisonkova, S.; Bedaiwy, M.A. Prevalence and Treatment Choices for Couples with Recurrent Pregnancy Loss Due to Structural Chromosomal Anomalies. *J. Obstet. Gynaecol. Can.* **2018**, *40*, 655–662. [CrossRef]
36. Ford, H.B.; Schust, D.J. Recurrent Pregnancy Loss: Etiology, Diagnosis, and Therapy. *Rev. Obstet. Gynecol.* **2009**, *2*, 76–83.
37. Robinson, W.P.; McFadden, D.E.; Stephenson, M.D. The Origin of Abnormalities in Recurrent Aneuploidy/Polyploidy. *Am. J. Hum. Genet.* **2001**, *69*, 1245–1254. [CrossRef]
38. Stephenson, M.D.; Awartani, K.A.; Robinson, W.P. Cytogenetic Analysis of Miscarriages from Couples with Recurrent Miscarriage: A Case–Control Study. *Hum. Reprod.* **2002**, *17*, 446–451. [CrossRef]
39. Brown, S. Miscarriage and Its Associations. *Semin. Reprod. Med.* **2008**, *26*, 391–400. [CrossRef]
40. Kalousek, D.K.; Vekemans, M. Confined Placental Mosaicism. *J. Med. Genet.* **1996**, *33*, 529–533. [CrossRef] [PubMed]
41. Yong, P.J.; Barrett, I.J.; Kalousek, D.K.; Robinson, W.P. Clinical Aspects, Prenatal Diagnosis, and Pathogenesis of Trisomy 16 Mosaicism. *J. Med. Genet.* **2003**, *40*, 175–182. [CrossRef]
42. Huether, C.A.; Martin, R.L.; Stoppelman, S.M.; D'Souza, S.; Bishop, J.K.; Torfs, C.P.; Lorey, F.; May, K.M.; Hanna, J.S.; Baird, P.A.; et al. Sex Ratios in Fetuses and Liveborn Infants with Autosomal Aneuploidy. *Am. J. Med. Genet.* **1996**, *63*, 492–500. [CrossRef]
43. Niedrist, D.; Riegel, M.; Achermann, J.; Rousson, V.; Schinzel, A. Trisomy 18: Changes in Sex Ratio during Intrauterine Life. *Am. J. Med. Genet. A* **2006**, *140A*, 2365–2367. [CrossRef]
44. Kalousek, D.K.; Barrett, I.J.; McGillivray, B.C. Placental Mosaicism and Intrauterine Survival of Trisomies 13 and 18. *Am. J. Hum. Genet.* **1989**, *44*, 338–343. [PubMed]
45. Hook, E.B.; Cross, P.K.; Mutton, D.E. Female Predominance (Low Sex Ratio) in 47, +21 Mosaics. *Am. J. Med. Genet.* **1999**, *84*, 316–319. [CrossRef]

46. Mutton, D.; Alberman, E.; Hook, E.B. Cytogenetic and Epidemiological Findings in Down Syndrome, England and Wales 1989 to 1993. National Down Syndrome Cytogenetic Register and the Association of Clinical Cytogeneticists. *J. Med. Genet.* **1996**, *33*, 387–394. [CrossRef]
47. Bastek, J.A.; Gómez, L.M.; Elovitz, M.A. The Role of Inflammation and Infection in Preterm Birth. *Clin. Perinatol.* **2011**, *38*, 385–406. [CrossRef]
48. Lawn, J.E.; Gravett, M.G.; Nunes, T.M.; Rubens, C.E.; Stanton, C.; The GAPPS Review Group. Global Report on Preterm Birth and Stillbirth (1 of 7): Definitions, Description of the Burden and Opportunities to Improve Data. *BMC Pregnancy Childbirth* **2010**, *10*, S1. [CrossRef]
49. Goldenberg, R.L.; Culhane, J.F.; Iams, J.D.; Romero, R. Epidemiology and Causes of Preterm Birth. *Lancet* **2008**, *371*, 75–84. [CrossRef]
50. Hall, M.H.; Carr-Hill, R. Impact of Sex Ratio on Onset and Management of Labour. *Br. Med. J. Clin. Res. Ed.* **1982**, *285*, 401–403. [CrossRef]
51. Cooperstock, M.; Campbell, J. Excess Males in Preterm Birth: Interactions with Gestational Age, Race, and Multiple Birth. *Obstet. Gynecol.* **1996**, *88*, 189–193. [CrossRef]
52. Astolfi, P.; Zonta, L.A. Risks of Preterm Delivery and Association with Maternal Age, Birth Order, and Fetal Gender. *Hum. Reprod.* **1999**, *14*, 2891–2894. [CrossRef] [PubMed]
53. Di Renzo, G.C.; Rosati, A.; Sarti, R.D.; Cruciani, L.; Cutuli, A.M. Does Fetal Sex Affect Pregnancy Outcome? *Gend. Med.* **2007**, *4*, 19–30. [CrossRef]
54. Zeitlin, J.; Saurel-Cubizolles, M.-J.; de Mouzon, J.; Rivera, L.; Ancel, P.-Y.; Blondel, B.; Kaminski, M. Fetal Sex and Preterm Birth: Are Males at Greater Risk? *Hum. Reprod.* **2002**, *17*, 2762–2768. [CrossRef]
55. Melamed, N.; Yogev, Y.; Glezerman, M. Fetal Gender and Pregnancy Outcome. *J. Matern. Fetal Neonatal Med. Off. J. Eur. Assoc. Perinat. Med. Fed. Asia Ocean. Perinat. Soc. Int. Soc. Perinat. Obstet.* **2010**, *23*, 338–344. [CrossRef] [PubMed]
56. Peelen, M.J.C.S.; Kazemier, B.M.; Ravelli, A.C.J.; Groot, C.J.M.D.; Post, J.A.M.V.D.; Mol, B.W.J.; Hajenius, P.J.; Kok, M. Impact of Fetal Gender on the Risk of Preterm Birth, a National Cohort Study. *Acta Obstet. Gynecol. Scand.* **2016**, *95*, 1034–1041. [CrossRef]
57. Aibar, L.; Puertas, A.; Valverde, M.; Carrillo, M.P.; Montoya, F. Fetal Sex and Perinatal Outcomes. *J. Perinat. Med.* **2012**, *40*, 271–276. [CrossRef] [PubMed]
58. Vatten, L.J.; Skjærven, R. Offspring Sex and Pregnancy Outcome by Length of Gestation. *Early Hum. Dev.* **2004**, *76*, 47–54. [CrossRef] [PubMed]
59. Brettell, R.; Yeh, P.S.; Impey, L.W.M. Examination of the Association between Male Gender and Preterm Delivery. *Eur. J. Obstet. Gynecol. Reprod. Biol.* **2008**, *141*, 123–126. [CrossRef]
60. Zeitlin, J.; Ancel, P.-Y.; Larroque, B.; Kaminski, M.; The EPIPAGE Group. Fetal Sex and Indicated Very Preterm Birth: Results of the EPIPAGE Study. *Am. J. Obstet. Gynecol.* **2004**, *190*, 1322–1325. [CrossRef]
61. Dehaene, I.; Scheire, E.; Steen, J.; De Coen, K.; Decruyenaere, J.; Smets, K.; Roelens, K. Obstetrical Characteristics and Neonatal Outcome According to Aetiology of Preterm Birth: A Cohort Study. *Arch. Gynecol. Obstet.* **2020**, *302*, 861–871. [CrossRef]
62. Verburg, P.E.; Tucker, G.; Scheil, W.; Erwich, J.J.H.M.; Dekker, G.A.; Roberts, C.T. Sexual Dimorphism in Adverse Pregnancy Outcomes—A Retrospective Australian Population Study 1981-2011. *PLoS ONE* **2016**, *11*, e0158807. [CrossRef]
63. Binet, M.-E.; Bujold, E.; Lefebvre, F.; Tremblay, Y.; Piedboeuf, B.; Canadian Neonatal Network™. Role of Gender in Morbidity and Mortality of Extremely Premature Neonates. *Am. J. Perinatol.* **2012**, *29*, 159–166. [CrossRef]
64. Shim, S.-Y.; Cho, S.J.; Kong, K.A.; Park, E.A. Gestational Age-Specific Sex Difference in Mortality and Morbidities of Preterm Infants: A Nationwide Study. *Sci. Rep.* **2017**, *7*, 6161. [CrossRef] [PubMed]
65. Ito, M.; Tamura, M.; Namba, F.; Neonatal Research Network of Japan. Role of Sex in Morbidity and Mortality of Very Premature Neonates. *Pediatr. Int. Off. J. Jpn. Pediatr. Soc.* **2017**, *59*, 898–905. [CrossRef] [PubMed]
66. Garfinkle, J.; Yoon, E.W.; Alvaro, R.; Nwaesei, C.; Claveau, M.; Lee, S.K.; Shah, P.S.; Canadian Neonatal Network Investigators. Trends in Sex-Specific Differences in Outcomes in Extreme Preterms: Progress or Natural Barriers? *Arch. Dis. Child. Fetal Neonatal Ed.* **2020**, *105*, 158–163. [CrossRef] [PubMed]
67. Teoh, P.J.; Ridout, A.; Seed, P.; Tribe, R.M.; Shennan, A.H. Gender and Preterm Birth: Is Male Fetal Gender a Clinically Important Risk Factor for Preterm Birth in High-Risk Women? *Eur. J. Obstet. Gynecol. Reprod. Biol.* **2018**, *225*, 155–159. [CrossRef]
68. Kildea, S.V.; Gao, Y.; Rolfe, M.; Boyle, J.; Tracy, S.; Barclay, L.M. Risk Factors for Preterm, Low Birthweight and Small for Gestational Age Births among Aboriginal Women from Remote Communities in Northern Australia. *Women Birth* **2017**, *30*, 398–405. [CrossRef]
69. Khalil, M.M.; Alzahra, E. Fetal Gender and Pregnancy Outcomes in Libya: A Retrospective Study. *Libyan J. Med.* **2013**, *8*, 20008. [CrossRef]
70. Peelen, M.J.C.S.; Kazemier, B.M.; Ravelli, A.C.J.; de Groot, C.J.M.; van der Post, J.A.M.; Mol, B.W.J.; Kok, M.; Hajenius, P.J. Ethnic Differences in the Impact of Male Fetal Gender on the Risk of Spontaneous Preterm Birth. *J. Perinatol.* **2021**. [CrossRef]
71. Ingemarsson, I. Gender Aspects of Preterm Birth. *BJOG Int. J. Obstet. Gynaecol.* **2003**, *110*, 34–38. [CrossRef]
72. Lao, T.T.; Sahota, D.S.; Suen, S.S.H.; Law, L.W.; Law, T.Y. The Impact of Fetal Gender on Preterm Birth in a Southern Chinese Population. *J. Matern. Fetal Neonatal Med.* **2011**, *24*, 1440–1443. [CrossRef]
73. Hou, L.; Wang, X.; Li, G.; Zou, L.; Chen, Y.; Zhang, W. Cross Sectional Study in China: Fetal Gender Has Adverse Perinatal Outcomes in Mainland China. *BMC Pregnancy Childbirth* **2014**, *14*, 372. [CrossRef] [PubMed]

74. Wilms, F.F.; Vis, J.Y.; Oudijk, M.A.; Kwee, A.; Porath, M.M.; Scheepers, H.C.J.; Spaanderman, M.E.A.; Bloemenkamp, K.W.M.; Bolte, A.C.; Bax, C.J.; et al. The Impact of Fetal Gender and Ethnicity on the Risk of Spontaneous Preterm Delivery in Women with Symptoms of Preterm Labor. *J. Matern. Fetal Neonatal Med. Off. J. Eur. Assoc. Perinat. Med. Fed. Asia Ocean. Perinat. Soc. Int. Soc. Perinat. Obstet.* **2016**, *29*, 3563–3569. [CrossRef]
75. Gordijn, S.J.; Beune, I.M.; Thilaganathan, B.; Papageorghiou, A.; Baschat, A.A.; Baker, P.N.; Silver, R.M.; Wynia, K.; Ganzevoort, W. Consensus Definition of Fetal Growth Restriction: A Delphi Procedure. *Ultrasound Obstet. Gynecol.* **2016**, *48*, 333–339. [CrossRef] [PubMed]
76. Alberry, M.; Soothill, P. Management of Fetal Growth Restriction. *Arch. Dis. Child. Fetal Neonatal Ed.* **2007**, *92*, F62–F67. [CrossRef]
77. Iams, J.D. Small for Gestational Age (SGA) and Fetal Growth Restriction (FGR). *Am. J. Obstet. Gynecol.* **2010**, *202*, 513. [CrossRef] [PubMed]
78. Kramer, M.S. Determinants of Low Birth Weight: Methodological Assessment and Meta-Analysis. *Bull. World Health Organ.* **1987**, *65*, 663–737.
79. Spinillo, A.; Capuzzo, E.; Nicola, S.; Colonna, L.; Iasci, A.; Zara, C. Interaction between Fetal Gender and Risk Factors for Fetal Growth Retardation. *Am. J. Obstet. Gynecol.* **1994**, *171*, 1273–1277. [CrossRef]
80. Yunis, K.A.; Beydoun, H.; Tamim, H.; Nassif, Y.; Khogali, M.; National Collaborative Perinatal Neonatal Network. Risk Factors for Term or Near-Term Fetal Growth Restriction in the Absence of Maternal Complications. *Am. J. Perinatol.* **2004**, *21*, 227–234. [CrossRef]
81. Voigt, M.; Hermanussen, M.; Wittwer-Backofen, U.; Fusch, C.; Hesse, V. Sex-Specific Differences in Birth Weight Due to Maternal Smoking during Pregnancy. *Eur. J. Pediatr.* **2006**, *165*, 757–761. [CrossRef]
82. Clifton, V.L. Sexually Dimorphic Effects of Maternal Asthma during Pregnancy on Placental Glucocorticoid Metabolism and Fetal Growth. *Cell Tissue Res.* **2005**, *322*, 63–71. [CrossRef]
83. Volpe, G.; Ioannou, C.; Cavallaro, A.; Vannuccini, S.; Ruiz-Martinez, S.; Impey, L. The Influence of Fetal Sex on the Antenatal Diagnosis of Small for Gestational Age. *J. Matern. Fetal Neonatal Med.* **2019**, *32*, 1832–1837. [CrossRef]
84. Vayssière, C.; Sentilhes, L.; Ego, A.; Bernard, C.; Cambourieu, D.; Flamant, C.; Gascoin, G.; Gaudineau, A.; Grangé, G.; Houfflin-Debarge, V.; et al. Fetal Growth Restriction and Intra-Uterine Growth Restriction: Guidelines for Clinical Practice from the French College of Gynaecologists and Obstetricians. *Eur. J. Obstet. Gynecol. Reprod. Biol.* **2015**, *193*, 10–18. [CrossRef] [PubMed]
85. Monier, I.; Blondel, B.; Ego, A.; Kaminski, M.; Goffinet, F.; Zeitlin, J. Does the Presence of Risk Factors for Fetal Growth Restriction Increase the Probability of Antenatal Detection? A French National Study. *Paediatr. Perinat. Epidemiol.* **2016**, *30*, 46–55. [CrossRef] [PubMed]
86. Sovio, U.; Smith, G.C.S. The Effect of Customization and Use of a Fetal Growth Standard on the Association between Birthweight Percentile and Adverse Perinatal Outcome. *Am. J. Obstet. Gynecol.* **2018**, *218*, S738–S744. [CrossRef] [PubMed]
87. Bernstein, I.M.; Horbar, J.D.; Badger, G.J.; Ohlsson, A.; Golan, A. Morbidity and Mortality among Very-Low-Birth-Weight Neonates with Intrauterine Growth Restriction. *Am. J. Obstet. Gynecol.* **2000**, *182*, 198–206. [CrossRef]
88. Quiñones, J.N.; Stamilio, D.M.; Coassolo, K.M.; Macones, G.A.; Odibo, A.O. Is Fetal Gender Associated with Adverse Perinatal Outcome in Intrauterine Growth Restriction (IUGR)? *Am. J. Obstet. Gynecol.* **2005**, *193*, 1233–1237. [CrossRef]
89. Magee, L.A.; Pels, A.; Helewa, M.; Rey, E.; von Dadelszen, P.; Magee, L.A.; Audibert, F.; Bujold, E.; Côté, A.-M.; Douglas, M.J.; et al. Diagnosis, Evaluation, and Management of the Hypertensive Disorders of Pregnancy: Executive Summary. *J. Obstet. Gynaecol. Can.* **2014**, *36*, 416–438. [CrossRef]
90. Brown, M.A.; Magee, L.A.; Kenny, L.C.; Karumanchi, S.A.; McCarthy, F.P.; Saito, S.; Hall, D.R.; Warren, C.E.; Adoyi, G.; Ishaku, S. Hypertensive Disorders of Pregnancy. *Hypertension* **2018**, *72*, 24–43. [CrossRef]
91. Redman, C.W. Early and Late Onset Preeclampsia: Two Sides of the Same Coin. *Pregnancy Hypertens. Int. J. Womens Cardiovasc. Health* **2017**, *7*, 58. [CrossRef]
92. Staff, A.C. The Two-Stage Placental Model of Preeclampsia: An Update. *J. Reprod. Immunol.* **2019**, *134–135*, 1–10. [CrossRef]
93. Elsmén, E.; Källén, K.; Maršál, K.; Hellström-Westas, L. Fetal Gender and Gestational-Age-Related Incidence of Pre-Eclampsia. *Acta Obstet. Gynecol. Scand.* **2006**, *85*, 1285–1291. [CrossRef] [PubMed]
94. Schalekamp-Timmermans, S.; Arends, L.R.; Alsaker, E.; Chappell, L.; Hansson, S.; Harsem, N.K.; Jälmby, M.; Jeyabalan, A.; Laivuori, H.; Lawlor, D.A.; et al. Fetal Sex-Specific Differences in Gestational Age at Delivery in Pre-Eclampsia: A Meta-Analysis. *Int. J. Epidemiol.* **2017**. [CrossRef]
95. Aliyu, M.H.; Salihu, H.M.; Lynch, O.; Alio, A.P.; Marty, P.J. Fetal Sex and Differential Survival in Preeclampsia and Eclampsia. *Arch. Gynecol. Obstet.* **2012**, *285*, 361–365. [CrossRef] [PubMed]
96. Basso, O.; Olsen, J. Sex Ratio and Twinning in Women With Hyperemesis or Pre-Eclampsia. *Epidemiology* **2001**, *12*, 747–749. [CrossRef] [PubMed]
97. Liu, Y.; Li, G.; Zhang, W. Effect of Fetal Gender on Pregnancy Outcomes in Northern China. *J. Matern. Fetal Neonatal Med.* **2017**, *30*, 858–863. [CrossRef] [PubMed]
98. Shiozaki, A.; Matsuda, Y.; Satoh, S.; Saito, S. Impact of Fetal Sex in Pregnancy-Induced Hypertension and Preeclampsia in Japan. *J. Reprod. Immunol.* **2011**, *89*, 133–139. [CrossRef] [PubMed]
99. Leduc, L. Guideline No. 394-Stillbirth Investigation. *J. Obstet. Gynaecol. Can.* **2020**, *42*, 92–99. [CrossRef]
100. Korteweg, F.J.; Gordijn, S.J.; Timmer, A.; Holm, J.P.; Ravisé, J.M.; Erwich, J.J.H.M. A Placental Cause of Intra-Uterine Fetal Death Depends on the Perinatal Mortality Classification System Used. *Placenta* **2008**, *29*, 71–80. [CrossRef]

101. Fretts, R.C. Etiology and Prevention of Stillbirth. *Am. J. Obstet. Gynecol.* **2005**, *193*, 1923–1935. [CrossRef]
102. Management of Stillbirth: Obstetric Care Consensus No, 10 Summary. *Obstet. Gynecol.* **2020**, *135*, 747–751. [CrossRef]
103. Smith, G.C.S. Sex, Birth Weight, and the Risk of Stillbirth in Scotland, 1980–1996. *Am. J. Epidemiol.* **2000**, *151*, 614–619. [CrossRef]
104. Dunn, L.; Prior, T.; Greer, R.; Kumar, S. Gender Specific Intrapartum and Neonatal Outcomes for Term Babies. *Eur. J. Obstet. Gynecol. Reprod. Biol.* **2015**, *185*, 19–22. [CrossRef]
105. Saleem, S.; Naqvi, F.; McClure, E.M.; Nowak, K.J.; Tikmani, S.S.; Garces, A.L.; Hibberd, P.L.; Moore, J.L.; Nolen, T.L.; Goudar, S.S.; et al. Neonatal Deaths in Infants Born Weighing ≥ 2500 g in Low and Middle-Income Countries. *Reprod. Health* **2020**, *17*, 158. [CrossRef] [PubMed]
106. Engel, P.J.; Smith, R.; Brinsmead, M.W.; Bowe, S.J.; Clifton, V.L. Male Sex and Pre-Existing Diabetes Are Independent Risk Factors for Stillbirth. *Aust. N. Z. J. Obstet. Gynaecol.* **2008**, *48*, 375–383. [CrossRef]
107. Aghai, Z.H.; Goudar, S.S.; Patel, A.; Saleem, S.; Dhaded, S.M.; Kavi, A.; Lalakia, P.; Naqvi, F.; Hibberd, P.L.; McClure, E.M.; et al. Gender Variations in Neonatal and Early Infant Mortality in India and Pakistan: A Secondary Analysis from the Global Network Maternal Newborn Health Registry. *Reprod. Health* **2020**, *17*, 178. [CrossRef] [PubMed]
108. Weng, Y.-H.; Yang, C.-Y.; Chiu, Y.-W. Neonatal Outcomes in Relation to Sex Differences: A National Cohort Survey in Taiwan. *Biol. Sex Differ.* **2015**, *6*, 30. [CrossRef]
109. Hadar, E.; Melamed, N.; Sharon-Weiner, M.; Hazan, S.; Rabinerson, D.; Glezerman, M.; Yogev, Y. The Association between Stillbirth and Fetal Gender. *J. Matern. Fetal Neonatal Med.* **2012**, *25*, 158–161. [CrossRef]
110. Nwosu, E.C.; Kumar, B.; El-Sayed, M.; Sa, E. Is Fetal Gender Significant in the Perinatal Outcome of Pregnancies Complicated by Placental Abruption? *J. Obstet. Gynaecol.* **1999**, *19*, 612–614. [CrossRef]
111. Tang, W.W.C.; Dietmann, S.; Irie, N.; Leitch, H.G.; Floros, V.I.; Bradshaw, C.R.; Hackett, J.A.; Chinnery, P.F.; Surani, M.A. A Unique Gene Regulatory Network Resets the Human Germline Epigenome for Development. *Cell* **2015**, *161*, 1453–1467. [CrossRef]
112. Zhou, Q.; Wang, T.; Leng, L.; Zheng, W.; Huang, J.; Fang, F.; Yang, L.; Chen, F.; Lin, G.; Wang, W.-J.; et al. Single-Cell RNA-Seq Reveals Distinct Dynamic Behavior of Sex Chromosomes during Early Human Embryogenesis. *Mol. Reprod. Dev.* **2019**, *86*, 871–882. [CrossRef] [PubMed]
113. Petropoulos, S.; Edsgärd, D.; Reinius, B.; Deng, Q.; Panula, S.P.; Codeluppi, S.; Plaza Reyes, A.; Linnarsson, S.; Sandberg, R.; Lanner, F. Single-Cell RNA-Seq Reveals Lineage and X Chromosome Dynamics in Human Preimplantation Embryos. *Cell* **2016**, *165*, 1012–1026. [CrossRef]
114. Ray, P.F.; Conaghan, J.; Winston, R.M.L.; Handyside, A.H. Increased Number of Cells and Metabolic Activity in Male Human Preimplantation Embryos Following in Vitro Fertilization. *Reproduction* **1995**, *104*, 165–171. [CrossRef]
115. Alfarawati, S.; Fragouli, E.; Colls, P.; Stevens, J.; Gutiérrez-Mateo, C.; Schoolcraft, W.B.; Katz-Jaffe, M.G.; Wells, D. The Relationship between Blastocyst Morphology, Chromosomal Abnormality, and Embryo Gender. *Fertil. Steril.* **2011**, *95*, 520–524. [CrossRef] [PubMed]
116. Hentemann, M.A.; Briskemyr, S.; Bertheussen, K. Blastocyst Transfer and Gender: IVF versus ICSI. *J. Assist. Reprod. Genet.* **2009**, *26*, 433–436. [CrossRef]
117. Luna, M.; Duke, M.; Copperman, A.; Grunfeld, L.; Sandler, B.; Barritt, J. Blastocyst Embryo Transfer Is Associated with a Sex-Ratio Imbalance in Favor of Male Offspring. *Fertil. Steril.* **2007**, *87*, 519–523. [CrossRef]
118. Peippo, J.; Bredbacka, P. Sex-Related Growth Rate Differences in Mouse Preimplantation Embryos in Vivo and in Vitro. *Mol. Reprod. Dev.* **1995**, *40*, 56–61. [CrossRef]
119. Kochhar, H.P.S.; Peippo, J.; King, W.A. Sex Related Embryo Development. *Theriogenology* **2001**, *55*, 3–14. [CrossRef]
120. Balaton, B.P.; Brown, C.J. Escape Artists of the X Chromosome. *Trends Genet.* **2016**, *32*, 348–359. [CrossRef]
121. Tukiainen, T.; Villani, A.-C.; Yen, A.; Rivas, M.A.; Marshall, J.L.; Satija, R.; Aguirre, M.; Gauthier, L.; Fleharty, M.; Kirby, A.; et al. Landscape of X Chromosome Inactivation across Human Tissues. *Nature* **2017**, *550*, 244–248. [CrossRef] [PubMed]
122. Carrel, L.; Willard, H.F. X-Inactivation Profile Reveals Extensive Variability in X-Linked Gene Expression in Females. *Nature* **2005**, *434*, 400–404. [CrossRef]
123. Sharp, A.J.; Stathaki, E.; Migliavacca, E.; Brahmachary, M.; Montgomery, S.B.; Dupre, Y.; Antonarakis, S.E. DNA Methylation Profiles of Human Active and Inactive X Chromosomes. *Genome Res.* **2011**, *21*, 1592–1600. [CrossRef] [PubMed]
124. Cotton, A.M.; Price, E.M.; Jones, M.J.; Balaton, B.P.; Kobor, M.S.; Brown, C.J. Landscape of DNA Methylation on the X Chromosome Reflects CpG Density, Functional Chromatin State and X-Chromosome Inactivation. *Hum. Mol. Genet.* **2015**, *24*, 1528–1539. [CrossRef] [PubMed]
125. Ehrlich, M.; Gama-Sosa, M.A.; Huang, L.H.; Midgett, R.M.; Kuo, K.C.; McCune, R.A.; Gehrke, C. Amount and Distribution of 5-Methylcytosine in Human DNA from Different Types of Tissues of Cells. *Nucleic Acids Res.* **1982**, *10*, 2709–2721. [CrossRef] [PubMed]
126. Cotton, A.M.; Avila, L.; Penaherrera, M.S.; Affleck, J.G.; Robinson, W.P.; Brown, C.J. Inactive X Chromosome-Specific Reduction in Placental DNA Methylation. *Hum. Mol. Genet.* **2009**, *18*, 3544–3552. [CrossRef]
127. de Mello, J.C.M.; de Araújo, É.S.S.; Stabellini, R.; Fraga, A.M.; de Souza, J.E.S.; Sumita, D.R.; Camargo, A.A.; Pereira, L.V. Random X Inactivation and Extensive Mosaicism in Human Placenta Revealed by Analysis of Allele-Specific Gene Expression along the X Chromosome. *PLoS ONE* **2010**, *5*, e10947. [CrossRef]

128. Peñaherrera, M.S.; Jiang, R.; Avila, L.; Yuen, R.K.C.; Brown, C.J.; Robinson, W.P. Patterns of Placental Development Evaluated by X Chromosome Inactivation Profiling Provide a Basis to Evaluate the Origin of Epigenetic Variation. *Hum. Reprod.* **2012**, *27*, 1745–1753. [CrossRef] [PubMed]
129. Brown, C.J.; Robinson, W.P. The Causes and Consequences of Random and Non-Random X Chromosome Inactivation in Humans. *Clin. Genet.* **2000**, *58*, 353–363. [CrossRef]
130. Peñaherrera, M.S.; Ma, S.; Ho Yuen, B.; Brown, C.J.; Robinson, W.P. X-Chromosome Inactivation (XCI) Patterns in Placental Tissues of a Paternally Derived Bal t(X;20) Case. *Am. J. Med. Genet. A* **2003**, *118A*, 29–34. [CrossRef]
131. Arnold, A.P. A General Theory of Sexual Differentiation. *J. Neurosci. Res.* **2017**, *95*, 291–300. [CrossRef]
132. Arnold, A.P.; Chen, X. What Does the "Four Core Genotypes" Mouse Model Tell Us about Sex Differences in the Brain and Other Tissues? *Front. Neuroendocrinol.* **2009**, *30*, 1–9. [CrossRef]
133. Ishikawa, H.; Rattigan, A.; Fundele, R.; Burgoyne, P.S. Effects of Sex Chromosome Dosage on Placental Size in Mice. *Biol. Reprod.* **2003**, *69*, 483–488. [CrossRef]
134. García-Acero, M.; Moreno, O.; Suárez, F.; Rojas, A. Disorders of Sexual Development: Current Status and Progress in the Diagnostic Approach. *Curr. Urol.* **2019**, *13*, 169–178. [CrossRef]
135. Case, L.K.; Teuscher, C. Y Genetic Variation and Phenotypic Diversity in Health and Disease. *Biol. Sex Differ.* **2015**, *6*. [CrossRef]
136. Case, L.K.; Wall, E.H.; Dragon, J.A.; Saligrama, N.; Krementsov, D.N.; Moussawi, M.; Zachary, J.F.; Huber, S.A.; Blankenhorn, E.P.; Teuscher, C. The Y Chromosome as a Regulatory Element Shaping Immune Cell Transcriptomes and Susceptibility to Autoimmune Disease. *Genome Res.* **2013**, *23*, 1474–1485. [CrossRef]
137. Graves, J.A.M. Review: Sex Chromosome Evolution and the Expression of Sex-Specific Genes in the Placenta. *Placenta* **2010**, *31*, S27–S32. [CrossRef]
138. Linscheid, C.; Petroff, M.G. Minor Histocompatibility Antigens and the Maternal Immune Response to the Fetus During Pregnancy. *Am. J. Reprod. Immunol.* **2013**, *69*, 304–314. [CrossRef] [PubMed]
139. Nielsen, H.S.; Steffensen, R.; Varming, K.; Van Halteren, A.G.S.; Spierings, E.; Ryder, L.P.; Goulmy, E.; Christiansen, O.B. Association of HY-Restricting HLA Class II Alleles with Pregnancy Outcome in Patients with Recurrent Miscarriage Subsequent to a Firstborn Boy. *Hum. Mol. Genet.* **2009**, *18*, 1684–1691. [CrossRef] [PubMed]
140. Christiansen, O.B.; Pedersen, B.; Nielsen, H.S.; Nybo Andersen, A.-M. Impact of the Sex of First Child on the Prognosis in Secondary Recurrent Miscarriage. *Hum. Reprod.* **2004**, *19*, 2946–2951. [CrossRef] [PubMed]
141. Ooi, P.V.; Russell, N.; O'Donoghue, K. Secondary Recurrent Miscarriage Is Associated with Previous Male Birth. *J. Reprod. Immunol.* **2011**, *88*, 38–41. [CrossRef]
142. Li, J.; Liu, L.; Liu, B.; Saravelos, S.; Li, T. Recurrent Miscarriage and Birth Sex Ratio. *Eur. J. Obstet. Gynecol. Reprod. Biol.* **2014**, *176*, 55–59. [CrossRef]
143. Recurrent Miscarriage and Birth Sex Ratio-ClinicalKey. Available online: https://www-clinicalkey-com.ezproxy.library.ubc.ca/#!/content/playContent/1-s2.0-S030121151400102X?returnurl=null&referrer=null (accessed on 23 April 2021).
144. Christiansen, O.B.; Steffensen, R.; Nielsen, H.S. Anti-HY Responses in Pregnancy Disorders. *Am. J. Reprod. Immunol.* **2011**, *66*, 93–100. [CrossRef]
145. Mucci, L.A.; Lagiou, P.; Tamimi, R.M.; Hsieh, C.-C.; Adami, H.-O.; Trichopoulos, D. Pregnancy Estriol, Estradiol, Progesterone and Prolactin in Relation to Birth Weight and Other Birth Size Variables (United States). *Cancer Causes Control* **2003**, *14*, 311–318. [CrossRef] [PubMed]
146. Kaludjerovic, J.; Ward, W.E. The Interplay between Estrogen and Fetal Adrenal Cortex. *J. Nutr. Metab.* **2012**, *2012*, e837901. [CrossRef] [PubMed]
147. Bazzett, L.B.; Yaron, Y.; O'Brien, J.E.; Critchfield, G.; Kramer, R.L.; Ayoub, M.; Johnson, M.P.; Evans, M.I. Fetal Gender Impact on Multiple-Marker Screening Results. *Am. J. Med. Genet.* **1998**, *76*, 369–371. [CrossRef]
148. Troisi, R.; Potischman, N.; Roberts, J.M.; Harger, G.; Markovic, N.; Cole, B.; Lykins, D.; Siiteri, P.; Hoover, R.N. Correlation of Serum Hormone Concentrations in Maternal and Umbilical Cord Samples. *Cancer Epidemiol. Prev. Biomark.* **2003**, *12*, 452–456.
149. Belgorosky, A.; Guercio, G.; Pepe, C.; Saraco, N.; Rivarola, M.A. Genetic and Clinical Spectrum of Aromatase Deficiency in Infancy, Childhood and Adolescence. *Horm. Res. Paediatr.* **2009**, *72*, 321–330. [CrossRef]
150. Berkane, N.; Liere, P.; Lefevre, G.; Alfaidy, N.; Nahed, R.A.; Vincent, J.; Oudinet, J.-P.; Pianos, A.; Cambourg, A.; Rozenberg, P.; et al. Abnormal Steroidogenesis and Aromatase Activity in Preeclampsia. *Placenta* **2018**, *69*, 40–49. [CrossRef]
151. Perez-Sepulveda, A.; Monteiro, L.J.; Dobierzewska, A.; España-Perrot, P.P.; Venegas-Araneda, P.; Guzmán-Rojas, A.M.; González, M.I.; Palominos-Rivera, M.; Irarrazabal, C.E.; Figueroa-Diesel, H.; et al. Placental Aromatase Is Deficient in Placental Ischemia and Preeclampsia. *PLoS ONE* **2015**, *10*, e0139682. [CrossRef]
152. Shimodaira, M.; Nakayama, T.; Sato, I.; Sato, N.; Izawa, N.; Mizutani, Y.; Furuya, K.; Yamamoto, T. Estrogen Synthesis Genes CYP19A1, HSD3B1, and HSD3B2 in Hypertensive Disorders of Pregnancy. *Endocrine* **2012**, *42*, 700–707. [CrossRef]
153. Mesiano, S.; Welsh, T.N. Steroid Hormone Control of Myometrial Contractility and Parturition. *Semin. Cell Dev. Biol.* **2007**, *18*, 321–331. [CrossRef] [PubMed]
154. Warne, G.L.; Faiman, C.; Reyes, F.I.; Winter, J.S.D. Studies on Human Sexual Development. V. Concentrations of Testosterone, 17-Hydroxyprogesterone and Progesterone in Human Amniotic Fluid Throughout Gestation. *J. Clin. Endocrinol. Metab.* **1977**, *44*, 934–938. [CrossRef]

155. Siemienowicz, K.J.; Wang, Y.; Marečková, M.; Nio-Kobayashi, J.; Fowler, P.A.; Rae, M.T.; Duncan, W.C. Early Pregnancy Maternal Progesterone Administration Alters Pituitary and Testis Function and Steroid Profile in Male Fetuses. *Sci. Rep.* **2020**, *10*, 21920. [CrossRef]
156. Lajic, S.; Nordenström, A.; Ritzén, E.M.; Wedell, A. Prenatal Treatment of Congenital Adrenal Hyperplasia. *Eur. J. Endocrinol.* **2004**, *151* (Suppl. 3), U63–U69. [CrossRef]
157. Garner, P.R. Congenital Adrenal Hyperplasia in Pregnancy. *Semin Perinatol* **1998**, *22*, 446–456. [CrossRef]
158. Reisch, N.; Taylor, A.E.; Nogueira, E.F.; Asby, D.J.; Dhir, V.; Berry, A.; Krone, N.; Auchus, R.J.; Shackleton, C.H.L.; Hanley, N.A.; et al. Alternative Pathway Androgen Biosynthesis and Human Fetal Female Virilization. *Proc. Natl. Acad. Sci. USA* **2019**, *116*, 22294–22299. [CrossRef] [PubMed]
159. Meakin, A.S.; Saif, Z.; Tuck, A.R.; Clifton, V.L. Human Placental Androgen Receptor Variants: Potential Regulators of Male Fetal Growth. *Placenta* **2019**, *80*, 18–26. [CrossRef] [PubMed]
160. Wilson, J.D.; George, F.W.; Griffin, J.E. The Hormonal Control of Sexual Development. *Science* **1981**, *211*, 1278–1284. [CrossRef] [PubMed]
161. Smail, P.J.; Reyes, F.I.; Winter, J.S.D.; Faiman, C. The Fetal Hormonal Environment and its Effect on the Morphogenesis of the Genital System. In *Pediatric Andrology*; Kogan, S.J., Hafez, E.S.E., Eds.; Clinics in Andrology; Springer: Dordrecht, The Netherlands, 1981; pp. 9–19. ISBN 978-94-010-3719-8.
162. Auyeung, B.; Baron-Cohen, S.; Ashwin, E.; Knickmeyer, R.; Taylor, K.; Hackett, G.; Hines, M. Fetal Testosterone Predicts Sexually Differentiated Childhood Behavior in Girls and in Boys. *Psychol. Sci.* **2009**, *20*, 144–148. [CrossRef]
163. van de Beek, C.; van Goozen, S.H.M.; Buitelaar, J.K.; Cohen-Kettenis, P.T. Prenatal Sex Hormones (Maternal and Amniotic Fluid) and Gender-Related Play Behavior in 13-Month-Old Infants. *Arch. Sex. Behav.* **2009**, *38*, 6–15. [CrossRef]
164. Carson, D.J.; Okuno, A.; Lee, P.A.; Stetten, G.; Didolkar, S.M.; Migeon, C.J. Amniotic Fluid Steroid Levels: Fetuses With Adrenal Hyperplasia, 46,XYY Fetuses, and Normal Fetuses. *Am. J. Dis. Child.* **1982**, *136*, 218–222. [CrossRef]
165. Gonzalez, T.L.; Sun, T.; Koeppel, A.F.; Lee, B.; Wang, E.T.; Farber, C.R.; Rich, S.S.; Sundheimer, L.W.; Buttle, R.A.; Chen, Y.-D.I.; et al. Sex Differences in the Late First Trimester Human Placenta Transcriptome. *Biol. Sex Differ.* **2018**, *9*, 4. [CrossRef]
166. Buckberry, S.; Bianco-Miotto, T.; Bent, S.J.; Dekker, G.A.; Roberts, C.T. Integrative Transcriptome Meta-Analysis Reveals Widespread Sex-Biased Gene Expression at the Human Fetal–Maternal Interface. *Mol. Hum. Reprod.* **2014**, *20*, 810–819. [CrossRef] [PubMed]
167. Raznahan, A.; Parikshak, N.N.; Chandran, V.; Blumenthal, J.D.; Clasen, L.S.; Alexander-Bloch, A.F.; Zinn, A.R.; Wangsa, D.; Wise, J.; Murphy, D.G.M.; et al. Sex-Chromosome Dosage Effects on Gene Expression in Humans. *Proc. Natl. Acad. Sci. USA* **2018**, *115*, 7398–7403. [CrossRef]
168. Itoh, Y.; Arnold, A.P. X Chromosome Regulation of Autosomal Gene Expression in Bovine Blastocysts. *Chromosoma* **2014**, *123*, 481–489. [CrossRef] [PubMed]
169. Carrel, L.; Brown, C.J. When the Lyon(Ized Chromosome) Roars: Ongoing Expression from an Inactive X Chromosome. *Philos. Trans. R. Soc. Lond. B. Biol. Sci.* **2017**, *372*. [CrossRef] [PubMed]
170. Yaron, Y.; Lehavi, O.; Orr-Urtreger, A.; Gull, I.; Lessing, J.B.; Amit, A.; Ben-Yosef, D. Maternal Serum HCG Is Higher in the Presence of a Female Fetus as Early as Week 3 Post-Fertilization. *Hum. Reprod.* **2002**, *17*, 485–489. [CrossRef] [PubMed]
171. Adibi, J.J.; Lee, M.K.; Saha, S.; Boscardin, W.J.; Apfel, A.; Currier, R.J. Fetal Sex Differences in Human Chorionic Gonadotropin Fluctuate by Maternal Race, Age, Weight and by Gestational Age. *J. Dev. Orig. Health Dis.* **2015**, *6*, 493–500. [CrossRef]
172. Brouillet, S.; Hoffmann, P.; Chauvet, S.; Salomon, A.; Chamboredon, S.; Sergent, F.; Benharouga, M.; Feige, J.J.; Alfaidy, N. Revisiting the Role of HCG: New Regulation of the Angiogenic Factor EG-VEGF and Its Receptors. *Cell. Mol. Life Sci.* **2012**, *69*, 1537–1550. [CrossRef]
173. Clifton, V.L.; Murphy, V.E. Maternal Asthma as a Model for Examining Fetal Sex-Specific Effects on Maternal Physiology and Placental Mechanisms That Regulate Human Fetal Growth. *Placenta* **2004**, *25*, S45–S52. [CrossRef]
174. Stark, M.J.; Wright, I.M.R.; Clifton, V.L. Sex-Specific Alterations in Placental 11β-Hydroxysteroid Dehydrogenase 2 Activity and Early Postnatal Clinical Course Following Antenatal Betamethasone. *Am. J. Physiol.-Regul. Integr. Comp. Physiol.* **2009**, *297*, R510–R514. [CrossRef]
175. Jahanfar, S.; Lim, V. Is There a Relationship between Fetal Sex and Placental Pathological Characteristics in Twin Gestations? *BMC Pregnancy Childbirth* **2018**, *18*, 285. [CrossRef]
176. Mitchell, A.M.; Palettas, M.; Christian, L.M. Fetal Sex Is Associated with Maternal Stimulated Cytokine Production, but Not Serum Cytokine Levels, in Human Pregnancy. *Brain. Behav. Immun.* **2017**, *60*, 32–37. [CrossRef] [PubMed]
177. Brown, Z.A.; Schalekamp-Timmermans, S.; Tiemeier, H.W.; Hofman, A.; Jaddoe, V.W.V.; Steegers, E.A.P. Fetal Sex Specific Differences in Human Placentation: A Prospective Cohort Study. *Placenta* **2014**, *35*, 359–364. [CrossRef] [PubMed]
178. Spencer, K. The Influence of Fetal Sex in Screening for Down Syndrome in the Second Trimester Using AFP and Free β-HCG. *Prenat. Diagn.* **2000**, *20*, 648–651. [CrossRef]
179. Knippel, A.J. Role of Fetal Sex in Amniotic Fluid Alphafetoprotein Screening. *Prenat. Diagn.* **2002**, *22*, 941–945. [CrossRef]
180. Santolaya-Forgas, J.; Mahoney, M.; Abdallah, M.; Duncan, J.; Delgado, A.; Stang, P.; Deleon, J.; Castracane, V.D. Fetal Gender and Maternal Serum Screening Markers. *Genet. Med.* **2006**, *8*, 671–672. [CrossRef] [PubMed]
181. Iruretagoyena, J.I.; Grady, M.; Shah, D. Discrepancy in Fetal Sex Assignment between Cell Free Fetal DNA and Ultrasound. *J. Perinatol.* **2015**, *35*, 229–230. [CrossRef] [PubMed]

182. Manokhina, I.; Singh, T.K.; Robinson, W.P. Cell-Free Placental DNA in Maternal Plasma in Relation to Placental Health and Function. *Fetal Diagn. Ther.* **2017**, *41*, 258–264. [CrossRef]
183. Moser, G.; Drewlo, S.; Huppertz, B.; Armant, D.R. Trophoblast Retrieval and Isolation from the Cervix: Origins of Cervical Trophoblasts and Their Potential Value for Risk Assessment of Ongoing Pregnancies. *Hum. Reprod. Update* **2018**, *24*, 484–496. [CrossRef]
184. Chitayat, D.; Langlois, S.; Wilson, R.D.; Audibert, F.; Blight, C.; Brock, J.A.; Cartier, L.; Carroll, J.; Désilets, V.A.; Gagnon, A.; et al. Prenatal Screening for Fetal Aneuploidy in Singleton Pregnancies. *J. Obstet. Gynaecol. Can.* **2011**, *33*, 736–750. [CrossRef]
185. Cowans, N.J.; Stamatopoulou, A.; Maiz, N.; Spencer, K.; Nicolaides, K.H. The Impact of Fetal Gender on First Trimester Nuchal Translucency and Maternal Serum Free Beta-HCG and PAPP-A MoM in Normal and Trisomy 21 Pregnancies. *Prenat. Diagn.* **2009**, *29*, 578–581. [CrossRef]
186. Spong, C.Y.; Ghidini, A.; Stanley-Christian, H.; Meck, J.M.; Seydel, F.D.; Pezzullo, J.C. Risk of Abnormal Triple Screen for Down Syndrome Is Significantly Higher in Patients with Female Fetuses. *Prenat. Diagn.* **1999**, *19*, 337–339. [CrossRef]
187. Tancrède, S.; Bujold, E.; Giguère, Y.; Renald, M.-H.; Girouard, J.; Forest, J.-C. Mid-Trimester Maternal Serum AFP and HCG as Markers of Preterm and Term Adverse Pregnancy Outcomes. *J. Obstet. Gynaecol. Can.* **2015**, *37*, 111–116. [CrossRef]
188. Gaccioli, F.; Sovio, U.; Cook, E.; Hund, M.; Charnock-Jones, D.S.; Smith, G.C.S. Screening for Fetal Growth Restriction Using Ultrasound and the SFLT1/PlGF Ratio in Nulliparous Women: A Prospective Cohort Study. *Lancet Child Adolesc. Health* **2018**, *2*, 569–581. [CrossRef]
189. Sovio, U.; Gaccioli, F.; Cook, E.; Hund, M.; Charnock-Jones, D.S.; Smith, G.C.S. Prediction of Preeclampsia Using the Soluble Fms-Like Tyrosine Kinase 1 to Placental Growth Factor Ratio: A Prospective Cohort Study of Unselected Nulliparous Women. *Hypertens. Dallas Tex 1979* **2017**, *69*, 731–738. [CrossRef] [PubMed]
190. Ong, C.Y.; Liao, A.W.; Cacho, A.M.; Spencer, K.; Nicolaides, K.H. First-Trimester Maternal Serum Levels of Placenta Growth Factor as Predictor of Preeclampsia and Fetal Growth Restriction. *Obstet. Gynecol.* **2001**, *98*, 608–611. [CrossRef] [PubMed]
191. Andersen, L.B.; Jørgensen, J.S.; Herse, F.; Andersen, M.S.; Christesen, H.T.; Dechend, R. The Association between Angiogenic Markers and Fetal Sex: Implications for Preeclampsia Research. *J. Reprod. Immunol.* **2016**, *117*, 24–29. [CrossRef]
192. Enninga, E.A.L.; Nevala, W.K.; Creedon, D.J.; Markovic, S.N.; Holtan, S.G. Fetal Sex-Based Differences in Maternal Hormones, Angiogenic Factors, and Immune Mediators during Pregnancy and the Postpartum Period. *Am. J. Reprod. Immunol.* **2015**, *73*, 251–262. [CrossRef] [PubMed]
193. Hogg, K.; Blair, J.D.; von Dadelszen, P.; Robinson, W.P. Hypomethylation of the LEP Gene in Placenta and Elevated Maternal Leptin Concentration in Early Onset Pre-Eclampsia. *Mol. Cell. Endocrinol.* **2013**, *367*, 64–73. [CrossRef]
194. McCarthy, M.M.; Arnold, A.P.; Ball, G.F.; Blaustein, J.D.; Vries, G.J.D. Sex Differences in the Brain: The Not So Inconvenient Truth. *J. Neurosci.* **2012**, *32*, 2241–2247. [CrossRef] [PubMed]
195. Joel, D.; McCarthy, M.M. Incorporating Sex as a Biological Variable in Neuropsychiatric Research: Where Are We Now and Where Should We Be? Neuropsychopharmacology. *Neuropsychopharmacology* **2016**, *42*, 379–385. [CrossRef] [PubMed]
196. Joel, D. Beyond the Binary: Rethinking Sex and the Brain. *Neurosci. Biobehav. Rev.* **2021**, *122*, 165–175. [CrossRef] [PubMed]
197. Maney, D.L. Perils and Pitfalls of Reporting Sex Differences. *Philos. Trans. R. Soc. B Biol. Sci.* **2016**, *371*, 20150119. [CrossRef]
198. Konwar, C.; Del Gobbo, G.F.; Terry, J.; Robinson, W.P. Association of a Placental Interleukin-6 Genetic Variant (Rs1800796) with DNA Methylation, Gene Expression and Risk of Acute Chorioamnionitis. *BMC Med. Genet.* **2019**, *20*, 36. [CrossRef] [PubMed]
199. Li, J.; Hong, X.; Mesiano, S.; Muglia, L.J.; Wang, X.; Snyder, M.; Stevenson, D.K.; Shaw, G.M. Natural Selection Has Differentiated the Progesterone Receptor among Human Populations. *Am. J. Hum. Genet.* **2018**, *103*, 45–57. [CrossRef]
200. Bublitz, M.H.; Vergara-Lopez, C.; Treter, M.O.; Stroud, L.R. Lower Socioeconomic Position in Pregnancy Is Associated with Lower Diurnal Cortisol Production and Lower Birth Weight in Male Infants. *Clin. Ther.* **2016**, *38*, 265–274. [CrossRef]

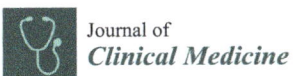

Review

Landscape of Preterm Birth Therapeutics and a Path Forward

Brahm Seymour Coler [1,2], Oksana Shynlova [3,4], Adam Boros-Rausch [3], Stephen Lye [3,4], Stephen McCartney [1], Kelycia B. Leimert [5], Wendy Xu [5], Sylvain Chemtob [6], David Olson [5,7], Miranda Li [1,8], Emily Huebner [1], Anna Curtin [1], Alisa Kachikis [1], Leah Savitsky [1], Jonathan W. Paul [9,10], Roger Smith [9,10,11] and Kristina M. Adams Waldorf [1,12,*]

1. Department of Obstetrics and Gynecology, University of Washington, Seattle, WA 98195, USA; brahm.coler@wsu.edu (B.S.C.); smccart@uw.edu (S.M.); miranda.li2@columbia.edu (M.L.); huebnem@uw.edu (E.H.); anna14@uw.edu (A.C.); abk26@uw.edu (A.K.); savitsky@uw.edu (L.S.)
2. Elson S. Floyd College of Medicine, Washington State University, Spokane, WA 99202, USA
3. Department of Physiology, University of Toronto, Toronto, ON M5S 1A8, Canada; shynlova@lunenfield.ca (O.S.); aboros@lunenfield.ca (A.B.-R.); lye@lunenfield.ca (S.L.)
4. Department of Obstetrics and Gynecology, University of Toronto, Toronto, ON M5G 1E2, Canada
5. Department of Obstetrics and Gynecology, University of Alberta, Edmonton, AB T6G 2R7, Canada; kelycia@ualberta.ca (K.B.L.); wendy2@ualberta.ca (W.X.); dmolson@ualberta.ca (D.O.)
6. Departments of Pediatrics, Université de Montréal, Montréal, QC H3T 1J4, Canada; sylvain.chemtob@gmail.com
7. Departments of Pediatrics and Physiology, University of Alberta, Edmonton, AB T6G 2S2, Canada
8. Department of Biological Sciences, Columbia University, New York, NY 10027, USA
9. Mothers and Babies Research Centre, School of Medicine and Public Health, College of Health, Medicine and Wellbeing, University of Newcastle, Callaghan, NSW 2308, Australia; jonathan.paul@newcastle.edu.au (J.W.P.); roger.smith@newcastle.edu.au (R.S.)
10. Hunter Medical Research Institute, 1 Kookaburra Circuit, New Lambton Heights, NSW 2305, Australia
11. John Hunter Hospital, New Lambton Heights, NSW 2305, Australia
12. Department of Global Health, University of Washington, Seattle, WA 98195, USA
* Correspondence: adamsk@uw.edu

Abstract: Preterm birth (PTB) remains the leading cause of infant morbidity and mortality. Despite 50 years of research, therapeutic options are limited and many lack clear efficacy. Tocolytic agents are drugs that briefly delay PTB, typically to allow antenatal corticosteroid administration for accelerating fetal lung maturity or to transfer patients to high-level care facilities. Globally, there is an unmet need for better tocolytic agents, particularly in low- and middle-income countries. Although most tocolytics, such as betamimetics and indomethacin, suppress downstream mediators of the parturition pathway, newer therapeutics are being designed to selectively target inflammatory checkpoints with the goal of providing broader and more effective tocolysis. However, the relatively small market for new PTB therapeutics and formidable regulatory hurdles have led to minimal pharmaceutical interest and a stagnant drug pipeline. In this review, we present the current landscape of PTB therapeutics, assessing the history of drug development, mechanisms of action, adverse effects, and the updated literature on drug efficacy. We also review the regulatory hurdles and other obstacles impairing novel tocolytic development. Ultimately, we present possible steps to expedite drug development and meet the growing need for effective preterm birth therapeutics.

Keywords: tocolytic; preterm birth; preterm labor; neonate; prematurity; pregnancy; therapeutic; progesterone; fetus

1. Introduction

Though preterm birth (PTB) is the leading cause of infant morbidity and mortality, it lacks clear therapeutic options. Approximately 15 million preterm neonates are born annually and more than 1 million die from subsequent complications within the following 5 years [1,2]. Adverse outcomes related to prematurity span a spectrum that includes neurodevelopmental (e.g., neurocognitive impairment, cerebral palsy, hearing impairments, and intellectual or motor disabilities), pulmonary (e.g., bronchopulmonary dysplasia) and ophthalmologic (e.g., retinopathy of immaturity) disorders that contribute to lifelong disability [3–5]. The earlier the gestational age at PTB, the greater the risk for prematurity-related adverse outcomes [6]. Thus, PTB presents a formidable health risk to the neonate and a compelling condition for which therapeutics could lessen the burden of disease and disability across a child's lifespan.

Tocolytic agents are drugs used to delay spontaneous preterm labor with intact membranes and comprise the focus of this review. We refer to tocolytic agents and select other drugs targeting other PTB pathways as 'preterm birth therapeutics'. Typically, these agents delay delivery only for a short time (i.e., 48 h or less; Table 1). The pathophysiology underlying PTB is multi-faceted yet largely predicated on premature activation of parturition pathways within the myometrium or placenta; many therapeutics are, therefore, tailored towards the specific etiologies of PTB. Historically, the approaches for reducing uterine contractions to delay PTB have followed two main pathways: (1) decreasing contractile proteins in the myometrium or (2) inhibiting the synthesis of myometrial stimulants [7]. A short delay prior to delivery can be crucial to provide an opportunity to administer antenatal corticosteroids to accelerate fetal lung development or to transfer the patient to a facility with neonatal intensive care [7]. Interestingly, most tocolytics have not been shown to be effective in improving neonatal outcomes, despite the efficacy in delaying PTB [8]. Combination therapies that involve tocolytic drugs and differing mechanisms of action are being studied, as it has been posited that combination therapy can not only improve the overall tocolytic impact but also reduce dosage, frequency of administration, and adverse effects [7]. Preliminary results from some studies, however, suggest no clear advantage for combination therapy over individual therapeutic administration [7]. Most tocolytics have been shown to be ineffective in further delaying PTB when used as maintenance therapy [9–13]. The choice for first-line tocolytic therapy is still controversial, as each class varies in effectiveness, safety profile, cost, and availability.

Globally, there is a significant need for better tocolytic agents to prevent PTB. The global PTB rate has risen steadily from 9.8% in 2000 to 10.6% in 2014 and ranges from 5–18%, depending on country and race/ethnicity [14,15]. The vast majority of PTBs occur in lower- and middle-income countries (LMICs)—particularly in southern Asia and sub-Saharan Africa [15]. LMICs in these regions account for 52% of global livebirths but more than 80% of PTBs [2,15]. In high-income countries, a neonate born very preterm (28–32 weeks) has a 95% chance of survival compared to only a 30% chance for neonates born in many low-income countries [16]. There are notable outliers, however, as some lower-income countries, such as Ecuador, have a low PTB rate of 5% [15]. Neighboring countries Uganda and Tanzania, of relatively similar economic standing and healthcare infrastructure, have strikingly different rates at 6.6% and 16.6%, respectively [15]. The United States is a high-income country and is another outlier, as it is included among the top ten countries with the highest numbers of PTBs [2].

Although the unmet need for new PTB therapeutics is significant, a combination of a relatively small market size and formidable regulatory hurdles has led to a stagnant drug pipeline with minimal pharmaceutical interest. Recently, discoveries using new therapeutic strategies and insights into the mechanism of parturition have increased the potential for new drugs with enhanced efficacy to be developed and approved for PTB. These discoveries have spurred the few ongoing pre-clinical and clinical trials currently studying the efficacy and safety profiles of novel therapeutics (Table 2). In this review, we focus on the dynamic landscape of PTB therapeutics, including drugs that have been used historically as well as new ones in development: ritodrine, terbutaline, atosiban, nifedipine, antibiotics, broad spectrum chemokine inhibitors (BSCIs), interleukin-1 (IL-1R) receptor antagonists, liposomes, and nanoparticle platforms. Agents administered to address more complex diseases associated with PTB (e.g., fetal growth restriction or emergent hypertensive disorders) are not discussed in this review. Discussion of mechanical therapies to prevent PTB, such as the cerclage and the cervical pessary, are outside the scope of this review [17–19]. When possible, we present the history of drug development, mechanism of action, side effects, and updated literature on drug efficacy. We also review the numerous regulatory hurdles and other obstacles for tocolytics in development and propose a path forward to expedite therapeutic advancements for the benefit of pregnant people and their neonates.

Table 1. Summary of preterm birth therapeutics.

Therapeutic	Route	Mechanism of Action	Stage of Development	Side Effects	Other Notes
Terbutaline (Bricanyl, Marex)	oral, IV	beta-2 adrenergic agonist	clinical use	Tremor, shakiness	
Atosiban (Tractocile, Antocin)	IV	oxytocin and vasopressin antagonist	clinical use	Nausea, vomiting, headache	
Nifedipine (Procardia, Adalat, Afeditab)	oral	calcium channel blocker	clinical use	Headache, flushing, constipation	
Antibiotics	oral, IV	dependent on the bacterial target	clinical use	Depends on antibiotic type	Used after PPROM
Aspirin [1]	oral	COX inhibitor	clinical use	Rash, peptic ulcers, abdominal pain, nausea	
Makena® (hydroxyprogesterone caproate) [2]	IM	17-OH-Progesterone	clinical use	Itching, nausea, diarrhea, injection site reaction	
OBE022 (Ebopiprant)	oral	prostaglandin receptor antagonist	Phase II	Headache, constipation	
Rytvela	IV, SC	IL-1 receptor allosteric modulator	pre-clinical	None noted in mothers or offspring	None noted in mothers or offspring
Kineret® (Anakinra)	SC	IL-1 receptor antagonist	clinically approved	Injection site reaction, immune suppression (increased infection risk)	Not approved (or used) to prevent preterm birth
BSCI Immunoliposome	IV	SSTR2	pre-clinical		

[1] ASA. [2] OHPC.

Table 2. Novel inflammatory therapeutics and ongoing clinical trials.

Company	Study (Type)	Drug	n, Target Population	Design	Primary Endpoint	Findings
AMAG	MEIS P2	Makena (17-OHP)	n = 463 16–21 week with history of PTB	RCT (US multi-center)	Reduction of PTB (<37 week, <35 week, <32 week)	PTB RR 0.66, 0.67, 0.58; Cl 0.54–0.81, 0.48–0.93, 0.37–0.91
AMAG	PROLONG P3	Makena (17-OHP)	n = 1708 16–21 week with history of PTB	RCT (international multi-center)	Reduction of PTB (<35 week), neonatal morbidity	No reduction in PTB or neonatal morbidity PTB RR 0.95, Cl 0.71, 1.26
ObsEva	TERM P2	OBE-001 (oxytocin receptor antagonist)	n = 10 34–36 week with PRETERM LABOR	RCT	Incidence of delivery within 7 days	terminated

Table 2. Cont.

Company	Study (Type)	Drug	n, Target Population	Design	Primary Endpoint	Findings
ObsEva	PROLONG P2	OBE-022 (PGF2$_\alpha$ receptor)	n = 120 28–34 week with PRETERM LABOR	RCT	Delivery < 2 days, Delivery < 7 days, delivery < 37 week, time to delivery	ongoing
GSK	P2	Retosiban (oxytocin receptor antagonist)	n = 64 30–35 week with PRETERM LABOR	RCT	Resolution of contractions	terminated
Ferring Pharma	P2	Barusiban (oxytocin receptor antagonist)	n = 163 34–36 week with PRETERM LABOR	RCT	Delivery within 48 h	No reduction in delivery within 48 h
Lipocine	P3	LPCN1107 (oral 17-OHP)	n = 1100	RCT 17OHP oral vs. IM	Reduction of PTB < 37 week	ongoing
Hadassah Medical Organization	P2	Indomethacin	n = 300 24–32 week with PRETERM LABOR	RCT Indometh vs. nifedipine	Time to delivery, GA at delivery	proposed
University of Hong Kong	P3	Oral dydrogesterone	n = 1714 <14 week	RCT	Rate of PTB < 37 week	ongoing
NICHD	ASPIRIN	Oral Aspirin	n = 11,976 6–14 week	RCT (international multi-center)	Rate of PTB < 37 week	PTB RR 0.89, CI 0.81–0.98

2. Pathophysiology of PTB

The pathophysiology of PTB is complex, brought on by a myriad of pathologic processes or underlying conditions that include activation of the fetal hypothalamic-pituitary-adrenal axis, infection and inflammation, decidual hemorrhage or thrombosis, uterine distension, premature placental senescence and oxidative stress, psychosocial stress and racism, and genomic variants at several loci [20–42]. Across these pathologic processes and conditions, inflammation is often a central mechanism triggering preterm labor or prematurely accelerating maturation of parturition pathways [3,43,44]. Although inflammation plays a critical role in the normal delivery process, dysregulated and pathologic inflammation can induce premature decidual and fetal membrane activation. Pathologic inflammation and the various other aforementioned processes thus comprise the 'upstream' initiators that confer fetal membrane activation, followed subsequently by the upregulation of 'downstream' effectors (e.g., cytokines, chemokines, contraction-associated proteins, prostaglandins, neuropeptides, matrix metalloproteinases, and receptors for inflammatory mediators) [20,45–52]. These pro-inflammatory initiators activate and potentiate a 'parturition cascade', leading to cervical shortening and dilation, chorioamniotic membrane rupture, and a contractile state in the myometrium. Most tocolytic agents act to directly suppress uterine contractility (e.g., betamimetics, magnesium sulfate) or inhibit the downstream mediators that stimulate the parturition pathway (e.g., indomethacin, atosiban). New therapeutics in pre-clinical development are shifting focus to address the upstream initiators (e.g., IL-1β receptor antagonists, BSCIs) to confer a broader delay of PTB. When possible, we have addressed specific mechanisms of action for each therapeutic in the parturition cascade.

3. The Earliest Tocolytic Agents: Betamimetics

Betamimetics were among the first drugs studied—in the 1960s—for potential use in tocolysis [53]. Some betamimetics, like terbutaline, were tested and approved as anti-asthmatic agents before having any widespread application as tocolytics [54,55]. Off-label use to prevent PTB began with terbutaline being labeled as category B under the prior Federal Drug Administration (FDA) labeling system, which indicated its potential to cause birth defects; category B drugs, however, included prenatal vitamins and use was thought to be routine and safe in pregnancy [54,55]. Terbutaline came under FDA scrutiny in 1997 and was labeled in 2011 as a category C drug; this class indicates that a drug is associated with adverse outcomes in animal studies. Well-controlled human studies, however, are lacking, and the therapeutic benefit may outweigh any risks [54]. Category C labeling of terbutaline was controversial, with many arguing that terbutaline's efficacy in delaying PTB outweighed its side effects and potential harms [54]. At present, terbutaline still lacks FDA approval for tocolysis but continues to be used in PTB management. In 1977, ritodrine was developed and granted FDA approval for intravenous administration to treat PTB [54,56]. Tocolytic efficacy of oral ritodrine was demonstrated in 1980. In 1995, both oral and IV ritodrine were discontinued and removed from the U.S. market due to adverse cardiovascular effects [56,57]. At present, ritodrine is still used internationally as a tocolytic. Hexoprenaline and salbutamol are other betamimetics that were never marketed in the U.S. but that have limited use internationally [58,59].

Betamimetics function as beta-2 adrenergic receptor agonists, binding to receptors on cell membranes of smooth muscle tissues, which ultimately inhibits myometrial contractions. Activation of these receptors stimulates G_s proteins that bind to adenyl cyclase, subsequently increasing cAMP concentrations [60]. Increased cAMP leads to activation of cAMP-dependent protein kinase (PRKA) which phosphorylates and inhibits myosin light chain kinase (MLCK) [60]. Inactivated MLCK is unable to phosphorylate smooth muscle myosin, which prevents interaction with actin, reducing contractile force in smooth muscle tissues [60]. PRKA can also inhibit phospholamban, an inhibitor of SERCA channels [60]. This allows for increased calcium uptake and reduced intracellular calcium, leading to less MLCK activation, calcium-calmodulin interaction, and cross-bridge interactions between myosin and actin [60]. Betamimetic tocolytics reduce uterine contractions through binding to beta-2 receptors located on myometrial cell membranes, slowing the progression of labor.

Despite their use as tocolytics, betamimetics have not been shown to reduce perinatal death or complications of neonatal prematurity compared with placebo [60]. Some studies comparing tocolytic efficacy and adverse outcomes between ritodrine and terbutaline have found no significant differences between them, though other trials have demonstrated an increased efficacy of oral terbutaline compared with oral ritodrine [60–64]. Despite generally similar side effect profiles, numerous studies have described an increased risk of hyperglycemia with oral terbutaline administration and tachycardia following intravenous ritodrine when compared with placebo [59,60,65]. In countries where both agents are available, terbutaline is infrequently used for tocolysis, largely due to a general preference for the safety profile of ritodrine [55,64]. In some instances, however, terbutaline is administered as a single dose subcutaneous injection to examine preliminary uterine reaction to tocolytics or as maintenance therapy following initial treatment with other tocolytics [55,59]. Maintenance therapy with either betamimetic, however, has not been found to further delay PTB or decrease perinatal mortality and morbidity [10,11]. A meta-analysis compared trials of intravenous ritodrine alone with combination therapies of IV ritodrine and other tocolytic agents (e.g., intravenous or oral magnesium sulfate, magnesium gluconate, and indomethacin) [7]. In nearly all trials, combination therapies with ritodrine showed no significant differences in efficacy or adverse effects compared to ritodrine alone [7]. In contrast, other studies have found that combination therapy with progesterone (P4) may allow for increased expression of beta-2 receptors on the myometrium and therefore may influence betamimetic impact [66,67].

Side effects of tocolytic betamimetics are extensive, as beta-adrenergic activity is responsible for a wide range of homeostatic functions. Stimulation of beta-adrenergic receptors upregulates sympathetic pathways, leading to tachycardia, palpitations, chest pain, arrhythmias, tremors, nausea, vomiting, headaches, nervousness, anxiety, and shortness of breath as well as hyperglycemia, hypokalemia, bronchodilation, hypotension, and pulmonary edema [59,60]. Mild beta-1 receptor binding activity contributes to an increased risk of maternal tachycardia [59]. Both terbutaline and ritodrine interact at the maternal-fetal interface and can cross the placenta to induce fetal tachycardia, hypoglycemia, and hyperinsulinism [60]. Recent studies have also suggested that exposure to ritodrine or terbutaline during pregnancy may be associated with an increased risk for autism in the child [57,68]. After adjusting for confounding variables, one study demonstrated that ritodrine administration for delaying PTB has been associated with a moderately increased risk of autism (HR 1.23, 95% CI 1.05–1.47) [57]. It is unclear whether this outcome is due to betamimetic exposure during preterm labor or more generally to PTB and significant fetal exposure to intrauterine inflammation that adversely impacts fetal neurodevelopment [57]. However, in rat models, administration of betamimetics has been associated with adverse neurobehavioral teratogenicity, and terbutaline, specifically, has been shown to alter fetal neurochemistry [57,68].

In a cost-effectiveness analysis comparing tocolytic drug classes, terbutaline and ritodrine were shown to be relatively expensive, costing hundreds of U.S. dollars compared to nifedipine or indomethacin, which are often available for less than 20 U.S. dollars [69]. Betamimetics have been shown to be less effective than numerous other therapeutic agents, and their side effect profile is sufficiently significant to warrant use of other therapeutics when available [60]. Despite the waning use of betamimetics as tocolytic agents in higher-income countries, they continue to be used significantly in countries where other tocolytic agents are not easily available [60].

4. Oxytocin Antagonism: Hope for Atosiban

Atosiban, an oxytocin receptor antagonist, was first described in the literature in 1985 and in 1994 was developed specifically as a tocolytic agent [70]. It is currently available for clinical use in Europe but not the U.S. [59,71,72]. Despite a promising maternal safety profile, the FDA failed to approve atosiban for clinical use due to the possible association between atosiban and death in premature infants [73,74]. The FDA also declined to approve atosiban because the studies available at the time were not well designed, ultimately failing to demonstrate improved neonatal outcomes compared to a placebo or other tocolytics [54]. While this decision was largely in accordance with the Kefauver-Harris Amendments, passed in 1962 in response to Germany's thalidomide scandal, this precedent crippled PTB therapeutic development [75]. The regulatory hurdles resulting from the final edict on atosiban continue to impact the field of PTB therapeutic development and will be expanded upon in a later section of this review (Box 1).

Box 1. U.S. regulatory hurdles for PTB therapeutics.

- Institutional Review Boards, participants, and physicians have heightened concern when dealing with any drug that has a potential effect on the fetus and on the mother
- Can people give adequate informed consent during active labor?
- No templates of successful study design in tocolytic studies, since the only drugs previously approved by the FDA were approved under standards that are now deemed inadequate
- No tocolytic drug presented to the FDA has consistently shown neonatal benefit in controlled trials
- Lack of standardization for disease risk, severity, and progression for common diagnoses
- Small market: sales for 'blockbuster drugs' in the U.S. for 2004 (~$5 billion) versus annual sales for a tocolytic agent, estimated at < $500 million

Oxytocin serves numerous roles in the body—namely the promotion of milk letdown for breastfeeding and the stimulation of myometrial contractions during labor. When activated, myometrial oxytocin receptors, which are G-protein-coupled receptors linked to phospholipase C (PLC), activate PLC to trigger a signaling cascade, beginning with increased IP_3 and diacyl glycerol (DAG), which ultimately leads to calcium release into the cytosol and muscle contraction. Estrogen upregulates myometrial oxytocin receptors to mature the contractile ability of the uterus [76,77]. Although typically produced in the hypothalamus and released from the posterior pituitary, oxytocin is also produced by the uterine decidua during late gestation in preparation for parturition [77]. As an oxytocin receptor antagonist, atosiban blocks this pathway to produce tocolytic effects. The full mechanism, however, has not been determined.

Additionally, atosiban acts as a vasopressin receptor antagonist and may impact prostaglandin F ($PGF_{2\alpha}$) signaling pathways, which normally contribute to the onset and maintenance of labor [78]. These other mechanisms may be involved in atosiban's tocolytic effects, though further research into these alternative pathways is needed [16]. Atosiban lacks oral bioavailability as a peptide antagonist and is administered subcutaneously or intravenously. Other oxytocin receptor antagonists, barusiban and retosiban, have been studied, but have not been used for tocolysis outside of clinical trials [16].

Atosiban has been shown to significantly reduce uterine contractions during PTB and delay labor by up to 48 h, without conferring significant maternal, fetal, or neonatal adverse effects [8,78,79]. One meta-analysis and multiple other studies have found no significant differences in rates of delivery at 48 h when comparing atosiban with a placebo, betamimetics, or calcium channel blockers (CCBs) [16,80,81]. Data are not available to suggest atosiban improves neonatal outcomes, but its lower discontinuation rate and safer side effect profile have led some studies to conclude that atosiban is preferable to betamimetics [16,80,81]. Like other tocolytic agents, long-term maintenance therapy with atosiban has generally not been shown to delay PTB beyond 48 h, and a meta-analysis suggested maintenance therapy was associated with a significantly higher incidence of injection site reaction when compared with a placebo [9,81]. One study found that, following successful initial intravenous administration of atosiban, continued subcutaneous therapy with atosiban reduced the need for subsequent intravenous atosiban therapy [82]. Combination therapies between intravenous atosiban and other tocolytic agents have demonstrated no significant superior effects compared to atosiban alone [7].

Atosiban is associated with fewer maternal adverse effects than other tocolytic agents, like betamimetics or calcium channel blockers (CCBs) [8]. Maternal side effects are infrequent and include adverse reactions at the site of injection, nausea, vomiting, headache, chest pain, and hypotension [8,16,79]. Atosiban crosses the placenta, but has not been shown to accumulate in the fetus [8]. Compared with a placebo and other tocolytics, Atosiban causes a similar range of possible adverse neonatal effects, and it has not been shown to reduce the incidence of respiratory distress syndrome in premature infants when compared to a placebo [8]. Though betamimetic agents predominate in the global market for tocolytics, atosiban is often considered a drug of choice for tocolysis in high-resource settings where it is available.

5. Calcium Channel Blockers (CCBs): Low Cost and Favorable Safety Profile

Nifedipine was first synthesized in 1966 as a coronary vasodilator [83]. Nifedipine and nicardipine (another calcium channel blocker) have been studied as first line tocolytic agents for nearly 20 years but have not been granted FDA approval for use as tocolytics [84].

CCBs act on voltage-gated L-type calcium channels (VGCCs) by binding to the dihydropyridine (DHP) site to block the calcium influx that follows membrane depolarization. Decreased intracellular calcium leads to reduced calcium-calmodulin interactions and reduces activation of MLCK. Similar to betamimetics, decreased MLCK activity inhibits myosin-actin crossbridge formation and reduces muscle contraction. VGCCs are upregulated in uterine myometrial tissue during pregnancy and labor, providing the impetus to study the use of nifedipine and nicardipine in reducing uterine contractions to delay labor [67].

CCBs are used off-label as tocolytic agents and are very popular in the U.S. Certain studies have demonstrated a comparable or increased benefit from CCBs over betamimetics, not only with regards to delay of preterm labor and delivery but also in improving neonatal morbidity and reducing maternal adverse complications [16,84]. Administration of CCBs has not been shown to improve perinatal mortality [16]. Nifedipine is equally efficacious when compared to atosiban, though the lower cost of nifedipine and the impact on reducing neonatal morbidity often makes it the preferred drug of choice [67]. Other CCBs, such as nicardipine, can be administered intravenously or orally; this flexible route of administration is a benefit over nifedipine, which is only orally or sublingually administered [85]. However, nicardipine may have reduced efficacy in prolonging the duration of pregnancy and may produce more side effects in neonates [67,85]. Though nifedipine is not FDA-approved for tocolysis, numerous meta-analyses have shown that CCBs may sometimes effectively delay PTB by up to 7 days, a significant increase in the extent of PTB delay when compared with the 24 h or 48 h delay conferred by most other therapeutics [59,86]. Maintenance tocolysis with nifedipine is ineffective in further delaying labor or reducing neonatal complications when compared to a placebo or observation [12,84].

CCBs and betamimetics have long been used in combination for treatment of cardiovascular diseases, and synergistic effects have been observed in myometrial tissue following combination therapy; interestingly, administration of nifedipine followed by terbutaline confers a synergistic efficacy, but the effect is diminished if administered in reverse order [67]. Combination therapy with these agents is sometimes contraindicated, especially in twin pregnancies and pre-existing maternal cardiovascular disorders, due to increased risk of myocardial infarction and pulmonary edema [67]. Animal studies have demonstrated that pre-treatment with progesterone (P4) can decrease the efficacy of nifedipine; the relationship between these tocolytics is still being assessed [67]. Emerging research on combination therapy with atosiban and nifedipine suggests a strong synergistic relationship, while combination therapy with nifedipine and celecoxib shows a decreased efficacy compared to the use of nifedipine alone [67].

Adverse effects following nifedipine and nicardipine use are typically mild [59]. The most common side effects are headaches, associated with the transient hypotension induced by these drugs. Reflexive tachycardia, anxiety, nausea, vomiting, skin flushing, and palpitations have also been described [67]. Side effects specific to CCB use in tocolysis include severe maternal dyspnea and pulmonary edema, though these manifestations are rare [67]. Nifedipine has not demonstrated any direct adverse fetal side effects [67].

In summary, the extended multi-day delay in labor and the favorable safety profile of nifedipine makes it an appealing agent for tocolysis; the low cost and oral route of administration also allows for implementation of nifedipine in low- and middle-income countries. Like most other PTB therapeutics, CCBs have shown negligible impact when used for maintenance tocolysis. Additional studies on long-term use of CCBs and combination therapy with CCBs and other tocolytic agents is needed [67].

6. Nonsteroidal Anti-Inflammatory Drugs as Tocolytic Agents: A Short-Term Prostaglandin Blockade

Non-steroidal anti-inflammatory drugs (NSAIDs), including indomethacin, ibuprofen, and aspirin, have a long history of use in the prevention of PTB; these vasoactive agents were first used as tocolytics in the 1970s [87]. The main mechanism of action of NSAIDs is inhibition of the cyclooxygenase (COX) enzyme, which facilitates the conversion of arachidonic acid to prostaglandins. Prostaglandins are involved in the parturition pathway and facilitate uterine contractions and cervical ripening. Certain NSAIDS, including indomethacin, are thought to inhibit neutrophil activation by suppressing inflammatory stimuli [88]. Indomethacin and ibuprofen reversibly bind to COX, while aspirin binds irreversibly; although each agent binds to both COX-1 and COX-2 isoforms, these drugs have been shown to bind to COX-1 with varying increased selectively [89–91]. In pregnancy, both COX-1 and COX-2 are expressed by the myometrium, decidua, and chorioamniotic membranes, and research is ongoing to evaluate the differential expression of those isoforms in these tissues [92–99].

There is little evidence to suggest COX-inhibitors should be prioritized as effective tocolytics when compared with other available therapeutics; however, some studies have indicated a potential use for NSAIDs in preventing PTB [100]. In 2015, a Cochrane review and meta-analysis evaluated the use of indomethacin for the prevention of PTB [101]. In one small study ($n = 36$), indomethacin reduced the risk of PTB before 37 weeks' gestation (relative risk (RR) 0.21, 95% Confidence Interval (CI) 0.07–0.62) [101]. Indomethacin administration was also associated with a greater gestational age at birth (two studies, $n = 66$; average mean difference (MD) 3.59 weeks, 95% CI 0.65–6.52) and higher birth weight (two studies, $n = 67$ infants; MD 716.3 g, 95% CI 425.5–1007.2) [101]. In this meta-analysis, two trials (total $n = 70$) compared indomethacin to placebo and determined that, with indomethacin, the risk of PTB within 48 h of treatment initiation was reduced, albeit with a wide confidence interval (relative risk (RR) 0.2, 95% CI 0.03–1.28). In trials comparing indomethacin to beta-mimetics, indomethacin reduced the risk of PTB less within 48 h (two trials, total $n = 100$; RR 0.27; 95% CI 0.08–0.96) and PTB before 37 weeks of gestation (two studies, $n = 80$; RR 0.53; 95% CI 0.28–0.99) compared to betamimetics [101]. There was no difference between indomethacin and magnesium sulfate (seven studies, $n = 792$) or CCB (two studies, $n = 230$) in terms of pregnancy prolongation or fetal/neonatal outcomes [101]. A selective COX-2 inhibitor, Rofecoxib, was studied for potential use in tocolysis and ultimately shown to not reduce the incidence of preterm birth [102].

Aspirin is also a COX-inhibitor and has been theorized to be useful in the prevention of PTB by decreasing the incidence of preeclampsia [103]. Recently, meta-analyses and secondary analyses of trials of women taking aspirin for the prevention of preeclampsia have shown a decreased rate of PTB, as preeclampsia is a risk factor for PTB [104–106]. A secondary analysis of an RCT examining aspirin for the prevention of preeclampsia showed that in nulliparous, low-risk women, there was a decreased rate of spontaneous PTB < 34 weeks among women who received aspirin ($n = 2543$; AOR 0.46; 95% CI 0.23–0.89) [106]. In a larger RCT comparing aspirin to placebo in nulliparous women, aspirin was associated with a decreased rate of preterm delivery ($n = 11,976$; RR 0.89; 95% CI 0.81–0.98) [104]. In this same study, among those who did deliver preterm, aspirin was associated with a decreased rate of early preterm delivery < 34 weeks (RR 0.75, 95% CI 0.61–0.93) [104]. Low-dose aspirin prophylaxis has been indicated for reducing risk of preeclampsia in women with particular high-risk factors; however, further evaluation of aspirin for use as a tocolytic is necessary to affirm current findings.

Maternal side effects of NSAID use generally depend on length of time of treatment. Serious side effects are uncommon if NSAIDS are used for less than 48 h. Common maternal reactions include nausea and heartburn but can also involve gastrointestinal bleeding and prolonged bleeding time [107,108]. Prolonged treatment with NSAIDS can also lead to renal injury [109]. In the 2015 Cochrane review, COX-inhibitors were found to have fewer maternal side effects compared to betamimetics and decreased cases of treatment cessation due to maternal adverse effects. Compared to magnesium sulfate, COX-inhibitors also had fewer maternal adverse effects [101]. Maternal contradictions to indomethacin include chronic renal or hepatic disease, peptic ulcer disease, and coagulation disorders [110].

NSAIDs cross the placenta and can result in premature closure of the ductus arteriosus leading to neonatal pulmonary hypertension. Constriction of the ductus arteriosus due to maternal NSAID use occurs via inhibition of prostacyclin and prostaglandin E2, which maintain vasodilation of the duct [111]. Additionally, NSAIDs may diminish prostaglandin inhibition of antidiuretic hormone and affect fetal renal blood flow, typically resulting in dose-dependent and reversible oligohydramnios [112]. These adverse effects are generally associated with use of COX-inhibitors for longer than 48 h before 32 weeks' gestation and for any length of time after 32 weeks [111,113–115]. The 2015 Cochrane review noted that data were insufficient to determine fetal safety [101]. As many NSAID-related side effects appear to be dose-dependent, low-dose aspirin and other NSAIDs are considered safe throughout much of pregnancy. Notable fetal complications, however, arise from the inappropriate use of higher-dose NSAIDs in the third trimester.

Despite a near fifty-year history of use in the management of PTB, there is a relative paucity of studies on NSAID use in tocolysis, particularly with regards to combination therapies or as a maintenance tocolytic. The significant adverse and sometimes life-threatening fetal complications induced by these drugs warrant careful administration of NSAID therapeutics later in pregnancy and present an important challenge to navigate when studying these agents in future PTB clinical trials.

7. Magnesium Sulfate: A Classic Tocolytic, Called into Question

As early as the 1940s, magnesium sulfate was shown to promote uterine quiescence [116,117]. It was originally studied for potential use in reducing abnormal uterine contractions underlying severe dysmenorrhea [116]. In 1977, magnesium sulfate was first described for use in tocolysis [118]. In 1983, a case series of 355 patients demonstrated a dose-dependent association between magnesium sulfate and tocolysis [119]. It has since become one of the most commonly used therapeutics for delaying PTB [120,121].

The mechanism for magnesium sulfate as a tocolytic has not been fully determined. Physiologically, magnesium regulates calcium uptake, which impacts muscle contraction and neuronal activity. This calcium regulation is thought to be due to both an extracellular effect of decreasing the intracellular calcium stores as well as an intracellular effect of blocking the release of intracellular calcium via IP_3 receptor/channels [120,122–125]. Magnesium sulfate also appears to impact the binding and distribution of calcium in smooth muscle, including uterine tissues, reducing the frequency of cellular depolarization to potentially reduce myometrial contractions [126]. Interestingly, magnesium sulfate must be kept at suprapharmacologic levels (4–10 mmol, 8–16 mEq/L) in vitro in order to effectively inhibit cyclic uterine activity [123].

Whether magnesium sulfate delays PTB significantly in comparison to other available tocolytics is unknown [127,128]. Comparisons of different studies of magnesium sulfate are challenged by the complexity of underlying PTB pathophysiology, sub-therapeutic dosing in some studies, and generally small sample populations [119]. In a meta-analysis of 19 randomized clinical trials, magnesium sulfate was not shown to reduce the frequency of delivery within 48 h when compared with a placebo (RR 0.75, 95% CI 0.54–1.03), and there was no significant reduction in delivery before 37 weeks' gestation (RR 1.18, 95% CI 0.93–1.51) [120]. Magnesium sulfate has also not been shown to provide improvements in neonatal morbidity or mortality [120]. Another meta-analysis of 95 trials of varying tocolytics (31 studies, encompassing 2653 patients, focused specifically on magnesium sulfate) found that magnesium sulfate was comparable to prostaglandin inhibitors in its probability of effectively delaying PTB by up to 48 h [129,130]. This meta-analysis, however, noted that other tocolytics (e.g., prostaglandin inhibitors and calcium channel blockers) provide a more effective delay of PTB, with better neonatal outcomes and safer side effect profiles. The 1983 case series study demonstrated significant differences in effective tocolysis among women who received varying doses of magnesium sulfate, with high doses associated with the greatest tocolysis [119,131]. More recent studies comparing high- and low-dose intravenous magnesium sulfate found no significant differences in fetal or neonatal death and were unable to verify a dose-dependent impact on delaying PTB when compared with a placebo [129]. Compared to short-term administration, long-term administration of magnesium sulfate is associated with the development of fetal osteopenia [119]. Despite conflicting and generally low-power studies of the efficacy of magnesium sulfate as a tocolytic, there is a known benefit to administering magnesium sulfate for fetal neurological protection to pregnant people at risk for PTB [128,129,132–135]. Magnesium sulfate supplementation may also provide protection against preeclampsia—a known risk factor for PTB—though more research is needed for confirmation [136].

The adverse effects of magnesium sulfate in mothers include respiratory arrest and pulmonary edema, nausea, flushing, gastrointestinal disturbance, lethargy, and blurred vision [137]. Common adverse effects in neonates include lethargy, poor suckling, and delayed time to onset of established respiration [138]. Prolonged magnesium sulfate administration has been suggested to increase risk of fetal hypocalcemia and osteopenia, as magnesium sulfate is known to cross the placenta and cause fetal hypermagnesemia; fetal bone calcification can be inhibited by magnesium sulfate, which may lead to changes in bone thickness [119,139]. High doses of magnesium sulfate have also been suggested to contribute to increased risk of fetal and neonatal death [140].

Magnesium sulfate has long served as one of the more well-known drugs employed for PTB management. There is, however, a significant lack of data to support therapeutic efficacy in delaying PTB, despite magnesium sulfate's extensive clinical use as a tocolytic agent. Both efficacy and adverse effects of magnesium sulfate appear to be at least partially dose-dependent. As other therapeutic classes gain prominence in the field of PTB management, magnesium sulfate may eventually decline in use.

8. Addressing Infection: Trials of Antibiotics to Prevent PTB

Infection and inflammation are frequent causes of early PTB, and infections are typically polymicrobial [24,141–144]. Numerous studies have sought to determine the specific associations between preterm labor and infectious states in order to elucidate the potential utility of antibiotic administration in preventing or delaying PTB. Multiple randomized clinical trials have failed to demonstrate a benefit from antibiotic therapy for women in preterm labor with intact membranes [145]. A key study in this area was the ORACLE II randomized controlled trial, which addressed the question of whether administration of broad-spectrum antibiotics might prolong pregnancy and prevent neonatal morbidity in women with preterm labor and intact membranes, who had no evidence of an amniotic fluid infection [146]. Antibiotic administration in the absence of an evident infection has long been understood to carry numerous risks, which include detrimental impacts on an individual's microbiome, increasing risk for antibiotic-resistant neonatal sepsis, and antibiotic resistance in the mother if undertreated or inappropriately treated [147]. In the ORACLE II trial, women were randomized to either co-amoxiclav, erythromycin, co-amoxiclav and erythromycin, or a placebo for 10 days or until delivery. Antibiotic therapy did not prolong pregnancy or improve neonatal outcomes; higher rates of necrotizing enterocolitis (0.6% vs. 0.3%) were observed in the neonates exposed to co-amoxiclav, but the data was not statistically significant [145,146]. In addition, higher rates of neonatal mortality and cerebral palsy were observed in infants and children who received both macrolide and beta-lactam antibiotics [145,146]. When the children initially included in the ORACLE II trial were reevaluated at 7 years of age, there were higher rates of cerebral palsy in children of women who received both antibiotics (3.3% vs. 1.7% for erythromycin, 3.2% vs. 1.9% for amoxiclav) and higher rates of functional impairment in those who received erythromycin (42.3% vs. 38.3%) [148]. Thus, the use of antibiotics as a PTB therapeutic is not recommended in GBS-negative women due to the lack of benefit in preventing PTB and concern regarding an elevated risk for the development of neonatal necrotizing enterocolitis or other adverse effects conferred by unnecessary antibiotic administration.

Preterm premature rupture of membranes (PPROM) is a major cause of PTB, and women with PPROM are highly likely to have a subclinical or overt intra-amniotic infection [149–152]. In contrast to the treatment of PTB with intact membranes, antibiotic therapy as a means of tocolysis is recommended and routinely used for women with PPROM in high-income countries [153]. There are, however, notable deficiencies in clinical knowledge regarding which antibiotic agents should be administered as well as the respective regimens and dosages to adequately address PTB in the setting of PPROM. Nevertheless, intravenous ampicillin and erythromycin, followed by oral amoxicillin and erythromycin, has been shown to significantly prolong pregnancy in GBS negative women and lower rates of neonatal respiratory distress (40.5% vs. 48.7%) and necrotizing enterocolitis (2.3% vs. 5.8%) in those with and without GBS colonization [154]. The use of broader spectrum antibiotics like co-amoxiclav is not recommended, however, due to an increased rate of neonatal necrotizing enterocolitis, similar to the findings in women with PTB and intact membranes [146,155]. In patients colonized with GBS, latency antibiotics were also associated with significantly decreased neonatal sepsis (8.4% vs. 15.6%) and pneumonia (2.9% vs. 7%) [154]. A review of 13 randomized controlled clinical trials that included more than 6000 women with PPROM before 37 weeks' gestational age found that the use of latency antibiotics was associated with decreased rates of chorioamnionitis (RR 0.66, 95% CI 0.46–0.96), neonatal infection (RR 0.67, CI 95% 0.52–0.850), oxygen requirements (RR 0.88, 95% CI 0.81–0.96), and abnormal cerebral ultrasound findings (RR 0.81, 95% CI 0.68–0.98) [156]. Based on this evidence, narrower spectrum antibiotics are routinely given to women with PPROM and have shown neonatal benefit. Conflicting data, however, complicate recommendations for employing a broader scope of tocolytic agents in managing patients with PPROM [157,158]. Numerous studies have demonstrated that tocolytic (e.g., betamimetics, CCBs, and COX-inhibitors) administration does not reduce perinatal mortality in women with PPROM and is instead associated with a potentially increased risk of chorioamnionitis as well as increased risk for subsequent need of respiratory support for neonates when compared with a placebo [157,158]. Therefore, although there is limited data to indicate the utility of antibiotics in managing PPROM-induced PTB, the clinical benefit of administering a broader range of therapeutics to delay PTB in patients with PPROM remains unproven.

Bacterial vaginosis (BV) is a complex, heterogenous vaginal infection associated with PTB [24,142,159–165]. Unfortunately, antibiotic treatment trials of BV have generally not reduced PTB [166–169]. The US Preventative Task Force Services released updated recommendations in 2020 regarding screening and treatment of BV in pregnancy. After reviewing results from 13 randomized clinical trials, they recommend against treatment of asymptomatic BV in pregnancy, as treatment does not seem to decrease adverse obstetrical outcomes including PTB, low birth weight, or PPROM [170–172]. The benefits of treating high-risk individuals with a history of PTB is less clear [170]. There are numerous problems associated with prior trials of BV in pregnancy to prevent PTB, which may have confounded these studies. First, BV treatment in pregnancy may be too late to prevent microbial trafficking into the uterus; pre-conception treatment may be necessary to optimize outcomes. The antibiotics tested may be ineffective against the many uncultivable pathogens associated with BV [173,174]. Finally, BV treatment may shift the vaginal microbiota from one BV-associated microbiota profile to another, and many clinical trials did not follow changes in the microbiota over time [175]. Understanding the gene-environment interaction of BV and PTB could broaden the approach to treatment or prenatal care. Pregnant people with BV who had certain genotypes of PRKCA, FLT1, and IL-6 genes were more likely to deliver preterm than people without BV [176]. Although screening and treatment of BV is not currently recommended to prevent PTB, research in this area continues to evolve.

Screening and treatment of sexually transmitted infections (STIs; e.g., *Chlamydia trachomatis, Neisseria gonorrhoeae, Trichomonas vaginalis*) is recommended to reduce the neonatal risks associated with maternal infection and reduce STI transmission in the community. Antibiotic treatment of STIs does not appear to prolong pregnancy and prevent PTB [177]. Likewise, treatment of asymptomatic urinary tract infections with antibiotics does not lower rates of PTB [178–180]. Nevertheless, urinary tract infection treatment is recommended to decrease rates of other high-risk outcomes, such as pyelonephritis and low birth weight. Metronidazole should be offered to people with a symptomatic *T. vaginalis* infection in pregnancy to relieve maternal symptoms and prevent spread of STIs. Although metronidazole is safe for use in the first trimester of pregnancy, there is concern that treatment of *T. vaginalis* with metronidazole in the late second or third trimester of pregnancy may increase rates of PTB [181,182]. Vaginal candidiasis has not been shown to be a risk factor for PTB, and treatment appears to be safe in pregnancy [183]. Overall, the treatment of STIs and UTIs has not been shown to reduce the rate of PTB, but treatment of UTIs in early pregnancy confers both maternal and neonatal benefit.

9. Progesterone (P4) Analogs

The first studies on the use of P4 to prevent PTB were in the 1960s, demonstrating a potential protective effect of P4 administration [184,185]. Studies of P4 as a PTB therapeutic dwindled throughout the 1990s, until two studies in 2003 reinvigorated interest in P4 as a viable preventative strategy [184,186–188]. In 2011, the FDA approved the use of hydroxyprogesterone caproate (17-OHPC) to reduce the risk of PTB [184]. The approval of 17-OHPC for use as a preventative agent marked the first drug approved for use in pregnancy in over 15 years [184]. However, significant controversy surrounds the use of P4 to prevent recurrent spontaneous PTB, and the FDA has proposed the withdrawal of this approval after post-market studies failed to verify clinical benefit [189]. Additional studies of P4 for use in tocolysis are ongoing (Table 2).

P4 is a pro-gestational hormone, which maintains uterine quiescence for most of pregnancy by inhibiting the transcription of labor-associated genes in the myometrium. These genes include *gja1* (Connexin 43), *otr* (oxytocin receptor), and *ptgs2* (cyclooxygenase), which encode uterine activation proteins; *nfkb* (nuclear factor kappa-B), *ilb1b* (IL-1β), *ccl2* (MCP-1), and *cxcl8* (IL-8), which encode proteins involved in cytokine and chemokine signaling. Myometrial activation and the initiation of labor requires withdrawal of P4, which in most viviparous species is achieved by a fall in peripheral P4, a key trigger of parturition. In contrast, circulating P4 levels remain elevated in women at term [190]. Yet, blocking P4 action at any time during human pregnancy by administration of the specific antagonist, RU486, induces preterm labor. Therefore, it has been hypothesized that a 'functional withdrawal' of P4 occurs in the human myometrium, whereby uterine smooth muscle cells become resistant to the pro-gestational actions of P4, inducing labor onset [191,192].

Although the molecular mechanism by which P4 controls the timing of labor onset is not well understood, recent studies have shed light on how a functional P4 withdrawal might occur in pregnant people. Recently, it was reported that during gestation, P4 signals predominantly through its nuclear receptor PRB, suppressing the transcription of labor-associated and inflammatory genes and promoting myometrial relaxation [193]. Further study found the truncated PR isoform, PRA (when not bound to P4, 'un-liganded'), antagonizes the action of PRB. At the end of gestation, the increased nuclear abundance of PRA relative to PRB may be an important factor in antagonizing the signaling of P4, which would promote CAP gene expression and labor initiation [193,194]. Importantly, despite the abundance of P4 in maternal blood during term labor, intracellular P4 concentration in myometrial cells decreases due to an increased expression of the P4-metabolizing enzyme 20α-hydroxysteroid dehydrogenase (AKR1C1/20α-HSD), which converts P4 into its inactive metabolite, 20alpha-hydroxyprogesterone (20α-OHP). Thus, it is possible that catabolism of P4 in myometrial cells leads to a local withdrawal of P4, the un-liganding of PRA from P4, which in turn switches PRA to an activator of CAP gene transcription, triggering labor onset. In summary, the P4/PR signaling pathway in the myometrium may represent a target for the development of novel therapeutic agents for PTB prevention. Administration of synthetic progestins that are not metabolized by 20α-HSD may maintain liganding of P4 to PRB and suppress the transcription of genes that otherwise would induce labor (Figure 1).

While P4 is required for the maintenance of human pregnancy, research on its use as a prophylactic therapeutic to prevent PTB has produced contradictory data [186,187,195–199]. In 2003, a small double-blind trial found that 17α-hydroxyprogesterone caproate (17-OHPC, weak progestin) significantly reduced the risk of PTB in people with a prior PTB [187]. However, other studies failed to find evidence that P4 can prevent recurrent PTB. For instance, larger trials have recently shown that the effectiveness of P4 is limited [200,201]. A double-blind, randomized, placebo-controlled trial of vaginal P4 prophylaxis in high-risk women with a previous spontaneous PTB was not associated with reduced risk of PTB or composite neonatal adverse outcomes [196]. A 2017 meta-analysis showed that administration of vaginal P4 to asymptomatic women with a twin gestation and a sonographic short cervix in the mid-trimester reduced the risk of PTB as well as neonatal mortality and morbidity [202]. However, only one study conducted in women with singleton pregnancies and a mid-gestation sonographic cervical length greater than 25 mm resulted in a positive outcome for prophylactic therapy against PTB using a vaginal suppository with micronized P4, with others showing no effect [203,204].

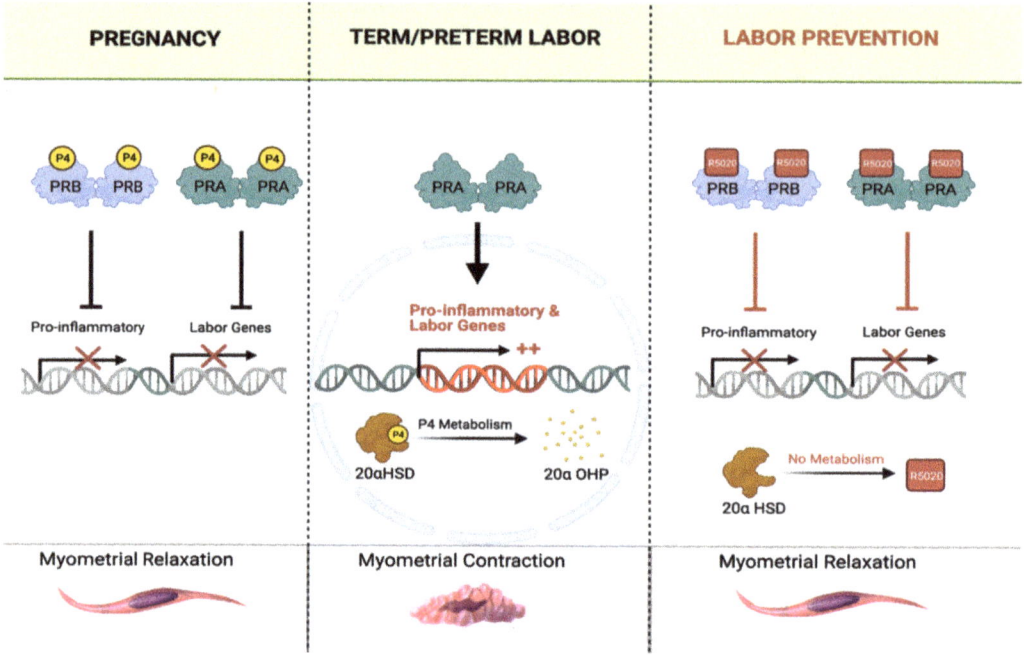

Figure 1. The potential mechanisms of selective P4 receptor modulator action on uterine muscle during pregnancy and term/preterm labor. (**Left panel**) During pregnancy, P4 liganding of P4 receptors (PR-A and PR-B) inhibits pro-inflammatory (cytokines and chemokines) and pro-contractile (CAPs) uterine genes, thereby maintaining myometrial relaxation. (**Middle panel**) During term and preterm labor, myometrial 20α-hydroxysteroid dehydrogenase (20α-HSD) enzyme expression and activity is upregulated, which results in local intracellular metabolism of P4 into its PR-inactive metabolite, 20α-hydroxyprogesterone (20αOHP). This leads to un-liganding of PRs (unbounding of P4). Un-liganded PR-A activates myometrial expression of pro-inflammatory and pro-contractile genes (i.e., *oxtr* and *gja1*) and induces labor contractions. (**Right panel**) Administration of SPRM compounds such as R5020 (aka: Promegestone), which is not a substrate for 20α-HSD, has higher affinity for PRs, longer half-life than P4, keeps the PRs constitutively liganded, maintains uterine quiescence, and prevents labor contractions. Note: this figure was created with Biorender.com.

A therapeutic strength of P4 is the excellent safety profile in pregnancy, underlying its FDA approval for use as a PTB therapeutic [184,188]. Endogenous P4 naturally induces a number of systemic side effects, including headache, moodiness, and loss of libido. These side effects are significantly reduced with the use of synthetic P4 [188,205]. Micronized P4 has been shown to eliminate these adverse effects entirely [188]. No risk to the neonate has been associated with P4 administration [188,206]. Other P4 formulations may have greater efficacy in preventing PTB than 17-OHPC. R5020 binds PRs with high affinity and is not a substrate for metabolism by 20α-HSD; a pilot study in pregnant rats was associated with inhibition of preterm labor [207]. R5020 or other steroidal or non-steroidal P4 analogs may represent an innovative approach to PTB prevention in people at risk for PTB.

10. Inhibiting Inflammation: Use of Broad-Spectrum Chemokine Inhibitors

Numerous studies over the past decade have focused on developing anti-inflammatory agents that target specific chemokines and chemokine receptors underlying pathologic inflammation in certain human diseases. Successes in the development of BSCIs for human immunodeficiency virus (HIV) treatment and prevention of cancer metastasis have spurred recent interest in studying the use of BSCIs in preventing or delaying PTB in high-risk pregnant women [208–210]. The exploration of BSCIs for use in addressing PTB is currently limited to animal models [210,211].

Leukocytes are an active component of the maternal immune system; therefore, they can provide relatively accessible means to interrupt the inflammatory pathway that leads to labor initiation. Studies indicate that circulating maternal leukocytes are not activated during most of gestation but become primed and migrate to the uterus before term labor or prematurely due to an infection process [212–215]. Whether these leukocytes act to help induce labor or represent a consequence of parturition is an active debate [216]. Chemokines mediate the recruitment of immune cells from the peripheral circulation to the site of inflammation by attracting and activating specific leukocyte subsets. There are approximately 50 chemokines that can bind to over 20 distinct chemokine receptors [217]. Blocking one specific receptor may prevent the actions of multiple chemokines, as they induce peripheral leukocyte infiltration into the target tissues. Importantly, the simultaneous blockage of multiple chemokines has not been associated with acute or chronic toxicity, signifying a possible new approach to developing potential PTB therapeutic candidates.

A BSCI can block multiple chemokine signaling pathways [218]. BSCIs specifically bind to the cell-surface somatostatin receptor type 2 (SSTR2) [208,219–225]. Somatostatin is a cyclic neuropeptide hormone that functions as a mediator between the nervous and the immune systems and regulates the immune response [226–230]. In addition to its role in inflammation, recent studies have explored the role of somatostatin and SSTR2 in myometrial cell contractility [231]. In a porcine model, an experimental *Escherichia coli* infection led to increased uterine expression of SSTR2 and an increased amplitude of somatostatin-stimulated uterine contractions [231]. Importantly, SSTR2 antagonists prevented the increase in contraction amplitude, suggesting a role for SSTR2 in mediating uterine contractility [231]. BSCIs are partial agonists of SSTR2 and inhibit pathways generated by multiple chemokine receptors without affecting classical SSTR2 agonist signaling. Mechanisms of BSCI action are not well understood, but it has been hypothesized that partial agonism of BSCI to SSTR2 enables binding to an inflammatory site, which inhibits directional signals from the receptor; consequently, cells become effectively 'blind' to the chemokine gradient. The ability of BSCIs to improve the outcome of many different inflammatory diseases (e.g., allergic asthma, surgical adhesion formation, rheumatoid arthritis, HIV replication, and endometriosis) has been demonstrated in animal models [208,219–224]. Targeting chemokine signaling to prevent pathologic uterine activation in high-risk pregnant people may represent a useful therapeutic approach for PTB prevention.

The first in vivo studies demonstrated that prophylactic administration of the BSCI compound 'BN83470' was able to prevent infection (LPS)-induced PTB in pregnant mice by blocking multiple inflammatory pathways in the uterus and leukocyte infiltration into uterine myometrium (Figure 2) [211]. As a proof of principle in a nonhuman primate model of Group B Streptococcus (GBS)-induced preterm labor, a novel BSCI compound 'FX125L' inhibited preterm labor and suppressed the cytokine response (Figure 2) [210]. Antibiotics were not administered in these experiments, and the GBS infection progressed and invaded the amniotic cavity and the fetus. Despite this invasive GBS infection, BSCI prophylaxis was associated with significantly lower cytokine levels in the amniotic fluid, fetal plasma, lung, and brain, demonstrating its power in suppressing an inflammatory response. However, this result also highlights the danger of administering a chemokine or cytokine inhibitor in the setting of an intrauterine infection without concomitant antibiotic administration; preterm labor may be inhibited, while an intrauterine infection silently invades and injures the fetus. Nevertheless, these data represent an important proof of principal that BSCIs may be highly effective in preventing PTB in humans. Current studies in animal models have suggested that BSCI compounds do not exhibit any significant fetal toxicity. Further study, particularly in human clinical trials, is required to elucidate the effect of BSCI on the fetal immune response and fetal development [210,211].

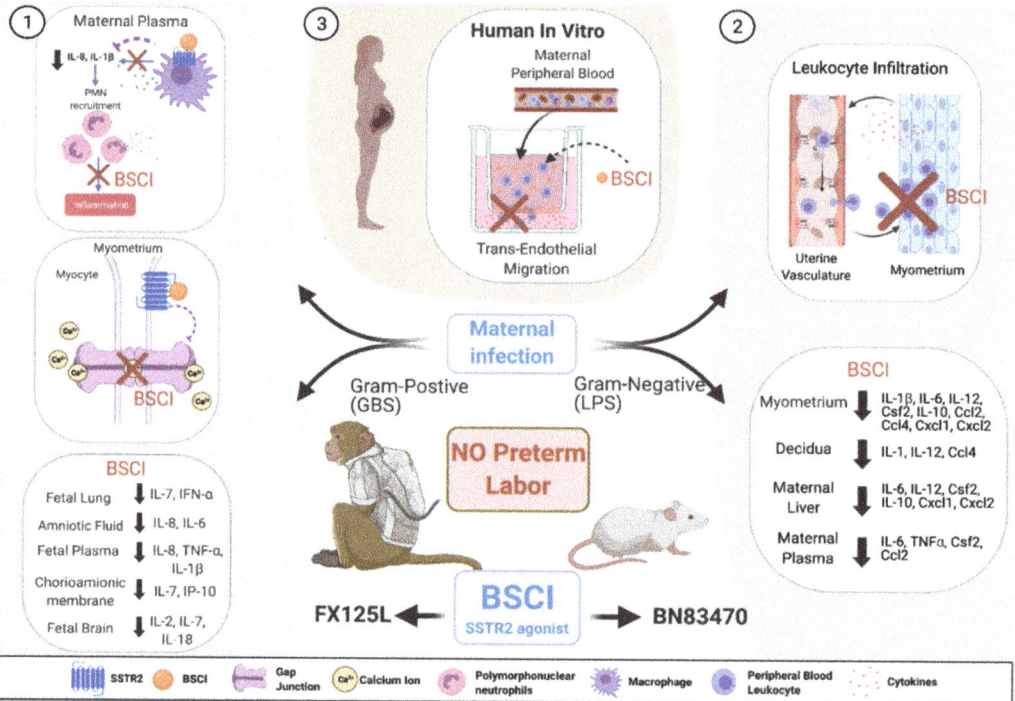

Figure 2. Conceptual model showing BSCI actions in vivo and in vitro as a preterm labor therapeutic. (**1**) In vivo administration of BSCI (FX125L) using a nonhuman primate model of preterm labor induced by Group B Streptococcus (GBS) led to the powerful suppression of uterine activity and a complete blockade of PTB. BSCI treatment led to reduced maternal plasma IL-8 and IL-1β inhibited myometrial gap junction protein connexin 43 mRNA levels and reduced pro-inflammatory cytokines in amniotic fluid, chorioamniotic membrane, fetal plasma, lungs, and brain compared to GBS alone [210]. (**2**) Prophylactic in vivo administration of BSCI (BN83470) decreased LPS-induced PTB in pregnant mice, significantly inhibited neutrophil infiltration in the mouse myometrium, and significantly attenuated multiple cytokine/chemokine expression in maternal tissues (myometrium, decidua, plasma, and liver) [211]. (**3**) We hypothesize that pre-treatment with BSCI (FX125L) of human primary leukocytes isolated from peripheral blood of pregnant people will also prevent the in vitro trans-endothelial migration of neutrophils towards media containing multiple cytokines secreted from the pregnant human decidua and myometrium. Note: this figure was created with Biorender.com.

11. Targeting the Prostaglandin F2 Alpha Receptor: OBE-022

The key role of prostaglandins (particularly PGE_2 and $PGF_{2\alpha}$) in the initiation and progression of labor has made them a target for therapeutics to prevent PTB [232]. Activation of the $PGF_{2\alpha}$ receptor stimulates myometrial contractions and upregulation of matrix metalloproteinases, which leads to cervical ripening and the rupture of membranes [233–236]. Since PGE_2 is the primary fetal prostaglandin, selective inhibition of $PGF_{2\alpha}$ has been proposed to provide effective tocolysis, with reduced fetal morbidity [237].

OBE-022 (ebopiprant) is a highly potent, competitive, reversible inhibitor of the prostaglandin F 2-alpha (PGF$_{2\alpha}$) receptor [238]. OBE-022 has been studied in both human tissues and pregnant animal models and is in Phase II clinical trials. In preclinical studies, OBE-022 inhibited human myometrial contraction in vitro and was more effective in combination with nifedipine or atosiban [238]. In an animal model, OBE-022 showed similar activity to nifedipine for reduction of parturition as well as synergistic effects when used together with nifedipine, without evidence of fetal ductus arteriosus constriction, impairment of fetal renal function, or platelet inhibition [238]. A Phase I trial was performed, which demonstrated that OBE-022 was well tolerated, with no significant side effects in the postmenopausal female population [239,240]. An additional Phase I trial was performed on non-pregnant premenopausal women and demonstrated that OBE-022 was well tolerated alone as well as in combination with nifedipine, magnesium sulfate, atosiban, and betamethasone [241]. Based on the favorable results in the Phase I trials, OBE-022 is currently under investigation in the PROLONG trial, an ongoing Phase 2a randomized, double-blind, placebo-controlled proof-of-concept study in pregnant persons with spontaneous preterm labor at 24–34 weeks' gestation.

OBE022 is also currently being studied for potential side effects similar to indomethacin, with particular focus on closure of the ductus arteriosus, impaired fetal renal function, and inhibition of platelet aggregation [238]. In preclinical studies, OBE-022 was not shown to increase these fetal adverse effects in rat models [238]. Some of the first studies in humans on the potential adverse effects of OBE-022 found favorable pharmacokinetic characteristics and no significant impact on prolonging the QT interval among a cohort of healthy postmenopausal women [239,240].

Additional study is required to examine the effects of co-administration of OBE-022 with other tocolytics [238]. Preliminary data from this study (and others) suggest an encouraging potential for the approach of selective targeting of prostaglandin receptors. Potent tocolytic effects, with reduced adverse fetal impact, may make OBE-022 a promising new therapeutic for delaying PTB [238].

12. Interleukin-1 Receptor Antagonism: Kineret and Rytvela

Early inflammatory events have become an intriguing target for delaying or blocking PTB while protecting the fetus from harmful inflammation [242–246]. A significant upstream target is IL-1β, a pro-inflammatory cytokine thought to be the apex initiator of the parturition cascade (Figure 3) [245]. IL-1β has been shown to induce preterm labor in a mouse model via intrauterine injection as well as in a nonhuman primate model when administered into the amniotic fluid [245,247].

Therapeutic inhibition studies have traditionally involved screening for ligands that bind to the natural ligand's receptor site (orthosteric binding site). Kineret, canakinumab, and rilonacept are large protein orthosteric antagonists to IL-1β that are approved for clinical treatment of inflammatory disorders but have shown limited efficacy for preventing PTB in animal models [245,248,249]. Of particular interest is kineret, a recombinant version of the endogenous IL-1 receptor antagonist (IL-1RA). In rodent, sheep, and nonhuman primate models, systemic administration of kineret at standard (low) doses reduced IL-1β- and LPS-induced fetal inflammation and injury, but much higher doses were required to inhibit inflammation in the uteroplacental unit and prevent PTB [245,246,248–251]. Conversely, standard doses of kineret reduced inflammatory signaling at uteroplacental tissues when directly administered to the amniotic fluid in nonhuman primates and primary cultures of human amnion and chorion [252,253]. This discrepancy is likely attributed to the large molecular size of kineret, which may have limited bioavailability to the placenta. As an orthosteric antagonist, kineret may induce undesired side effects by exerting nonspecific inhibition of all IL-1β signaling pathways, including the immunoregulatory NF-κB pathway [254]. Indeed, kineret, canakinumab, and rilonacept have been associated with injection site reactions, upper respiratory tract infections, vertigo, gastrointestinal disorders, and immune suppression [255,256]. Given these limitations, the alternative is to identify ligands that bind to remote allosteric sites with greater selectivity by affecting the conformational dynamics of the receptor and biasing receptor signaling pathways [257–259].

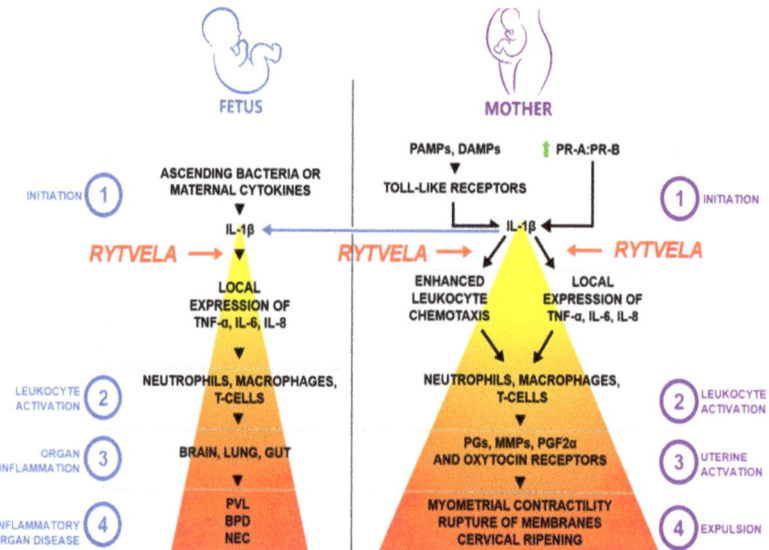

Figure 3. Conceptual model for the role of IL-1β in preterm labor and fetal inflammation. This model illustrates that IL-1β is the apex cytokine in the inflammatory cascade of preterm birth and fetal inflammatory injury, thereby presenting an attractive molecular target for drug discovery. PR-A/PR-B, P4 receptors A and B; PGs, prostaglandins; MMPs, matrix metalloproteinases; $PGF_{2\alpha}$, prostaglandin $F_{2\alpha}$; PLV, periventricular leukomalacia; BPD, bronchopulmonary dysplasia; and NEC, necrotizing enterocolitis. Increasing color intensity represents increasing inflammatory response. The level where Rytvela acts is identified by red arrows. Courtesy of Han Lee.

Rytvela is an example of an allosteric inhibitor of the IL-1R. Rytvela was designed to target the structural region of the IL-1R adjacent to the extracellular juxtamembranous domain of the IL-1RacP (accessory protein), because of its importance to tyrosine kinase receptor activation [260,261]. Rytvela is a 7-amino-acid peptide (each letter refers to the amino acid nomenclature), which was made resistant to hydrolysis by using all d-amino acids. Rytvela has been shown to potently inhibit IL-1β-induced PGE_2 generation, whereas a scrambled peptide (verytla) was ineffective [262]. Furthermore, Rytvela specifically inhibits IL-1R but not homologous IL-1 family cytokines IL-18 or IL-33, the latter of which shares IL-1RacP; acute effects of other pro-inflammatory cytokines (TNFα, IL-6) are also not affected. In contrast to kineret, rytvela does not inhibit IL-1β-induced NF-κB activation and dependent monocyte phagocytosis, preserving immunosurveillance. However, rytvela does inhibit RhoA kinase, p38 and JNK phosphorylation, which inhibits IL-1β from generating more IL-1β—a mechanism that likely leads to blocking PTB but requires further study [243–245]. Hence, consistent with IL-1β-induced inflammation independent of NF-κB, rytvela preserves the NF-κB pathway [245,263–265]. Rytvela exhibits anti-inflammatory properties in several in vivo disease models (e.g., acute dermatitis, chronic rheumatoid arthritis, acute bowel inflammation, ischemic retinopathy and encephalopathy, and degenerative inflammatory retinopathies) [262,266–268].

In rodent models, rytvela has been shown to markedly reduce the uteroplacental surge in inflammatory cytokines and inhibit PTB induced by sterile inflammation from either IL-1β or bacterial-like inflammation triggered by lipoteichoic acid or lipopolysaccharide [245,246]. In these models, rytvela also yielded significant improvements in fetal outcomes. These included reductions in inflammatory signals in the plasma, brain, lungs, retina, and intestines and the associated protection of the fetal brain parenchyma, lung alveolarization, retinal vascular development, and gut mucosal integrity [245,246,266,269–272]. Rytvela will soon be entering a formal pre-clinical phase for toxicity evaluation.

13. Nanoparticles

Nanocarrier systems are aimed at improving the safety profile of tocolytics, and where uterine targeting is included, also improving tocolytic efficacy. These are potentially deliverable benefits, as targeted delivery increases the proportion of a drug that reaches a target tissue while simultaneously reducing localization to non-target tissues. This reduces the amount of drug required to achieve therapeutic efficacy and reduces off-target side effects, which together improve patient safety [273].

Early applications of nanoparticles for improving tocolysis utilized non-targeted liposomes, which are organic, nano-scale lipid vesicles that can be loaded with a broad array of drugs. In 2015, liposomal administration of indomethacin was tested as a method of reducing placental transfer and avoiding adverse effects on the fetus [274–276]. Studies in mice showed strong liposome localization to the pregnant uterus, weak localization to the placenta, and no liposomal transfer to fetuses [274]. Moreover, liposomal encapsulation significantly reduced indomethacin fetal transfer (7.6-fold) [274]. The study did not examine liposome localization to other maternal tissues; however, it provided promising insight into the potential benefits of nanoparticle-facilitated tocolysis.

The first targeted nanoparticles for improving tocolysis were reported in 2015, which were nanoliposomes coated with an antibody that recognized an extracellular domain of the oxytocin receptor (OTR; Figure 4) [277]. The rationale was that the high levels of OTR expression on uterine myocytes during pregnancy could serve as a means of targeting therapeutics to the pregnant myometrium [278,279].

Using spontaneously contracting strips of pregnant human myometrium suspended in organ baths, OTR-targeted nanoliposomes were shown to either abolish or significantly enhance contractions when they were loaded with contraction-blocking or contraction-enhancing drugs, respectively [277,280]. This demonstrated the versatility of the approach. Soon after, the same group reported on the in vivo biodistribution of OTR-targeted nanoliposomes in pregnant mice and evaluated their application toward delivering indomethacin for preventing lipopolysaccharide (LPS)-induced PTB [281]. Less than two months later, a complementary analysis by another lab reported on the benefits of administering indomethacin via OTR-targeted nanoliposomes [282]. These two studies provided compelling proof-of-concept data that demonstrated effective targeting of the pregnant mouse uterus in vivo, enhanced drug delivery to the pregnant mouse uterus, reduced fetal transfer of the drug, and significant reductions in rates of LPS-induced PTB. A key difference between the two studies' OTR-targeted nanoliposomes was their respective OTR targeting moiety, with the former utilizing antibody targeting and the latter utilizing the OTR antagonist peptide, atosiban [281,282]. In a comprehensive in vitro comparison of the two systems, no difference was found in OTR binding, stability, or cellular toxicity [283]. Moreover, both types of OTR-targeted nanoliposomes were shown to be internalized by clathrin- and caveolin-mediated endocytosis, which provided valuable insight into the mechanism of action of OTR-targeted nanoliposomes.

Vaginally administered nanoformulations have also emerged as a promising avenue for preterm birth therapeutics. Uterine efficacy of vaginally administered drugs is facilitated by the uterine first-pass effect; however, vaginally administered drugs must first penetrate the cervicovaginal mucus [284]. To facilitate this, mucus-penetrating particles were developed; they are approximately 200 nm in diameter, with a net neutral surface charge, making them mucoinert (non-adhesive to mucus) and able to penetrate the cervicovaginal mucus [285]. These mucoinert nanosuspensions have been shown to improve the vaginal administration of progesterone and prevent progesterone withdrawal (RU486)-induced preterm birth in mice, while avoiding stimulating myometrial expression of inflammatory cytokines [286]. Other studies have demonstrated successful vaginal administration of the histone deacetylase inhibitors trichostatin-A (TSA) and suberoylanilide hydroxamic acid

(SAHA) via mucoinert nanosuspensions [287]. Nanosuspensions of TSA in combination with progesterone had anti-inflammatory effects on myometrial gene expression and were effective in significantly reducing rates of LPS-induced preterm birth in mice, whereas nanosuspensions of progesterone alone were not effective [287].

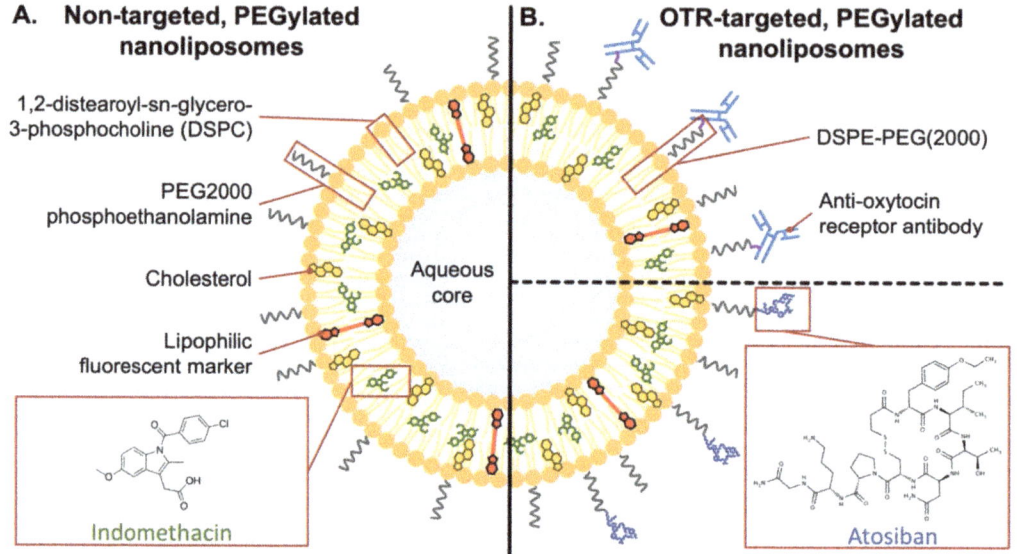

Figure 4. Schematic of non-targeted and uterine-targeted nanoliposomes. (**A**) The nanoliposomes are composed primarily of 1,2-distearoyl-sn-glycero-3-phosphocholine (DSPC) and cholesterol but also include PEGylated lipid (PEG2000 phosphoethanolamine; ~2% of total lipids), which produces steric hindrance that improves circulation time, but without a targeting moiety. Indomethacin and lipophilic markers partition into the lipid bilayer. (**B**) Oxytocin receptor (OTR)-targeted nanoliposomes, whereby PEGylated 1,2-distearoyl-sn-glycero-3-phosphoethanolamine (DSPE, ~2% of total lipids) is conjugated to either an OTR-binding antibody (via maleimide linkage) or peptide (Atosiban, via amine linkage).

Similarly, nanoformulations of the sphingosine kinase (SphK) inhibitor (SKI II) were developed, as SphK inhibition was previously shown to prevent LPS-induced preterm birth in mice [288]. To facilitate the use of SKI II, which has extremely low aqueous solubility, it was incorporated into a self-nanoemulsifying drug delivery system (SNEDDS), which is an isotropic mixture of oil, surfactant, and solvent that forms a stable nanoemulsion when dispersed in aqueous media [289,290]. The SNEDDS increased SKI II solubility over 500-fold, and when vaginally administered, it was effective in significantly reducing rates of LPS-induced preterm birth in mice [289].

Nanoparticle-based systems for improving tocolysis have yet to progress beyond preclinical studies. As such, there are only limited data available from which to speculate on a safety profile respective to mothers or their neonates. Nonetheless, the data generated thus far is promising. For liposome-based systems, OTR-targeted nanoliposomes showed no significant impact on myocyte viability in vitro, while ex vivo, drug-free, OTR-targeted nanoliposomes had no effect on contracting pregnant human myometrial tissue strips, and contractions resumed when drug-loaded OTR-targeted nanoliposomes were washed away [281,283]. In vivo, OTR-targeted nanoliposomes produced no adverse effects upon repeated intravenous administration to pregnant mice [281]. The nanoliposomes were not detected in the maternal brain, kidneys, lung, or heart and were only detected at low levels in mammary tissue and placentae [281,282]. Neither of the landmark studies detected fetal transfer of non-targeted or OTR-targeted nanoliposomes [281,282]. For the vaginal nanoformulations, nanosuspensions of progesterone were found to produce no significant inflammation or toxicity and actually avoided the cervical and myometrial inflammatory signaling induced by a clinical progesterone gel, while nanosuspensions of TSA and progesterone led to delivery of live pups that exhibited neurotypical development [286,287]. Moreover, vaginal delivery of SKI II via SNEDDS had no toxic effect on cultured human cervical cells (HeLa) after 24 h, and a teratogenicity study revealed no effect on birth weight or the prevalence of congenital anomalies among pups born to treated dams. Collectively, these data support low toxicity of both OTR nanoliposomes and vaginal nanoformulations; however, more in-depth studies are required as technologies advance toward clinical translation.

14. Challenges in Therapeutic Development

Historically, the ability to study medication use in pregnancy has been limited by the ethical challenges of enrolling pregnant people in research studies and regulatory hurdles posed by the U.S. FDA edict on atosiban in 1998 (Box 1). Atosiban was not given FDA approval due to concerns regarding the number of infant deaths among pregnant people treated with atosiban compared to a placebo. That ruling generated tremendous challenges in designing studies to clinically test potential tocolytic drugs. Novel agents now require a placebo-controlled trial to show efficacy, an option that few U.S. centers would consider, and one that some U.S. IRBs resist as contradictory to the standard of care. Attempts to circumvent stringent regulations on therapeutic research have led to many studies being exported to other countries with fewer restrictions [291]. This emerging practice raises numerous ethical concerns regarding the potential exploitation of local residents. An alternative to a purely placebo-controlled trial is 'rescue therapy', in which researchers administer a community-standard tocolytic (e.g., magnesium sulfate) one hour after administration of the study drug. However, as seen in the Atosiban-096 trial, rescue therapy diminishes the chance of demonstrating the full benefits of the novel drug and complicates interpretation of the results [71,73]. Furthermore, because there are no FDA-approved drugs for tocolysis that are still marketed, it is not possible to conduct an active control trial for a new tocolytic therapeutic in the U.S. In a given subset of pregnant patients, the accepted standard of care to administer off-label use of tocolytics confounds the study results, as the intervention in practice may have taken place before patients meet the definition of preterm labor necessary for enrollment.

Compounding these challenges, the FDA further insisted that future approval of tocolytic drugs be contingent upon improving neonatal outcomes. Delaying PTB is not sufficient by itself for a novel drug to obtain FDA approval, and perinatal mortality occurs too infrequently to use as a measurable outcome [54]. This poses a significant logistical burden for subject enrollment. The Atosiban-096 randomized control trial ran for longer than three years and involved 35 centers in North and South America, but it only enrolled 513 women, despite broad diagnostic criteria for spontaneous preterm labor [74]. Additionally, the field of obstetrics currently lacks a laboratory measure that can be tightly linked to PTB or neonatal outcomes, making it difficult to measure the ability of a PTB therapeutic to prevent a surrogate endpoint [6].

15. Pathway Forward toward New PTB Therapeutics

Identifying and finding solutions to navigate the obstacles for tocolytic development is a profound challenge. The solution is most likely to come from a coordinated, unified effort between PTB researchers, regulatory agencies, tocolytic pharmaceutical companies, obstetricians and other clinicians, funding bodies—both private foundations and government agencies—academic organizations, and patient advocacy groups. A model for this kind of collaboration already exists: the International Neonatal Consortium [292]. Developed in 2015, the International Neonatal Consortium is focused on standardizing criteria and methods for regulating both neonatal medicine development and administration in collaboration with regulatory agencies [292]. This organization has already demonstrated progress in addressing the regulatory science of two other common neonatal disorders, neonatal seizures and bronchopulmonary dysplasia, for which various therapeutics have long been employed off-label [292]. A similar global and coordinated effort could be applied to advancing the regulatory science of PTB therapeutics. Without a well-defined path to regulatory approval for novel tocolytics in the U.S., workshops are needed to debate the requirements for tocolytic approval. Should neonatal morbidity and mortality remain an imperative outcome of study to earn FDA approval, alternative study designs should be considered to achieve practical and timely study execution. Global collaboration would allow for data pooling and could accelerate study completion [292]. Finally, pregnant people are crucial stakeholders in this process and should be involved in the study design.

16. Conclusions

PTB is a multi-faceted obstetric problem and a major cause of neonatal morbidity and mortality. At present, there are numerous tocolytics employed in the management of PTB, providing a short delay in order to transfer patients to high-level care facilities or, rarely, to effectively reduce neonatal morbidities. There is an urgent need to develop tocolytic agents that can provide a longer-lasting delay of PTB that clearly impacts neonatal and child health. These novel agents in pre-clinical development or in clinical trials include BSCI, OBE-022, IL1-R antagonist (e.g., Rytvela, Kineret), and nanoparticle delivery systems. Significant regulatory hurdles exist for bringing any new therapeutic in pregnancy to market. The few tocolytic studies that previously garnered FDA approval are no longer adequate or appropriate as a model for testing new PTB therapeutics, hindering the ability of novel therapeutic research to follow a standardized study design. A new coordinated approach between clinicians, scientists, drug development agencies, pharmaceutical companies, funding organizations, and patient advocacy groups is necessary to accelerate the development of PTB therapeutics. This collaboration will aid in developing more effective study designs and will cultivate data pooling to allow for practical and timely evaluation of novel therapeutic agents.

Author Contributions: All authors have contributed to writing the first draft of the manuscript: B.S.C. (Abstract, Sections 1–5, Sections 7 and 16 and contributed to Sections 6 and 8, Sections 9–15), A.K. (contributed to Sections 6 and 7), L.S. (contributed to Section 6), A.C. (Section 8). O.S., A.B.-R. and S.L. (Sections 9 and 10 and Figure 1), S.M. (Section 11 and Figure 2), K.B.L., W.X., S.C. and D.O. (Section 12, Figure 3). J.W.P. and R.S. (Section 13 and Figure 4), M.L. (Sections 4 and 14), E.H. (Section 15, Table 2, and Box 1). Subsequent critical revisions were made by B.S.C. and K.M.A.W. All authors agree to be accountable for the content of the work. All authors have read and agreed to the published version of the manuscript.

Funding: This work was supported primarily by funding from the University of Washington Population Health Initiative, Department of Obstetrics & Gynecology and philanthropic gift funds. This work was also supported by the National Institute of Allergy and Infectious Diseases (grant numbers AI133976, AI145890, AI143265, and HD098713 to K.M.A.W. and HD001264 to A.K.) and the National Health and Medical Research Council, Australia (grant numbers APP1162684 to J.W.P. and APP1113847 to R.S.). This work was also supported by the Canadian Institute of Health Research Foundation Grant to S.L. (CIHR: FDN-143262), March of Dimes Foundation to S.L. and O.S. (MOD-6-FY17-647) and the Burroughs Wellcome Fund to S.L., O.S. and K.M.A.W. (#1013759). D. Olson, K.B. Leimert, W. Xu, and S. Chemtob are supported by the Canadian Institutes of Health Research #168858; a portion of the work presented, conducted by S. Chemtob and D. Olson, was also partly supported by the Ministry of Economy and Innovation, Quebec. K. Leimert is also supported by the generosity of the Stollery Children's Hospital Foundation and supporters of the Alberta Women's Health Foundation through the Women and Children's Health Research Institute. S. Chemtob is recipient of a Canada Research Chair and the Leopoldine Wolfe Chair. The content is solely the responsibility of the authors and does not necessarily represent the official views of the National Institutes of Health or other funders.

Institutional Review Board Statement: Not applicable.

Informed Consent Statement: Not applicable.

Data Availability Statement: Not applicable.

Conflicts of Interest: Alisa Kachikis is on a Pfizer and GlaxoSmithKline Advisory Board for Immunizations, which is unrelated to the content of this manuscript. David Olson and Sylvain Chemtob are founders of Maternica Therapeutics, Inc., and David Olson is founder and CEO of Livmor Therapeutics, Inc. David Olson and Sylvain Chemtob were the primary authors of the following section(s) of this manuscript: Section 12. Jonathan W. Paul and Roger Smith hold patents in the United States, Europe, and Australia related to reproductive medical applications of uterine-targeted nanoparticles. Jonathan Paul and Roger Smith were the primary authors of the following section(s) of this manuscript: Section 13. The remaining authors report no conflict of interest.

References

1. Howson, C.P.; Kinney, M.V.; McDougall, L.; Lawn, J.E.; The Born Too Soon Preterm Birth Action Group. Born too soon: Preterm birth matters. *Repro. Health* **2013**, *10* (Suppl. 1), 1–9. [CrossRef]
2. Blencowe, H.; Cousens, S.; Oestergaard, M.Z.; Chou, D.; Moller, A.B.; Narwal, R.; Adler, A.; Vera Garcia, C.; Rohde, S.; Say, L.; et al. National, regional, and worldwide estimates of preterm birth rates in the year 2010 with time trends since 1990 for selected countries: A systematic analysis and implications. *Lancet* **2012**, *379*, 2162–2172. [CrossRef]
3. Romero, R.; Dey, S.K.; Fisher, S.J. Preterm labor: One syndrome, many causes. *Science* **2014**, *345*, 760–765. [CrossRef] [PubMed]
4. Suman, V.; Luther, E.E. Preterm Labor. In *StatPearls*; StatPearls Publishing: Treasure Island, FL, USA, 2021.
5. Kramer, M.S.; Demissie, K.; Yang, H.; Platt, R.W.; Sauve, R.; Liston, R. The contribution of mild and moderate preterm birth to infant mortality. Fetal and Infant Health Study Group of the Canadian Perinatal Surveillance System. *JAMA* **2000**, *284*, 843–849. [CrossRef] [PubMed]
6. Behrman, R.E.; Butler, A.S. *Preterm Birth: Causes, Consequences, and Prevention*; National Academies Press (US): Washington, DC, USA, 2007. [CrossRef]
7. Vogel, J.P.; Nardin, J.M.; Dowswell, T.; West, H.M.; Oladapo, O.T. Combination of tocolytic agents for inhibiting preterm labour. *Cochrane Database Syst. Rev.* **2014**, CD006169. [CrossRef]
8. De Heus, R.; Mulder, E.J.; Visser, G.H. Management of preterm labor: Atosiban or nifedipine? *Int. J. Womens Health* **2010**, *2*, 137–142. [CrossRef]
9. Papatsonis, D.N.; Flenady, V.; Liley, H.G. Maintenance therapy with oxytocin antagonists for inhibiting preterm birth after threatened preterm labour. *Cochrane Database Syst. Rev.* **2013**, CD005938. [CrossRef]
10. Dodd, J.M.; Crowther, C.A.; Middleton, P. Oral betamimetics for maintenance therapy after threatened preterm labour. *Cochrane Database Syst. Rev.* **2012**, *12*, CD003927. [CrossRef]
11. Nanda, K.; Cook, L.A.; Gallo, M.F.; Grimes, D.A. Terbutaline pump maintenance therapy after threatened preterm labor for preventing preterm birth. *Cochrane Database Syst. Rev.* **2002**, CD003933. [CrossRef]
12. Naik Gaunekar, N.; Raman, P.; Bain, E.; Crowther, C.A. Maintenance therapy with calcium channel blockers for preventing preterm birth after threatened preterm labour. *Cochrane Database Syst. Rev.* **2013**. [CrossRef]
13. Han, S.; Crowther, C.A.; Moore, V. Magnesium maintenance therapy for preventing preterm birth after threatened preterm labour. *Cochrane Database Syst. Rev.* **2013**. [CrossRef]
14. Chawanpaiboon, S.; Vogel, J.P.; Moller, A.B.; Lumbiganon, P.; Petzold, M.; Hogan, D.; Landoulsi, S.; Jampathong, N.; Kongwattanakul, K.; Laopaiboon, M.; et al. Global, regional, and national estimates of levels of preterm birth in 2014: A systematic review and modelling analysis. *Lancet Glob. Health* **2019**, *7*, e37–e46. [CrossRef]
15. Walani, S.R. Global burden of preterm birth. *Int. J. Gynaecol. Obstet.* **2020**, *150*, 31–33. [CrossRef]
16. Flenady, V.; Reinebrant, H.E.; Liley, H.G.; Tambimuttu, E.G.; Papatsonis, D.N. Oxytocin receptor antagonists for inhibiting preterm labour. *Cochrane Database Syst. Rev.* **2014**, CD004452. [CrossRef]
17. Ples, L.; Sima, R.M.; Ricu, A.; Moga, M.A.; Ionescu, A.C. The efficacy of cervical cerclage combined with a pessary for the prevention of spontaneous preterm birth. *J. Matern Fetal Neonatal Med.* **2019**, 1–5. [CrossRef]
18. Care, A.; Jackson, R.; O'Brien, E.; Leigh, S.; Cornforth, C.; Haycox, A.; Whitworth, M.; Lavender, T.; Alfirevic, Z. Cervical cerclage, pessary, or vaginal progesterone in high-risk pregnant women with short cervix: A randomized feasibility study. *J. Matern Fetal Neonatal Med.* **2021**, *34*, 49–57. [CrossRef]
19. Saccone, G.; Maruotti, G.M.; Giudicepietro, A.; Martinelli, P.; The Italian Preterm Birth Prevention Working Group. Effect of Cervical Pessary on Spontaneous Preterm Birth in Women With Singleton Pregnancies and Short Cervical Length: A Randomized Clinical Trial. *JAMA* **2017**, *318*, 2317–2324. [CrossRef]
20. Adams Waldorf, K.M.; Singh, N.; Mohan, A.R.; Young, R.C.; Ngo, L.; Das, A.; Tsai, J.; Bansal, A.; Paolella, L.; Herbert, B.R.; et al. Uterine overdistention induces preterm labor mediated by inflammation: Observations in pregnant women and nonhuman primates. *Am. J. Obstet. Gynecol.* **2015**, *213*, 830.e1–830.e19. [CrossRef]
21. Lye, S.J.; Mitchell, J.; Nashman, N.; Oldenhof, A.; Ou, R.; Shynlova, O.; Langille, L. Role of mechanical signals in the onset of term and preterm labor. *Front. Horm Res.* **2001**, *27*, 165–178.
22. McLean, M.; Bisits, A.; Davies, J.; Woods, R.; Lowry, P.; Smith, R. A placental clock controlling the length of human pregnancy. *Nat. Med.* **1995**, *1*, 460–463. [CrossRef]
23. Gravett, M.G.; Novy, M.J. Endocrine-immune interactions in pregnant non-human primates with intrauterine infection. *Infect. Dis. Obstet. Gynecol.* **1997**, *5*, 142–153. [CrossRef] [PubMed]

24. Hillier, S.L.; Krohn, M.A.; Kiviat, N.B.; Watts, D.H.; Eschenbach, D.A. Microbiologic causes and neonatal outcomes associated with chorioamnion infection. *Am. J. Obstet. Gynecol.* **1991**, *165*, 955–961. [CrossRef]
25. Hillier, S.L.; Witkin, S.S.; Krohn, M.A.; Watts, D.H.; Kiviat, N.B.; Eschenbach, D.A. The relationship of amniotic fluid cytokines and preterm delivery, amniotic fluid infection, histologic chorioamnionitis, and chorioamnion infection. *Obstet. Gynecol.* **1993**, *81*, 941–948. [PubMed]
26. Romero, R.; Sepulveda, W.; Kenney, J.S.; Archer, L.E.; Allison, A.C.; Sehgal, P.B. Interleukin 6 determination in the detection of microbial invasion of the amniotic cavity. *Ciba Found. Symp.* **1992**, *167*, 205–220, discussion 220–203.
27. Yoon, B.H.; Romero, R.; Kim, C.J.; Jun, J.K.; Gomez, R.; Choi, J.H.; Syn, H.C. Amniotic fluid interleukin-6: A sensitive test for antenatal diagnosis of acute inflammatory lesions of preterm placenta and prediction of perinatal morbidity. *Am. J. Obstet. Gynecol.* **1995**, *172*, 960–970. [CrossRef]
28. Rosen, T.; Kuczynski, E.; O'Neill, L.M.; Funai, E.F.; Lockwood, C.J. Plasma levels of thrombin-antithrombin complexes predict preterm premature rupture of the fetal membranes. *J. Matern. Fetal Med.* **2001**, *10*, 297–300. [CrossRef]
29. Stephenson, C.D.; Lockwood, C.J.; Ma, Y.; Guller, S. Thrombin-dependent regulation of matrix metalloproteinase (MMP)-9 levels in human fetal membranes. *J. Matern Fetal Neona* **2005**, *18*, 17–22. [CrossRef]
30. Chai, M.; Barker, G.; Menon, R.; Lappas, M. Increased oxidative stress in human fetal membranes overlying the cervix from term non-labouring and post labour deliveries. *Placenta* **2012**, *33*, 604–610. [CrossRef]
31. Menon, R.; Fortunato, S.J.; Yu, J.; Milne, G.L.; Sanchez, S.; Drobek, C.O.; Lappas, M.; Taylor, R.N. Cigarette smoke induces oxidative stress and apoptosis in normal term fetal membranes. *Placenta* **2011**, *32*, 317–322. [CrossRef]
32. Menon, R.; Yu, J.; Basanta-Henry, P.; Brou, L.; Berga, S.L.; Fortunato, S.J.; Taylor, R.N. Short fetal leukocyte telomere length and preterm prelabor rupture of the membranes. *PLoS ONE* **2012**, *7*, e31136. [CrossRef]
33. Bredeson, S.; Papaconstantinou, J.; Deford, J.H.; Kechichian, T.; Syed, T.A.; Saade, G.R.; Menon, R. HMGB1 promotes a p38MAPK associated non-infectious inflammatory response pathway in human fetal membranes. *PLoS ONE* **2014**, *9*, e113799. [CrossRef]
34. Menon, R. Oxidative stress damage as a detrimental factor in preterm birth pathology. *Front. Immunol.* **2014**, *5*, 567. [CrossRef]
35. Menon, R.; Behnia, F.; Polettini, J.; Saade, G.R.; Campisi, J.; Velarde, M. Placental membrane aging and HMGB1 signaling associated with human parturition. *Aging* **2016**, *8*, 216–230. [CrossRef]
36. Menon, R.; Boldogh, I.; Hawkins, H.K.; Woodson, M.; Polettini, J.; Syed, T.A.; Fortunato, S.J.; Saade, G.R.; Papaconstantinou, J.; Taylor, R.N. Histological evidence of oxidative stress and premature senescence in preterm premature rupture of the human fetal membranes recapitulated in vitro. *Am. J. Pathol* **2014**, *184*, 1740–1751. [CrossRef]
37. Zhang, G.; Feenstra, B.; Bacelis, J.; Liu, X.; Muglia, L.M.; Juodakis, J.; Miller, D.E.; Litterman, N.; Jiang, P.P.; Russell, L.; et al. Genetic Associations with Gestational Duration and Spontaneous Preterm Birth. *N. Engl. J. Med.* **2017**, *377*, 1156–1167. [CrossRef]
38. Bower, K.M.; Geller, R.J.; Perrin, N.A.; Alhusen, J. Experiences of Racism and Preterm Birth: Findings from a Pregnancy Risk Assessment Monitoring System, 2004 through 2012. *Womens Health Issues* **2018**, *28*, 495–501. [CrossRef]
39. Krieger, N.; Van Wye, G.; Huynh, M.; Waterman, P.D.; Maduro, G.; Li, W.; Gwynn, R.C.; Barbot, O.; Bassett, M.T. Structural Racism, Historical Redlining, and Risk of Preterm Birth in New York City, 2013-2017. *Am. J. Public Health* **2020**, *110*, 1046–1053. [CrossRef]
40. Mendez, D.D.; Hogan, V.K.; Culhane, J.F. Institutional racism, neighborhood factors, stress, and preterm birth. *Ethn Health* **2014**, *19*, 479–499. [CrossRef]
41. Rich-Edwards, J.; Krieger, N.; Majzoub, J.; Zierler, S.; Lieberman, E.; Gillman, M. Maternal experiences of racism and violence as predictors of preterm birth: Rationale and study design. *Paediatr. Perinat Epidemiol.* **2001**, *15* (Suppl. 2), 124–135. [CrossRef]
42. Slaughter-Acey, J.C.; Sealy-Jefferson, S.; Helmkamp, L.; Caldwell, C.H.; Osypuk, T.L.; Platt, R.W.; Straughen, J.K.; Dailey-Okezie, R.K.; Abeysekara, P.; Misra, D.P. Racism in the form of micro aggressions and the risk of preterm birth among black women. *Ann. Epidemiol.* **2016**, *26*, 7–13.e11. [CrossRef]
43. Cappelletti, M.; Della Bella, S.; Ferrazzi, E.; Mavilio, D.; Divanovic, S. Inflammation and preterm birth. *J. Leukoc Biol.* **2016**, *99*, 67–78. [CrossRef]
44. Kemp, M.W. Preterm birth, intrauterine infection, and fetal inflammation. *Front. Immunol.* **2014**, *5*, 574. [CrossRef]
45. Fortunato, S.J.; Menon, R.P.; Swan, K.F.; Menon, R. Inflammatory cytokine (interleukins 1, 6 and 8 and tumor necrosis factor-alpha) release from cultured human fetal membranes in response to endotoxic lipopolysaccharide mirrors amniotic fluid concentrations. *Am. J. Obstet. Gynecol.* **1996**, *174*, 1855–1861, discussion 1861–1852. [CrossRef]
46. Menon, R.; Peltier, M.R.; Eckardt, J.; Fortunato, S.J. Diversity in cytokine response to bacteria associated with preterm birth by fetal membranes. *Am. J. Obstet. Gynecol.* **2009**, *201*, 306.e1–306.e6. [CrossRef]
47. Romero, R.; Ceska, M.; Avila, C.; Mazor, M.; Behnke, E.; Lindley, I. Neutrophil attractant/activating peptide-1/interleukin-8 in term and preterm parturition. *Am. J. Obstet. Gynecol.* **1991**, *165*, 813–820. [CrossRef]
48. Romero, R.; Gomez, R.; Ghezzi, F.; Yoon, B.H.; Mazor, M.; Edwin, S.S.; Berry, S.M. A fetal systemic inflammatory response is followed by the spontaneous onset of preterm parturition. *Am. J. Obstet. Gynecol.* **1998**, *179*, 186–193. [CrossRef]
49. Romero, R.; Gomez, R.; Galasso, M.; Mazor, M.; Berry, S.M.; Quintero, R.A.; Cotton, D.B. The natural interleukin-1 receptor antagonist in the fetal, maternal, and amniotic fluid compartments: The effect of gestational age, fetal gender, and intrauterine infection. *Am. J. Obstet. Gynecol.* **1994**, *171*, 912–921. [CrossRef]
50. Nadeau-Vallee, M.; Obari, D.; Quiniou, C.; Lubell, W.D.; Olson, D.M.; Girard, S.; Chemtob, S. A critical role of interleukin-1 in preterm labor. *Cytokine Growth Factor Rev.* **2016**, *28*, 37–51. [CrossRef]

51. Gomez-Lopez, N.; Laresgoiti-Servitje, E.; Olson, D.M.; Estrada-Gutierrez, G.; Vadillo-Ortega, F. The role of chemokines in term and premature rupture of the fetal membranes: A review. *Biol. Reprod* **2010**, *82*, 809–814. [CrossRef]
52. Vadillo-Ortega, F.; Estrada-Gutierrez, G. Role of matrix metalloproteinases in preterm labour. *BJOG* **2005**, *112* (Suppl. 1), 19–22. [CrossRef] [PubMed]
53. Keirse, M.J. The history of tocolysis. *BJOG* **2003**, *110* (Suppl. 20), 94–97. [CrossRef]
54. Elliott, J.P.; Morrison, J.C. The evidence regarding maintenance tocolysis. *Obstet. Gynecol. Int.* **2013**, *2013*, 708023. [CrossRef] [PubMed]
55. Chawanpaiboon, S.; Laopaiboon, M.; Lumbiganon, P.; Sangkomkamhang, U.S.; Dowswell, T. Terbutaline pump maintenance therapy after threatened preterm labour for reducing adverse neonatal outcomes. *Cochrane Database Syst. Rev.* **2014**, CD010800. [CrossRef] [PubMed]
56. Creasy, R.K.; Golbus, M.S.; Laros, R.K., Jr.; Parer, J.T.; Roberts, J.M. Oral ritodrine maintenance in the treatment of preterm labor. *Am. J. Obstet. Gynecol.* **1980**, *137*, 212–219. [CrossRef]
57. Chae, J.; Cho, G.J.; Oh, M.J.; Park, K.; Han, S.W.; Choi, S.J.; Oh, S.-Y.; Roh, C.R. In utero exposure to ritodrine during pregnancy and risk of autism in their offspring until 8 years of age. *Sci. Rep.* **2021**, [CrossRef]
58. Woyton, J.; Zimmer, M.; Fuchs, T. The use of Gynipral (hexoprenaline) in suppression of uterus contractions. *Ginekol. Pol.* **1999**, *70*, 896–900.
59. Haas, D.M.; Benjamin, T.; Sawyer, R.; Quinney, S.K. Short-term tocolytics for preterm delivery—Current perspectives. *Int. J. Womens Health* **2014**, *6*, 343–349. [CrossRef]
60. Neilson, J.P.; West, H.M.; Dowswell, T. Betamimetics for inhibiting preterm labour. *Cochrane Database Syst Rev.* **2014**, CD004352. [CrossRef]
61. Kosasa, T.S.; Nakayama, R.T.; Hale, R.W.; Rinzler, G.S.; Freitas, C.A. Ritodrine and terbutaline compared for the treatment of preterm labor. *Acta Obstet. Gynecol. Scand.* **1985**, *64*, 421–426. [CrossRef]
62. Beall, M.H.; Edgar, B.W.; Paul, R.H.; Smith-Wallace, T. A comparison of ritodrine, terbutaline, and magnesium sulfate for the suppression of preterm labor. *Am. J. Obstet. Gynecol.* **1985**, *153*, 854–859. [CrossRef]
63. Kopelman, J.N.; Duff, P.; Read, J.A. Randomized comparison of oral terbutaline and ritodrine for preventing recurrent preterm labor. *J. Reprod Med.* **1989**, *34*, 225–230. [PubMed]
64. Weiss, M.A. Retrospective analysis of the effects of ritodrine and terbutaline in the management of preterm labor. *Clin. Pharm.* **1982**, *1*, 453–456. [PubMed]
65. Caritis, S.N.; Toig, G.; Heddinger, L.A.; Ashmead, G. A double-blind study comparing ritodrine and terbutaline in the treatment of preterm labor. *Am. J. Obstet. Gynecol.* **1984**, *150*, 7–14. [CrossRef]
66. Galik, M.; Gaspar, R.; Kolarovszki-Sipiczki, Z.; Falkay, G. Gestagen treatment enhances the tocolytic effect of salmeterol in hormone-induced preterm labor in the rat in vivo. *Am. J. Obstet. Gynecol.* **2008**, *198*, 319.e1–319.e5. [CrossRef]
67. Gaspar, R.; Hajagos-Toth, J. Calcium channel blockers as tocolytics: Principles of their actions, adverse effects and therapeutic combinations. *Pharmaceuticals* **2013**, *6*, 689–699. [CrossRef]
68. Perna, R.; Loughan, A.; Perkey, H.; Tyson, K. Terbutaline and Associated Risks for Neurodevelopmental Disorders. *Child. Dev. Res.* **2014**, *2014*. [CrossRef]
69. Hayes, E.; Moroz, L.; Pizzi, L.; Baxter, J. A cost decision analysis of 4 tocolytic drugs. *Am. J. Obstet. Gynecol.* **2007**, *197*, 383.e1–383.e6. [CrossRef]
70. Akerlund, M.; Carlsson, A.M.; Melin, P.; Trojnar, J. The effect on the human uterus of two newly developed competitive inhibitors of oxytocin and vasopressin. *Acta Obstet. Gynecol. Scand.* **1985**, *64*, 499–504. [CrossRef]
71. Goodwin, T.M.; Paul, R.; Silver, H.; Spellacy, W.; Parsons, M.; Chez, R.; Hayashi, R.; Valenzuela, G.; Creasy, G.W.; Merriman, R. The effect of the oxytocin antagonist atosiban on preterm uterine activity in the human. *Am. J. Obstet. Gynecol.* **1994**, *170*, 474–478. [CrossRef]
72. Goodwin, T.M.; Valenzuela, G.J.; Silver, H.; Creasy, G. Dose ranging study of the oxytocin antagonist atosiban in the treatment of preterm labor. Atosiban Study Group. *Obstet. Gynecol.* **1996**, *88*, 331–336. [CrossRef]
73. Romero, R.; Sibai, B.M.; Sanchez-Ramos, L.; Valenzuela, G.J.; Veille, J.C.; Tabor, B.; Perry, K.G.; Varner, M.; Goodwin, T.M.; Lane, R.; et al. An oxytocin receptor antagonist (atosiban) in the treatment of preterm labor: A randomized, double-blind, placebo-controlled trial with tocolytic rescue. *Am. J. Obstet. Gynecol.* **2000**, *182*, 1173–1183. [CrossRef]
74. Valenzuela, G.J.; Sanchez-Ramos, L.; Romero, R.; Silver, H.M.; Koltun, W.D.; Millar, L.; Hobbins, J.; Rayburn, W.; Shangold, G.; Wang, J.; et al. Maintenance treatment of preterm labor with the oxytocin antagonist atosiban. The Atosiban PTL-098 Study Group. *Am. J. Obstet. Gynecol.* **2000**, *182*, 1184–1190. [CrossRef]
75. Greene, J.A.; Podolsky, S.H. Reform, regulation, and pharmaceuticals—The Kefauver-Harris Amendments at 50. *N. Engl. J. Med.* **2012**, *367*, 1481–1483. [CrossRef]
76. Veiga, G.A.; Milazzotto, M.P.; Nichi, M.; Lucio, C.F.; Silva, L.C.; Angrimani, D.S.; Vannucchi, C.I. Gene expression of estrogen and oxytocin receptors in the uterus of pregnant and parturient bitches. *Braz. J. Med. Biol. Res.* **2015**, *48*, 339–343. [CrossRef]
77. Arthur, P.; Taggart, M.J.; Mitchell, B.F. Oxytocin and parturition: A role for increased myometrial calcium and calcium sensitization? *Front. Biosci.* **2007**, *12*, 619–633. [CrossRef]

78. Kim, S.H.; Riaposova, L.; Ahmed, H.; Pohl, O.; Chollet, A.; Gotteland, J.P.; Hanyaloglu, A.; Bennett, P.R.; Terzidou, V. Oxytocin Receptor Antagonists, Atosiban and Nolasiban, Inhibit Prostaglandin F2alpha-induced Contractions and Inflammatory Responses in Human Myometrium. *Sci. Rep.* **2019**, *9*, 5792. [CrossRef]
79. Moutquin, J.M.; Sherman, D.; Cohen, H.; Mohide, P.T.; Hochner-Celnikier, D.; Fejgin, M.; Liston, R.M.; Dansereau, J.; Mazor, M.; Shalev, E.; et al. Double-blind, randomized, controlled trial of atosiban and ritodrine in the treatment of preterm labor: A multicenter effectiveness and safety study. *Am. J. Obstet. Gynecol.* **2000**, *182*, 1191–1199. [CrossRef]
80. Papatsonis, D.; Flenady, V.; Cole, S.; Liley, H. Oxytocin receptor antagonists for inhibiting preterm labour. *Cochrane Database Syst. Rev.* **2005**, CD004452. [CrossRef]
81. Fullerton, M.B.G.M.; Shetty, A.; Bhattacharya, S. Atosiban in the Management of Preterm Labor. *Clin. Med. Insights: Women's Health* **2011**, *4*. [CrossRef]
82. Sanchez-Ramos, L. A double-blind placebo-controlled trial of oxytocin receptor antagonist (antocin) maintenance therapy in patients with preterm labor. *Pediatric Res.* **1997**, *41*. [CrossRef]
83. Taira, N. Nifedipine: A novel vasodilator. *Drugs* **2006**, *66*, 1–3. [CrossRef] [PubMed]
84. Conde-Agudelo, A.; Romero, R.; Kusanovic, J.P. Nifedipine in the management of preterm labor: A systematic review and metaanalysis. *Am. J. Obstet. Gynecol.* **2011**, *204*, 134.e1–134.e20. [CrossRef] [PubMed]
85. Le Ray, C.; Maillard, F.; Carbonne, B.; Verspyck, E.; Cabrol, D.; Goffinet, F.; EVAPRIMA Group. Nifedipine or nicardipine in management of threatened preterm delivery: An observational population-based study. *J. Gynecol. Obstet. Biol. Reprod* **2010**, *39*, 490–497. [CrossRef] [PubMed]
86. Papatsonis, D.N.; Van Geijn, H.P.; Ader, H.J.; Lange, F.M.; Bleker, O.P.; Dekker, G.A. Nifedipine and ritodrine in the management of preterm labor: A randomized multicenter trial. *Obstet. Gynecol.* **1997**, *90*, 230–234. [CrossRef]
87. Habli, M.; Clifford, C.C.; Brady, T.M.; Rodriguez, Z.; Eschenbacher, M.; Wu, M.; DeFranco, E.; Gresh, J.; Kamath-Rayne, B.D. Antenatal exposure to nonsteroidal anti-inflammatory drugs and risk of neonatal hypertension. *J. Clin. Hypertens* **2018**, *20*, 1334–1341. [CrossRef]
88. Abramson, S.; Korchak, H.; Ludewig, R.; Edelson, H.; Haines, K.; Levin, R.I.; Herman, R.; Rider, L.; Kimmel, S.; Weissmann, G. Modes of action of aspirin-like drugs. *Proc. Natl. Acad. Sci. USA* **1985**, *82*, 7227–7231. [CrossRef]
89. Orlando, B.J.; Lucido, M.J.; Malkowski, M.G. The structure of ibuprofen bound to cyclooxygenase-2. *J. Struct. Biol.* **2015**, *189*, 62–66. [CrossRef]
90. Al-Mondhiri, H.M.A.; Spaet, T.H. Acetylation of human platelets by aspirin. *Fed. Proc.* **1969**, *28*, 576.
91. Mitchell, J.A.; Akarasereenont, P.; Thiemermann, C.; Flower, R.J.; Vane, J.R. Selectivity of nonsteroidal antiinflammatory drugs as inhibitors of constitutive and inducible cyclooxygenase. *Proc. Natl. Acad. Sci. USA* **1993**, *90*, 11693–11697. [CrossRef]
92. Sadovsky, Y.; Nelson, D.M.; Muglia, L.J.; Gross, G.A.; Harris, K.C.; Koki, A.; Masferrer, J.L.; Olson, L.M. Effective diminution of amniotic prostaglandin production by selective inhibitors of cyclooxygenase type 2. *Am. J. Obstet. Gynecol.* **2000**, *182*, 370–376. [CrossRef]
93. Gross, G.; Imamura, T.; Vogt, S.K.; Wozniak, D.F.; Nelson, D.M.; Sadovsky, Y.; Muglia, L.J. Inhibition of cyclooxygenase-2 prevents inflammation-mediated preterm labor in the mouse. *Am. J. Physiol. Regul. Integr. Comp. Physiol.* **2000**, *278*, R1415–R1423. [CrossRef]
94. Yousif, M.H.; Thulesius, O. Tocolytic effect of the cyclooxygenase-2 inhibitor, meloxicam: Studies on uterine contractions in the rat. *J. Pharm. Pharmacol.* **1998**, *50*, 681–685. [CrossRef]
95. Hirst, J.J.; Mijovic, J.E.; Zakar, T.; Olson, D.M. Prostaglandin endoperoxide H synthase-1 and -2 mRNA levels and enzyme activity in human decidua at term labor. *J. Soc. Gynecol. Investig.* **1998**, *5*, 13–20. [CrossRef]
96. Hirst, J.J.; Teixeira, F.J.; Zakar, T.; Olson, D.M. Prostaglandin endoperoxide-H synthase-1 and -2 messenger ribonucleic acid levels in human amnion with spontaneous labor onset. *J. Clin. Endocrinol. Metab.* **1995**, *80*, 517–523. [CrossRef]
97. Hirst, J.J.; Teixeira, F.J.; Zakar, T.; Olson, D.M. Prostaglandin H synthase-2 expression increases in human gestational tissues with spontaneous labour onset. *Reprod. Fertil. Dev.* **1995**, *7*, 633–637. [CrossRef]
98. Mijovic, J.E.; Zakar, T.; Nairn, T.K.; Olson, D.M. Prostaglandin-endoperoxide H synthase-2 expression and activity increases with term labor in human chorion. *Am. J. Physiol.* **1997**, *272*, E832–E840. [CrossRef]
99. Mijovic, J.E.; Zakar, T.; Angelova, J.; Olson, D.M. Prostaglandin endoperoxide H synthase mRNA expression in the human amnion and decidua during pregnancy and in the amnion at preterm labour. *Mol. Hum. Reprod.* **1999**, *5*, 182–187. [CrossRef]
100. Khanprakob, T.; Laopaiboon, M.; Lumbiganon, P.; Sangkomkamhang, U.S. Cyclo-oxygenase (COX) inhibitors for preventing preterm labour. *Cochrane Database Syst. Rev.* **2012**, *10*, CD007748. [CrossRef]
101. Reinebrant, H.E.; Pileggi-Castro, C.; Romero, C.L.; Dos Santos, R.A.; Kumar, S.; Souza, J.P.; Flenady, V. Cyclo-oxygenase (COX) inhibitors for treating preterm labour. *Cochrane Database Syst. Rev.* **2015**, CD001992. [CrossRef]
102. Groom, K.M.; Shennan, A.H.; Jones, B.A.; Seed, P.; Bennett, P.R. TOCOX–a randomised, double-blind, placebo-controlled trial of rofecoxib (a COX-2-specific prostaglandin inhibitor) for the prevention of preterm delivery in women at high risk. *BJOG* **2005**, *112*, 725–730. [CrossRef]
103. Rolnik, D.L.; Wright, D.; Poon, L.C.; O'Gorman, N.; Syngelaki, A.; de Paco Matallana, C.; Akolekar, R.; Cicero, S.; Janga, D.; Singh, M.; et al. Aspirin versus Placebo in Pregnancies at High Risk for Preterm Preeclampsia. *N. Engl. J. Med.* **2017**, *377*, 613–622. [CrossRef] [PubMed]

104. Hoffman, M.K.; Goudar, S.S.; Kodkany, B.S.; Metgud, M.; Somannavar, M.; Okitawutshu, J.; Lokangaka, A.; Tshefu, A.; Bose, C.L.; Mwapule, A.; et al. Low-dose aspirin for the prevention of preterm delivery in nulliparous women with a singleton pregnancy (ASPIRIN): A randomised, double-blind, placebo-controlled trial. *Lancet* **2020**, *395*, 285–293. [CrossRef]
105. Henderson, J.T.; Whitlock, E.P.; O'Connor, E.; Senger, C.A.; Thompson, J.H.; Rowland, M.G. Low-dose aspirin for prevention of morbidity and mortality from preeclampsia: A systematic evidence review for the U.S. Preventive Services Task Force. *Ann. Intern. Med.* **2014**, *160*, 695–703. [CrossRef] [PubMed]
106. Andrikopoulou, M.; Purisch, S.E.; Handal-Orefice, R.; Gyamfi-Bannerman, C. Low-dose aspirin is associated with reduced spontaneous preterm birth in nulliparous women. *Am. J. Obstet. Gynecol.* **2018**, *219*, 399.e1–399.e6. [CrossRef]
107. Lunt, C.C.; Satin, A.J.; Barth, W.H., Jr.; Hankins, G.D. The effect of indomethacin tocolysis on maternal coagulation status. *Obstet. Gynecol.* **1994**, *84*, 820–822.
108. Shah, A.A.; Thjodleifsson, B.; Murray, F.E.; Kay, E.; Barry, M.; Sigthorsson, G.; Gudjonsson, H.; Oddsson, E.; Price, A.B.; Fitzgerald, D.J.; et al. Selective inhibition of COX-2 in humans is associated with less gastrointestinal injury: A comparison of nimesulide and naproxen. *Gut* **2001**, *48*, 339–346. [CrossRef]
109. Ungprasert, P.; Cheungpasitporn, W.; Crowson, C.S.; Matteson, E.L. Individual non-steroidal anti-inflammatory drugs and risk of acute kidney injury: A systematic review and meta-analysis of observational studies. *Eur. J. Intern. Med.* **2015**, *26*, 285–291. [CrossRef]
110. American College of Obstetricians and Gynecologists; Committee on Practice Bulletins—Obstetrics. Practice Bulletin No. 171: Management of Preterm Labor. *Obstet. Gynecol.* **2016**, *128*, e155–e164. [CrossRef]
111. Moise, K.J., Jr. Effect of advancing gestational age on the frequency of fetal ductal constriction in association with maternal indomethacin use. *Am. J. Obstet. Gynecol.* **1993**, *168*, 1350–1353. [CrossRef]
112. Sawdy, R.J.; Lye, S.; Fisk, N.M.; Bennett, P.R. A double-blind randomized study of fetal side effects during and after the short-term maternal administration of indomethacin, sulindac, and nimesulide for the treatment of preterm labor. *Am. J. Obstet. Gynecol.* **2003**, *188*, 1046–1051. [CrossRef]
113. Moise, K.J., Jr.; Huhta, J.C.; Sharif, D.S.; Ou, C.N.; Kirshon, B.; Wasserstrum, N.; Cano, L. Indomethacin in the treatment of premature labor. Effects on the fetal ductus arteriosus. *N. Engl. J. Med.* **1988**, *319*, 327–331. [CrossRef]
114. Dudley, D.K.; Hardie, M.J. Fetal and neonatal effects of indomethacin used as a tocolytic agent. *Am. J. Obstet. Gynecol.* **1985**, *151*, 181–184. [CrossRef]
115. Niebyl, J.R.; Witter, F.R. Neonatal outcome after indomethacin treatment for preterm labor. *Am. J. Obstet. Gynecol.* **1986**, *155*, 747–749. [CrossRef]
116. Abarbanel, A.R. The spasmolysant action of magnesium ions on the tetanically contracting human gravid uterus. *Am. J. Obstet. Gynecol.* **1945**, 473–483. [CrossRef]
117. Hall, D.G. Serum magnesium in pregnancy. *Obstet. Gynecol.* **1957**, *9*, 158–162.
118. Gordon, M.C.; Iams, J.D. Magnesium sulfate. *Clin. Obstet. Gynecol.* **1995**, *38*, 706–712. [CrossRef]
119. Elliott, J.P.; Morrison, J.C.; Bofill, J.A. Risks and Benefits of Magnesium Sulfate Tocolysis in Preterm Labor (PTL). *AIMS Public Health* **2016**, *3*, 348–356. [CrossRef]
120. Mercer, B.M.; Merlino, A.A.; Society for Maternal-Fetal Medicine. Magnesium sulfate for preterm labor and preterm birth. *Obstet. Gynecol.* **2009**, *114*, 650–668. [CrossRef]
121. Crowther, C.A.; Brown, J.; McKinlay, C.J.; Middleton, P. Magnesium sulphate for preventing preterm birth in threatened preterm labour. *Cochrane Database Syst. Rev.* **2014**, CD001060. [CrossRef]
122. Hall, D.G.; Mc, G.H., Jr.; Corey, E.L.; Thornton, W.N., Jr. The effects of magnesium therapy on the duration of labor. *Am. J. Obstet. Gynecol.* **1959**, *78*, 27–32. [CrossRef]
123. Fomin, V.P.; Gibbs, S.G.; Vanam, R.; Morimiya, A.; Hurd, W.W. Effect of magnesium sulfate on contractile force and intracellular calcium concentration in pregnant human myometrium. *Am. J. Obstet. Gynecol.* **2006**, *194*, 1384–1390. [CrossRef]
124. Phillippe, M. Cellular mechanisms underlying magnesium sulfate inhibition of phasic myometrial contractions. *Biochem. Biophys. Res. Commun.* **1998**, *252*, 502–507. [CrossRef]
125. Tica, V.I.; Tica, A.A.; Carlig, V.; Banica, O.S. Magnesium ion inhibits spontaneous and induced contractions of isolated uterine muscle. *Gynecol. Endocrinol.* **2007**, *23*, 368–372. [CrossRef]
126. Lewis, D.F. Magnesium sulfate: The first-line tocolytic. *Obstet. Gynecol. Clin. North. Am.* **2005**, *32*, 485–500. [CrossRef]
127. Han, S.; Crowther, C.A.; Moore, V. Magnesium maintenance therapy for preventing preterm birth after threatened preterm labour. *Cochrane Database Syst. Rev.* **2010**. [CrossRef]
128. Committee Opinion No. 455: Magnesium sulfate before anticipated preterm birth for neuroprotection. *Obstet. Gynecol.* **2010**, *115*, 669–671. [CrossRef]
129. McNamara, H.C.; Crowther, C.A.; Brown, J. Different treatment regimens of magnesium sulphate for tocolysis in women in preterm labour. *Cochrane Database Syst. Rev.* **2015**, CD011200. [CrossRef]
130. Haas, D.M.; Caldwell, D.M.; Kirkpatrick, P.; McIntosh, J.J.; Welton, N.J. Tocolytic therapy for preterm delivery: Systematic review and network meta-analysis. *BMJ* **2012**, *345*, e6226. [CrossRef]
131. Makrides, M.; Crosby, D.D.; Bain, E.; Crowther, C.A. Magnesium supplementation in pregnancy. *Cochrane Database Syst. Rev.* **2014**, CD000937. [CrossRef]

132. Crowther, C.A.; Hiller, J.E.; Doyle, L.W.; Haslam, R.R.; Australasian Collaborative Trial of Magnesium Sulphate Collaborative Group. Effect of magnesium sulfate given for neuroprotection before preterm birth: A randomized controlled trial. *JAMA* 2003, *290*, 2669–2676. [CrossRef]
133. Rouse, D.J.; Hirtz, D.G.; Thom, E.; Varner, M.W.; Spong, C.Y.; Mercer, B.M.; Iams, J.D.; Wapner, R.J.; Sorokin, Y.; Alexander, J.M.; et al. A randomized, controlled trial of magnesium sulfate for the prevention of cerebral palsy. *N. Engl. J. Med.* 2008, *359*, 895–905. [CrossRef] [PubMed]
134. Marret, S.; Marpeau, L.; Follet-Bouhamed, C.; Cambonie, G.; Astruc, D.; Delaporte, B.; Bruel, H.; Guillois, B.; Pinquier, D.; Zupan-Simunek, V.; et al. Effect of magnesium sulphate on mortality and neurologic morbidity of the very-preterm newborn (of less than 33 weeks) with two-year neurological outcome: Results of the prospective PREMAG trial. *Gynecol. Obstet. Fertil.* 2008, *36*, 278–288. [CrossRef] [PubMed]
135. Marret, S.; Marpeau, L.; Zupan-Simunek, V.; Eurin, D.; Leveque, C.; Hellot, M.F.; Benichou, J.; PREMAG Trial Group. Magnesium sulphate given before very-preterm birth to protect infant brain: The randomised controlled PREMAG trial*. *BJOG* 2007, *114*, 310–318. [CrossRef] [PubMed]
136. Doyle, L.W.; Crowther, C.A.; Middleton, P.; Marret, S.; Rouse, D. Magnesium sulphate for women at risk of preterm birth for neuroprotection of the fetus. *Cochrane Database Syst. Rev.* 2009, CD004661. [CrossRef]
137. Grimes, D.A.; Nanda, K. Magnesium sulfate tocolysis: Time to quit. *Obstet. Gynecol.* 2006, *108*, 986–989. [CrossRef]
138. Klauser, C.K.; Briery, C.M.; Keiser, S.D.; Martin, R.W.; Kosek, M.A.; Morrison, J.C. Effect of antenatal tocolysis on neonatal outcomes. *J. Matern Fetal Neonatal Med.* 2012, *25*, 2778–2781. [CrossRef]
139. Nassar, A.H.; Sakhel, K.; Maarouf, H.; Naassan, G.R.; Usta, I.M. Adverse maternal and neonatal outcome of prolonged course of magnesium sulfate tocolysis. *Acta Obstet. Gynecol. Scand.* 2006, *85*, 1099–1103. [CrossRef]
140. Mittendorf, R.; Covert, R.; Boman, J.; Khoshnood, B.; Lee, K.S.; Siegler, M. Is tocolytic magnesium sulphate associated with increased total paediatric mortality? *Lancet* 1997, *350*, 1517–1518. [CrossRef]
141. Romero, R.; Espinoza, J.; Kusanovic, J.P.; Gotsch, F.; Hassan, S.; Erez, O.; Chaiworapongsa, T.; Mazor, M. The preterm parturition syndrome. *BJOG* 2006, *113* (Suppl. 3), 17–42. [CrossRef]
142. Hillier, S.L.; Krohn, M.A.; Cassen, E.; Easterling, T.R.; Rabe, L.K.; Eschenbach, D.A. The role of bacterial vaginosis and vaginal bacteria in amniotic fluid infection in women in preterm labor with intact fetal membranes. *Clin. Infect. Dis. Off. Publ. Infect. Dis. Soc. Am.* 1995, *20* (Suppl. 2), S276–S278. [CrossRef]
143. DiGiulio, D.B.; Romero, R.; Kusanovic, J.P.; Gomez, R.; Kim, C.J.; Seok, K.S.; Gotsch, F.; Mazaki-Tovi, S.; Vaisbuch, E.; Sanders, K.; et al. Prevalence and diversity of microbes in the amniotic fluid, the fetal inflammatory response, and pregnancy outcome in women with preterm pre-labor rupture of membranes. *Am. J. Reprod. Immunol.* 2010, *64*, 38–57. [CrossRef]
144. Romero, R.; Espinoza, J.; Goncalves, L.F.; Kusanovic, J.P.; Friel, L.; Hassan, S. The role of inflammation and infection in preterm birth. *Semin. Reprod. Med.* 2007, *25*, 21–39. [CrossRef]
145. Flenady, V.; Hawley, G.; Stock, O.M.; Kenyon, S.; Badawi, N. Prophylactic antibiotics for inhibiting preterm labour with intact membranes. *Cochrane Database Syst. Rev.* 2013, CD000246. [CrossRef]
146. Kenyon, S.L.; Taylor, D.J.; Tarnow-Mordi, W. Broad-spectrum antibiotics for spontaneous preterm labour: The ORACLE II randomised trial. ORACLE Collaborative Group. *Lancet* 2001, *357*, 989–994. [CrossRef]
147. Stetzer, B.P.; Mercer, B.M. Antibiotics and preterm labor. *Clin. Obstet. Gynecol.* 2000, *43*, 809–817. [CrossRef]
148. Kenyon, S.; Pike, K.; Jones, D.R.; Brocklehurst, P.; Marlow, N.; Salt, A.; Taylor, D.J. Childhood outcomes after prescription of antibiotics to pregnant women with spontaneous preterm labour: 7-year follow-up of the ORACLE II trial. *Lancet* 2008, *372*, 1319–1327. [CrossRef]
149. Goldenberg, R.L.; Culhane, J.F.; Iams, J.D.; Romero, R. Epidemiology and causes of preterm birth. *Lancet* 2008, *371*, 75–84. [CrossRef]
150. Menon, R.; Fortunato, S.J. Infection and the role of inflammation in preterm premature rupture of the membranes. *Best Pract. Res. Clin. Obstet. Gynaecol.* 2007, *21*, 467–478. [CrossRef]
151. Lannon, S.M.; Vanderhoeven, J.P.; Eschenbach, D.A.; Gravett, M.G.; Adams Waldorf, K.M. Synergy and interactions among biological pathways leading to preterm premature rupture of membranes. *Reprod. Sci.* 2014, *21*, 1215–1227. [CrossRef]
152. Ehsanipoor, R. ACOG Practice Bulletin No. 188: Prelabor Rupture of Membranes. *Obstet. Gynecol.* 2018, *131*, e1–e14. [CrossRef]
153. Prelabor Rupture of Membranes: ACOG Practice Bulletin, Number 217. *Obstet. Gynecol.* 2020, *135*, e80–e97. [CrossRef]
154. Mercer, B.M.; Miodovnik, M.; Thurnau, G.R.; Goldenberg, R.L.; Das, A.F.; Ramsey, R.D.; Rabello, Y.A.; Meis, P.J.; Moawad, A.H.; Iams, J.D.; et al. Antibiotic therapy for reduction of infant morbidity after preterm premature rupture of the membranes. A randomized controlled trial. National Institute of Child Health and Human Development Maternal-Fetal Medicine Units Network. *JAMA J. Am. Med. Assoc.* 1997, *278*, 989–995. [CrossRef]
155. Kenyon, S.L.; Taylor, D.J.; Tarnow-Mordi, W. Broad-spectrum antibiotics for preterm, prelabour rupture of fetal membranes: The ORACLE I randomised trial. ORACLE Collaborative Group. *Lancet* 2001, *357*, 979–988. [CrossRef]
156. Lee, J.; Romero, R.; Kim, S.M.; Chaemsaithong, P.; Park, C.W.; Park, J.S.; Jun, J.K.; Yoon, B.H. A new anti-microbial combination prolongs the latency period, reduces acute histologic chorioamnionitis as well as funisitis, and improves neonatal outcomes in preterm PROM. *J. Matern Fetal Neonatal Med.* 2016, *29*, 707–720. [CrossRef]
157. Mackeen, A.D.; Seibel-Seamon, J.; Muhammad, J.; Baxter, J.K.; Berghella, V. Tocolytics for preterm premature rupture of membranes. *Cochrane Database Syst. Rev.* 2014, CD007062. [CrossRef]

158. Lorthe, E.; Goffinet, F.; Marret, S.; Vayssiere, C.; Flamant, C.; Quere, M.; Benhammou, V.; Ancel, P.Y.; Kayem, G. Tocolysis after preterm premature rupture of membranes and neonatal outcome: A propensity-score analysis. *Am. J. Obstet. Gynecol.* **2017**, *217*, 212.e1–212.e12. [CrossRef]
159. Hillier, S.L.; Krohn, M.A.; Rabe, L.K.; Klebanoff, S.J.; Eschenbach, D.A. The normal vaginal flora, H2O2-producing lactobacilli, and bacterial vaginosis in pregnant women. *Clin. Infect. Dis. Off. Publ. Infect. Dis. Soc. Am.* **1993**, *16* (Suppl. 4), S273–S281. [CrossRef]
160. Hillier, S.L.; Martius, J.; Krohn, M.; Kiviat, N.; Holmes, K.K.; Eschenbach, D.A. A case-control study of chorioamnionic infection and histologic chorioamnionitis in prematurity. *N. Engl. J. Med.* **1988**, *319*, 972–978. [CrossRef] [PubMed]
161. Hillier, S.L.; Nugent, R.P.; Eschenbach, D.A.; Krohn, M.A.; Gibbs, R.S.; Martin, D.H.; Cotch, M.F.; Edelman, R.; Pastorek, J.G., 2nd; Rao, A.V.; et al. Association between bacterial vaginosis and preterm delivery of a low-birth-weight infant. The Vaginal Infections and Prematurity Study Group. *N. Engl. J. Med.* **1995**, *333*, 1737–1742. [CrossRef] [PubMed]
162. Hitti, J.; Hillier, S.L.; Agnew, K.J.; Krohn, M.A.; Reisner, D.P.; Eschenbach, D.A. Vaginal indicators of amniotic fluid infection in preterm labor. *Obstet. Gynecol.* **2001**, *97*, 211–219. [CrossRef] [PubMed]
163. Hitti, J.; Lapidus, J.A.; Lu, X.; Reddy, A.P.; Jacob, T.; Dasari, S.; Eschenbach, D.A.; Gravett, M.G.; Nagalla, S.R. Noninvasive diagnosis of intraamniotic infection: Proteomic biomarkers in vaginal fluid. *Am. J. Obstet. Gynecol.* **2010**, *203*, 32.e1–32.e8. [CrossRef]
164. Krohn, M.A.; Hillier, S.L.; Lee, M.L.; Rabe, L.K.; Eschenbach, D.A. Vaginal Bacteroides species are associated with an increased rate of preterm delivery among women in preterm labor. *J. Infect. Dis.* **1991**, *164*, 88–93. [CrossRef]
165. Krohn, M.A.; Hillier, S.L.; Nugent, R.P.; Cotch, M.F.; Carey, J.C.; Gibbs, R.S.; Eschenbach, D.A. The genital flora of women with intraamniotic infection. Vaginal Infection and Prematurity Study Group. *J. Infect. Dis.* **1995**, *171*, 1475–1480. [CrossRef]
166. Meis, P.J.; Goldenberg, R.L.; Mercer, B.; Moawad, A.; Das, A.; McNellis, D.; Johnson, F.; Iams, J.D.; Thom, E.; Andrews, W.W. The preterm prediction study: Significance of vaginal infections. National Institute of Child Health and Human Development Maternal-Fetal Medicine Units Network. *Am. J. Obstet. Gynecol.* **1995**, *173*, 1231–1235. [CrossRef]
167. Carey, J.C.; Klebanoff, M.A.; Hauth, J.C.; Hillier, S.L.; Thom, E.A.; Ernest, J.M.; Heine, R.P.; Nugent, R.P.; Fischer, M.L.; Leveno, K.J.; et al. Metronidazole to prevent preterm delivery in pregnant women with asymptomatic bacterial vaginosis. National Institute of Child Health and Human Development Network of Maternal-Fetal Medicine Units. *N. Engl. J. Med.* **2000**, *342*, 534–540. [CrossRef]
168. Joesoef, M.R.; Hillier, S.L.; Wiknjosastro, G.; Sumampouw, H.; Linnan, M.; Norojono, W.; Idajadi, A.; Utomo, B. Intravaginal clindamycin treatment for bacterial vaginosis: Effects on preterm delivery and low birth weight. *Am. J. Obstet. Gynecol.* **1995**, *173*, 1527–1531. [CrossRef]
169. McGregor, J.A.; French, J.I.; Jones, W.; Milligan, K.; McKinney, P.J.; Patterson, E.; Parker, R. Bacterial vaginosis is associated with prematurity and vaginal fluid mucinase and sialidase: Results of a controlled trial of topical clindamycin cream. *Am. J. Obstet. Gynecol.* **1994**, *170*, 1048–1059, discussion 1059–1060. [CrossRef]
170. US Preventive Services Task Force; Owens, D.K.; Davidson, K.W.; Krist, A.H.; Barry, M.J.; Cabana, M.; Caughey, A.B.; Donahue, K.; Doubeni, C.A.; Epling, J.W., Jr.; et al. Screening for Bacterial Vaginosis in Pregnant Persons to Prevent Preterm Delivery: US Preventive Services Task Force Recommendation Statement. *JAMA* **2020**, *323*, 1286–1292. [CrossRef]
171. Kahwati, L.C.; Clark, R.; Berkman, N.; Urrutia, R.; Patel, S.V.; Zeng, J.; Viswanathan, M. Screening for Bacterial Vaginosis in Pregnant Adolescents and Women to Prevent Preterm Delivery: Updated Evidence Report and Systematic Review for the US Preventive Services Task Force. *JAMA* **2020**, *323*, 1293–1309. [CrossRef]
172. Subtil, D.; Brabant, G.; Tilloy, E.; Devos, P.; Canis, F.; Fruchart, A.; Bissinger, M.C.; Dugimont, J.C.; Nolf, C.; Hacot, C.; et al. Early clindamycin for bacterial vaginosis in pregnancy (PREMEVA): A multicentre, double-blind, randomised controlled trial. *Lancet* **2018**, *392*, 2171–2179. [CrossRef]
173. Mitchell, C.; Balkus, J.; Agnew, K.; Lawler, R.; Hitti, J. Changes in the vaginal microenvironment with metronidazole treatment for bacterial vaginosis in early pregnancy. *J. Women's Health* **2009**, *18*, 1817–1824. [CrossRef] [PubMed]
174. Mitchell, C.M.; Hitti, J.E.; Agnew, K.J.; Fredricks, D.N. Comparison of oral and vaginal metronidazole for treatment of bacterial vaginosis in pregnancy: Impact on fastidious bacteria. *BMC Infect. Dis.* **2009**, *9*, 89. [CrossRef] [PubMed]
175. Hummelen, R.; Fernandes, A.D.; Macklaim, J.M.; Dickson, R.J.; Changalucha, J.; Gloor, G.B.; Reid, G. Deep sequencing of the vaginal microbiota of women with HIV. *PLoS ONE* **2010**, *5*, e12078. [CrossRef]
176. Gomez, L.M.; Sammel, M.D.; Appleby, D.H.; Elovitz, M.A.; Baldwin, D.A.; Jeffcoat, M.K.; Macones, G.A.; Parry, S. Evidence of a gene-environment interaction that predisposes to spontaneous preterm birth: A role for asymptomatic bacterial vaginosis and DNA variants in genes that control the inflammatory response. *Am. J. Obstet. Gynecol.* **2010**, *202*, 386.e1–386.e6. [CrossRef]
177. Andrews, W.W.; Klebanoff, M.A.; Thom, E.A.; Hauth, J.C.; Carey, J.C.; Meis, P.J.; Caritis, S.N.; Leveno, K.J.; Wapner, R.J.; Varner, M.W.; et al. Midpregnancy genitourinary tract infection with Chlamydia trachomatis: Association with subsequent preterm delivery in women with bacterial vaginosis and Trichomonas vaginalis. *Am. J. Obstet. Gynecol.* **2006**, *194*, 493–500. [CrossRef]
178. Meis, P.J.; Michielutte, R.; Peters, T.J.; Wells, H.B.; Sands, R.E.; Coles, E.C.; Johns, K.A. Factors associated with preterm birth in Cardiff, Wales. I. Univariable and multivariable analysis. *Am. J. Obstet. Gynecol.* **1995**, *173*, 590–596. [CrossRef]
179. Meis, P.J.; Michielutte, R.; Peters, T.J.; Wells, H.B.; Sands, R.E.; Coles, E.C.; Johns, K.A. Factors associated with preterm birth in Cardiff, Wales. II. Indicated and spontaneous preterm birth. *Am. J. Obstet. Gynecol.* **1995**, *173*, 597–602. [CrossRef]

180. Tilton, R.C.; Steingrimsson, O.; Ryan, R.W. Susceptibilities of Pseudomonas species to tetracycline, minocycline, gentamicin, and tobramycin. *Am. J. Clin. Pathol* **1978**, *69*, 410–413. [CrossRef] [PubMed]
181. Burtin, P.; Taddio, A.; Ariburnu, O.; Einarson, T.R.; Koren, G. Safety of metronidazole in pregnancy: A meta-analysis. *Am. J. Obstet. Gynecol.* **1995**, *172*, 525–529. [CrossRef]
182. Klebanoff, M.A.; Carey, J.C.; Hauth, J.C.; Hillier, S.L.; Nugent, R.P.; Thom, E.A.; Ernest, J.M.; Heine, R.P.; Wapner, R.J.; Trout, W.; et al. Failure of metronidazole to prevent preterm delivery among pregnant women with asymptomatic Trichomonas vaginalis infection. *N. Engl. J. Med.* **2001**, *345*, 487–493. [CrossRef]
183. Schuster, H.J.; de Jonghe, B.A.; Limpens, J.; Budding, A.E.; Painter, R.C. Asymptomatic vaginal Candida colonization and adverse pregnancy outcomes including preterm birth: A systematic review and meta-analysis. *Am. J. Obstet. Gynecol. MFM* **2020**, *2*, 100163. [CrossRef]
184. Norwitz, E.R.; Caughey, A.B. Progesterone supplementation and the prevention of preterm birth. *Rev. Obstet. Gynecol.* **2011**, *4*, 60–72.
185. Mesiano, S.A.; Peters, G.A.; Amini, P.; Wilson, R.A.; Tochtrop, G.P.; van Den Akker, F. Progestin therapy to prevent preterm birth: History and effectiveness of current strategies and development of novel approaches. *Placenta* **2019**, *79*, 46–52. [CrossRef]
186. Da Fonseca, E.B.; Bittar, R.E.; Carvalho, M.H.; Zugaib, M. Prophylactic administration of progesterone by vaginal suppository to reduce the incidence of spontaneous preterm birth in women at increased risk: A randomized placebo-controlled double-blind study. *Am. J. Obstet. Gynecol.* **2003**, *188*, 419–424. [CrossRef]
187. Meis, P.J.; Klebanoff, M.; Thom, E.; Dombrowski, M.P.; Sibai, B.; Moawad, A.H.; Spong, C.Y.; Hauth, J.C.; Miodovnik, M.; Varner, M.W.; et al. Prevention of recurrent preterm delivery by 17 alpha-hydroxyprogesterone caproate. *N. Engl. J. Med.* **2003**, *348*, 2379–2385. [CrossRef]
188. Choi, S.J. Use of progesterone supplement therapy for prevention of preterm birth: Review of literatures. *Obstet. Gynecol. Sci.* **2017**, *60*, 405–420. [CrossRef]
189. Chang, C.Y.; Nguyen, C.P.; Wesley, B.; Guo, J.; Johnson, L.L.; Joffe, H.V. Withdrawing Approval of Makena—A Proposal from the FDA Center for Drug Evaluation and Research. *N. Engl. J. Med.* **2020**, *383*, e131. [CrossRef]
190. Astle, S.; Slater, D.M.; Thornton, S. The involvement of progesterone in the onset of human labour. *Eur. J. Obstet. Gynecol. Reprod. Biol.* **2003**, *108*, 177–181. [CrossRef]
191. Brown, A.G.; Leite, R.S.; Strauss, J.F., 3rd. Mechanisms underlying "functional" progesterone withdrawal at parturition. *Ann. N. Y. Acad. Sci.* **2004**, *1034*, 36–49. [CrossRef]
192. Mesiano, S.; Chan, E.C.; Fitter, J.T.; Kwek, K.; Yeo, G.; Smith, R. Progesterone withdrawal and estrogen activation in human parturition are coordinated by progesterone receptor A expression in the myometrium. *J. Clin. Endocrinol. Metab.* **2002**, *87*, 2924–2930. [CrossRef]
193. Nadeem, L.; Shynlova, O.; Matysiak-Zablocki, E.; Mesiano, S.; Dong, X.; Lye, S. Molecular evidence of functional progesterone withdrawal in human myometrium. *Nat. Commun.* **2016**, *7*, 11565. [CrossRef]
194. Nadeem, L.; Shynlova, O.; Mesiano, S.; Lye, S. Progesterone Via its Type-A Receptor Promotes Myometrial Gap Junction Coupling. *Sci. Rep.* **2017**, *7*, 13357. [CrossRef]
195. Hassan, S.S.; Romero, R.; Vidyadhari, D.; Fusey, S.; Baxter, J.K.; Khandelwal, M.; Vijayaraghavan, J.; Trivedi, Y.; Soma-Pillay, P.; Sambarey, P.; et al. Vaginal progesterone reduces the rate of preterm birth in women with a sonographic short cervix: A multicenter, randomized, double-blind, placebo-controlled trial. *Ultrasound. Obstet. Gynecol.* **2011**, *38*, 18–31. [CrossRef]
196. Norman, J.E.; Marlow, N.; Messow, C.M.; Shennan, A.; Bennett, P.R.; Thornton, S.; Robson, S.C.; McConnachie, A.; Petrou, S.; Sebire, N.J.; et al. Vaginal progesterone prophylaxis for preterm birth (the OPPTIMUM study): A multicentre, randomised, double-blind trial. *Lancet* **2016**, *387*, 2106–2116. [CrossRef]
197. O'Brien, J.M.; Adair, C.D.; Lewis, D.F.; Hall, D.R.; Defranco, E.A.; Fusey, S.; Soma-Pillay, P.; Porter, K.; How, H.; Schackis, R.; et al. Progesterone vaginal gel for the reduction of recurrent preterm birth: Primary results from a randomized, double-blind, placebo-controlled trial. *Ultrasound Obstet. Gynecol.* **2007**, *30*, 687–696. [CrossRef]
198. Romero, R.; Nicolaides, K.; Conde-Agudelo, A.; Tabor, A.; O'Brien, J.M.; Cetingoz, E.; Da Fonseca, E.; Creasy, G.W.; Klein, K.; Rode, L.; et al. Vaginal progesterone in women with an asymptomatic sonographic short cervix in the midtrimester decreases preterm delivery and neonatal morbidity: A systematic review and metaanalysis of individual patient data. *Am. J. Obstet. Gynecol.* **2012**, *206*, 124.e1–124.e19. [CrossRef]
199. Fonseca, E.B.; Celik, E.; Parra, M.; Singh, M.; Nicolaides, K.H.; Fetal Medicine Foundation Second Trimester Screening, G. Progesterone and the risk of preterm birth among women with a short cervix. *N. Engl. J. Med.* **2007**, *357*, 462–469. [CrossRef]
200. Nelson, D.B.; McIntire, D.D.; McDonald, J.; Gard, J.; Turrichi, P.; Leveno, K.J. 17-alpha Hydroxyprogesterone caproate did not reduce the rate of recurrent preterm birth in a prospective cohort study. *Am. J. Obstet. Gynecol.* **2017**, *216*, 600.e1–600.e9. [CrossRef]
201. Blackwell, S.C.; Gyamfi-Bannerman, C.; Biggio, J.R., Jr.; Chauhan, S.P.; Hughes, B.L.; Louis, J.M.; Manuck, T.A.; Miller, H.S.; Das, A.F.; Saade, G.R.; et al. 17-OHPC to Prevent Recurrent Preterm Birth in Singleton Gestations (PROLONG Study): A Multicenter, International, Randomized Double-Blind Trial. *Am. J. Perinatol.* **2020**, *37*, 127–136. [CrossRef]
202. Romero, R.; Conde-Agudelo, A.; El-Refaie, W.; Rode, L.; Brizot, M.L.; Cetingoz, E.; Serra, V.; Da Fonseca, E.; Abdelhafez, M.S.; Tabor, A.; et al. Vaginal progesterone decreases preterm birth and neonatal morbidity and mortality in women with a twin gestation and a short cervix: An updated meta-analysis of individual patient data. *Ultrasound Obstet. Gynecol.* **2017**, *49*, 303–314. [CrossRef]

203. Shambhavi, S.; Bagga, R.; Bansal, P.; Kalra, J.; Kumar, P. A randomised trial to compare 200 mg micronised progesterone effervescent vaginal tablet daily with 250 mg intramuscular 17 alpha hydroxy progesterone caproate weekly for prevention of recurrent preterm birth. *J. Obstet. Gynaecol.* **2018**, *38*, 800–806. [CrossRef] [PubMed]
204. American College of Obstetricians and Gynecologists. Practice bulletin no. 130: Prediction and prevention of preterm birth. *Obstet. Gynecol.* **2012**, *120*, 964–973. [CrossRef] [PubMed]
205. How, H.Y.; Sibai, B.M. Progesterone for the prevention of preterm birth: Indications, when to initiate, efficacy and safety. *Ther. Clin. Risk Manag.* **2009**, *5*, 55–64. [CrossRef] [PubMed]
206. Ahn, K.H.; Bae, N.Y.; Hong, S.C.; Lee, J.S.; Lee, E.H.; Jee, H.J.; Cho, G.J.; Oh, M.J.; Kim, H.J. The safety of progestogen in the prevention of preterm birth: Meta-analysis of neonatal mortality. *J. Perinat Med.* **2017**, *45*, 11–20. [CrossRef]
207. Kuon, R.J.; Shi, S.Q.; Maul, H.; Sohn, C.; Balducci, J.; Maner, W.L.; Garfield, R.E. Pharmacologic actions of progestins to inhibit cervical ripening and prevent delivery depend on their properties, the route of administration, and the vehicle. *Am. J. Obstet. Gynecol.* **2010**, *202*, 455.e1–455.e9. [CrossRef]
208. Grainger, D.J.; Lever, A.M. Blockade of chemokine-induced signalling inhibits CCR5-dependent HIV infection in vitro without blocking gp120/CCR5 interaction. *Retrovirology* **2005**, *2*, 23. [CrossRef]
209. Larena, M.; Regner, M.; Lobigs, M. The Chemokine Receptor CCR5, a Therapeutic Target for HIV/AIDS Antagonists, Is Critical for Recovery in a Mouse Model of Japanese Encephalitis. *PLoS ONE* **2012**, *7*, 10. [CrossRef]
210. Coleman, M.; Orvis, A.; Wu, T.Y.; Dacanay, M.; Merillat, S.; Ogle, J.; Baldessari, A.; Kretzer, N.M.; Munson, J.; Boros-Rausch, A.J.; et al. A Broad Spectrum Chemokine Inhibitor Prevents Preterm Labor but Not Microbial Invasion of the Amniotic Cavity or Neonatal Morbidity in a Non-human Primate Model. *Front. Immunol.* **2020**, *11*, 770. [CrossRef]
211. Shynlova, O.; Dorogin, A.; Li, Y.; Lye, S. Inhibition of infection-mediated preterm birth by administration of broad spectrum chemokine inhibitor in mice. *J. Cell Mol. Med.* **2014**, *18*, 1816–1829. [CrossRef]
212. Yuan, M.; Jordan, F.; McInnes, I.B.; Harnett, M.M.; Norman, J.E. Leukocytes are primed in peripheral blood for activation during term and preterm labour. *Mol. Hum. Reprod* **2009**, *15*, 713–724. [CrossRef]
213. Thomson, A.J.; Telfer, J.F.; Young, A.; Campbell, S.; Stewart, C.J.; Cameron, I.T.; Greer, I.A.; Norman, J.E. Leukocytes infiltrate the myometrium during human parturition: Further evidence that labour is an inflammatory process. *Hum. Reprod.* **1999**, *14*, 229–236. [CrossRef]
214. Shynlova, O.; Tsui, P.; Dorogin, A.; Lye, S.J. Monocyte chemoattractant protein-1 (CCL-2) integrates mechanical and endocrine signals that mediate term and preterm labor. *J. Immunol.* **2008**, *181*, 1470–1479. [CrossRef]
215. Keski-Nisula, L.T.; Aalto, M.L.; Kirkinen, P.P.; Kosma, V.M.; Heinonen, S.T. Myometrial inflammation in human delivery and its association with labor and infection. *Am. J. Clin. Pathol.* **2003**, *120*, 217–224. [CrossRef]
216. Singh, N.; Herbert, B.; Sooranna, G.R.; Orsi, N.M.; Edey, L.; Dasgupta, T.; Sooranna, S.R.; Yellon, S.M.; Johnson, M.R. Is myometrial inflammation a cause or a consequence of term human labour? *J. Endocrinol.* **2017**, *235*, 69–83. [CrossRef]
217. Grainger, D.J.; Reckless, J. Broad-spectrum chemokine inhibitors (BSCIs) and their anti-inflammatory effects in vivo. *Biochem. Pharmacol.* **2003**, *65*, 1027–1034. [CrossRef]
218. Fox, D.J.; Reckless, J.; Lingard, H.; Warren, S.; Grainger, D.J. Highly potent, orally available anti-inflammatory broad-spectrum chemokine inhibitors. *J. Med. Chem.* **2009**, *52*, 3591–3595. [CrossRef]
219. Reckless, J.; Tatalick, L.; Wilbert, S.; McKilligin, E.; Grainger, D.J. Broad-spectrum chemokine inhibition reduces vascular macrophage accumulation and collagenolysis consistent with plaque stabilization in mice. *J. Vasc Res.* **2005**, *42*, 492–502. [CrossRef]
220. Naidu, B.V.; Farivar, A.S.; Krishnadasan, B.; Woolley, S.M.; Grainger, D.J.; Verrier, E.D.; Mulligan, M.S. Broad-spectrum chemokine inhibition ameliorates experimental obliterative bronchiolitis. *Ann. Thorac. Surg.* **2003**, *75*, 1118–1122. [CrossRef]
221. Miklos, S.; Mueller, G.; Chang, Y.; Bouazzaoui, A.; Spacenko, E.; Schubert, T.E.O.; Grainger, D.J.; Holler, E.; Andreesen, R.; Hildebrandt, G.C. Preventive usage of broad spectrum chemokine inhibitor NR58-3.14.3 reduces the severity of pulmonary and hepatic graft-versus-host disease. *Int. J. Hematol.* **2009**, *89*, 383–397. [CrossRef]
222. Berkkanoglu, M.; Zhang, L.; Ulukus, M.; Cakmak, H.; Kayisli, U.A.; Kursun, S.; Arici, A. Inhibition of chemokines prevents intraperitoneal adhesions in mice. *Hum. Reprod.* **2005**, *20*, 3047–3052. [CrossRef]
223. Fox, D.J.; Reckless, J.; Wilbert, S.M.; Greig, I.; Warren, S.; Grainger, D.J. Identification of 3-(acylamino)azepan-2-ones as stable broad-spectrum chemokine inhibitors resistant to metabolism in vivo. *J. Med. Chem.* **2005**, *48*, 867–874. [CrossRef] [PubMed]
224. Reckless, J.; Tatalick, L.M.; Grainger, D.J. The pan-chemokine inhibitor NR58-3.14.3 abolishes tumour necrosis factor-alpha accumulation and leucocyte recruitment induced by lipopolysaccharide in vivo. *Immunology* **2001**, *103*, 244–254. [CrossRef] [PubMed]
225. Elliott, D.E.; Li, J.; Blum, A.M.; Metwali, A.; Patel, Y.C.; Weinstock, J.V. SSTR2A is the dominant somatostatin receptor subtype expressed by inflammatory cells, is widely expressed and directly regulates T cell IFN-gamma release. *Eur. J. Immunol.* **1999**, *29*, 2454–2463. [CrossRef]
226. Olias, G.; Viollet, C.; Kusserow, H.; Epelbaum, J.; Meyerhof, W. Regulation and function of somatostatin receptors. *J. Neurochem.* **2004**, *89*, 1057–1091. [CrossRef] [PubMed]
227. Armani, C.; Catalani, E.; Balbarini, A.; Bagnoli, P.; Cervia, D. Expression, pharmacology, and functional role of somatostatin receptor subtypes 1 and 2 in human macrophages. *J. Leukoc. Biol.* **2007**, *81*, 845–855. [CrossRef] [PubMed]
228. Cervia, D.; Nunn, C.; Bagnoli, P. Multiple Signalling Transduction Mechanisms Differentially Coupled to Somatostatin Receptor Subtypes: A Current View. *Curr. Enzym. Inhib.* **2005**, *1*. [CrossRef]

229. Krantic, S. Peptides as regulators of the immune system: Emphasis on somatostatin. *Peptides* **2000**, *21*, 1941–1964. [CrossRef]
230. Lichtenauer-Kaligis, E.G.; van Hagen, P.M.; Lamberts, S.W.; Hofland, L.J. Somatostatin receptor subtypes in human immune cells. *Eur. J. Endocrinol.* **2000**, *143* (Suppl. 1), S21–S25. [CrossRef]
231. Jana, B.; Calka, J.; Czajkowska, M. The role of somatostatin and its receptors (sstr2, sstr5) in the contractility of gilt inflamed uterus. *Res. Vet. Sci.* **2020**, *133*, 163–173. [CrossRef]
232. Olson, D.M.; Ammann, C. Role of the prostaglandins in labour and prostaglandin receptor inhibitors in the prevention of preterm labour. *Front. Biosci.* **2007**, *12*, 1329–1343. [CrossRef]
233. Senior, J.; Marshall, K.; Sangha, R.; Clayton, J.K. In vitro characterization of prostanoid receptors on human myometrium at term pregnancy. *Br. J. Pharmacol.* **1993**, *108*, 501–506. [CrossRef]
234. Grigsby, P.L.; Sooranna, S.R.; Adu-Amankwa, B.; Pitzer, B.; Brockman, D.E.; Johnson, M.R.; Myatt, L. Regional expression of prostaglandin E2 and F2alpha receptors in human myometrium, amnion, and choriodecidua with advancing gestation and labor. *Biol. Reprod.* **2006**, *75*, 297–305. [CrossRef]
235. Ulug, U.; Goldman, S.; Ben-Shlomo, I.; Shalev, E. Matrix metalloproteinase (MMP)-2 and MMP-9 and their inhibitor, TIMP-1, in human term decidua and fetal membranes: The effect of prostaglandin F(2alpha) and indomethacin. *Mol. Hum. Reprod.* **2001**, *7*, 1187–1193. [CrossRef]
236. Yoshida, M.; Sagawa, N.; Itoh, H.; Yura, S.; Takemura, M.; Wada, Y.; Sato, T.; Ito, A.; Fujii, S. Prostaglandin F(2alpha), cytokines and cyclic mechanical stretch augment matrix metalloproteinase-1 secretion from cultured human uterine cervical fibroblast cells. *Mol. Hum. Reprod.* **2002**, *8*, 681–687. [CrossRef]
237. Slater, D.M.; Zervou, S.; Thornton, S. Prostaglandins and prostanoid receptors in human pregnancy and parturition. *J. Soc. Gynecol. Investig.* **2002**, *9*, 118–124. [CrossRef]
238. Pohl, O.; Chollet, A.; Kim, S.H.; Riaposova, L.; Spezia, F.; Gervais, F.; Guillaume, P.; Lluel, P.; Meen, M.; Lemaux, F.; et al. OBE022, an Oral and Selective Prostaglandin F2alpha Receptor Antagonist as an Effective and Safe Modality for the Treatment of Preterm Labor. *J. Pharmacol. Exp. Ther.* **2018**, *366*, 349–364. [CrossRef]
239. Pohl, O.; Marchand, L.; Gotteland, J.P.; Coates, S.; Taubel, J.; Lorch, U. Pharmacokinetics, safety and tolerability of OBE022, a selective prostaglandin F2alpha receptor antagonist tocolytic: A first-in-human trial in healthy postmenopausal women. *Br. J. Clin. Pharmacol.* **2018**, *84*, 1839–1855. [CrossRef]
240. Taubel, J.; Lorch, U.; Coates, S.; Fernandes, S.; Foley, P.; Ferber, G.; Gotteland, J.P.; Pohl, O. Confirmation of the Cardiac Safety of PGF2alpha Receptor Antagonist OBE022 in a First-in-Human Study in Healthy Subjects, Using Intensive ECG Assessments. *Clin. Pharmacol. Drug Dev.* **2018**, *7*, 889–900. [CrossRef]
241. Pohl, O.; Marchand, L.; Gotteland, J.P.; Coates, S.; Taubel, J.; Lorch, U. Coadministration of the prostaglandin F2alpha receptor antagonist preterm labour drug candidate OBE022 with magnesium sulfate, atosiban, nifedipine and betamethasone. *Br. J. Clin. Pharmacol.* **2019**, *85*, 1516–1527. [CrossRef]
242. Romero, R.; Miranda, J.; Chaiworapongsa, T.; Korzeniewski, S.J.; Chaemsaithong, P.; Gotsch, F.; Dong, Z.; Ahmed, A.I.; Yoon, B.H.; Hassan, S.S.; et al. Prevalence and clinical significance of sterile intra-amniotic inflammation in patients with preterm labor and intact membranes. *Am. J. Reprod. Immunol.* **2014**, *72*, 458–474. [CrossRef]
243. Leimert, K.B.; Messer, A.; Gray, T.; Fang, X.; Chemtob, S.; Olson, D.M. Maternal and fetal intrauterine tissue crosstalk promotes proinflammatory amplification and uterine transitiondagger. *Biol. Reprod.* **2019**, *100*, 783–797. [CrossRef]
244. Leimert, K.B.; Verstraeten, B.S.E.; Messer, A.; Nemati, R.; Blackadar, K.; Fang, X.; Robertson, S.A.; Chemtob, S.; Olson, D.M. Cooperative effects of sequential PGF2alpha and IL-1beta on IL-6 and COX-2 expression in human myometrial cellsdagger. *Biol. Reprod.* **2019**, *100*, 1370–1385. [CrossRef]
245. Nadeau-Vallee, M.; Quiniou, C.; Palacios, J.; Hou, X.; Erfani, A.; Madaan, A.; Sanchez, M.; Leimert, K.; Boudreault, A.; Duhamel, F.; et al. Novel Noncompetitive IL-1 Receptor-Biased Ligand Prevents Infection- and Inflammation-Induced Preterm Birth. *J. Immunol.* **2015**, *195*, 3402–3415. [CrossRef]
246. Nadeau-Vallee, M.; Chin, P.Y.; Belarbi, L.; Brien, M.E.; Pundir, S.; Berryer, M.H.; Beaudry-Richard, A.; Madaan, A.; Sharkey, D.J.; Lupien-Meilleur, A.; et al. Antenatal Suppression of IL-1 Protects against Inflammation-Induced Fetal Injury and Improves Neonatal and Developmental Outcomes in Mice. *J. Immunol.* **2017**, *198*, 2047–2062. [CrossRef]
247. Sadowsky, D.W.; Adams, K.M.; Gravett, M.G.; Witkin, S.S.; Novy, M.J. Preterm labor is induced by intraamniotic infusions of interleukin-1beta and tumor necrosis factor-alpha but not by interleukin-6 or interleukin-8 in a nonhuman primate model. *Am. J. Obstet. Gynecol.* **2006**, *195*, 1578–1589. [CrossRef]
248. Leitner, K.; Al Shammary, M.; McLane, M.; Johnston, M.V.; Elovitz, M.A.; Burd, I. IL-1 receptor blockade prevents fetal cortical brain injury but not preterm birth in a mouse model of inflammation-induced preterm birth and perinatal brain injury. *Am. J. Reprod. Immunol.* **2014**, *71*, 418–426. [CrossRef]
249. Fidel, P.L., Jr.; Romero, R.; Cutright, J.; Wolf, N.; Gomez, R.; Araneda, H.; Ramirez, M.; Yoon, B.H. Treatment with the interleukin-I receptor antagonist and soluble tumor necrosis factor receptor Fc fusion protein does not prevent endotoxin-induced preterm parturition in mice. *J. Soc. Gynecol. Investig.* **1997**, *4*, 22–26. [CrossRef]
250. Kallapur, S.G.; Nitsos, I.; Moss, T.J.; Polglase, G.R.; Pillow, J.J.; Cheah, F.C.; Kramer, B.W.; Newnham, J.P.; Ikegami, M.; Jobe, A.H. IL-1 mediates pulmonary and systemic inflammatory responses to chorioamnionitis induced by lipopolysaccharide. *Am. J. Respir. Crit. Care Med.* **2009**, *179*, 955–961. [CrossRef]

251. Boonkasidecha, S.; Kannan, P.S.; Kallapur, S.G.; Jobe, A.H.; Kemp, M.W. Fetal skin as a pro-inflammatory organ: Evidence from a primate model of chorioamnionitis. *PLoS ONE* **2017**, *12*, e0184938. [CrossRef]
252. Presicce, P.; Park, C.W.; Senthamaraikannan, P.; Bhattacharyya, S.; Jackson, C.; Kong, F.; Rueda, C.M.; DeFranco, E.; Miller, L.A.; Hildeman, D.A.; et al. IL-1 signaling mediates intrauterine inflammation and chorio-decidua neutrophil recruitment and activation. *JCI Insight* **2018**, *3*. [CrossRef]
253. Romero, R.; Sepulveda, W.; Mazor, M.; Brandt, F.; Cotton, D.B.; Dinarello, C.A.; Mitchell, M.D. The natural interleukin-1 receptor antagonist in term and preterm parturition. *Am. J. Obstet. Gynecol.* **1992**, *167*, 863–872. [CrossRef]
254. Girard, S.; Sebire, G. Transplacental Transfer of Interleukin-1 Receptor Agonist and Antagonist Following Maternal Immune Activation. *Am. J. Reprod. Immunol.* **2016**, *75*, 8–12. [CrossRef] [PubMed]
255. Kaiser, C.; Knight, A.; Nordstrom, D.; Pettersson, T.; Fransson, J.; Florin-Robertsson, E.; Pilstrom, B. Injection-site reactions upon Kineret (anakinra) administration: Experiences and explanations. *Rheumatol. Int.* **2012**, *32*, 295–299. [CrossRef] [PubMed]
256. Dhimolea, E. Canakinumab. *MAbs* **2010**, *2*, 3–13. [CrossRef]
257. Christopoulos, A.; May, L.T.; Avlani, V.A.; Sexton, P.M. G-protein-coupled receptor allosterism: The promise and the problem(s). *Biochem. Soc. Trans.* **2004**, *32*, 873–877. [CrossRef]
258. Terrillon, S.; Bouvier, M. Roles of G-protein-coupled receptor dimerization. *EMBO Rep.* **2004**, *5*, 30–34. [CrossRef]
259. Kenakin, T. Allosteric modulators: The new generation of receptor antagonist. *Mol. Interv.* **2004**, *4*, 222–229. [CrossRef]
260. Kubatzky, K.F.; Liu, W.; Goldgraben, K.; Simmerling, C.; Smith, S.O.; Constantinescu, S.N. Structural requirements of the extracellular to transmembrane domain junction for erythropoietin receptor function. *J. Biol. Chem.* **2005**, *280*, 14844–14854. [CrossRef]
261. Remy, I.; Wilson, I.A.; Michnick, S.W. Erythropoietin receptor activation by a ligand-induced conformation change. *Science* **1999**, *283*, 990–993. [CrossRef]
262. Quiniou, C.; Sapieha, P.; Lahaie, I.; Hou, X.; Brault, S.; Beauchamp, M.; Leduc, M.; Rihakova, L.; Joyal, J.S.; Nadeau, S.; et al. Development of a novel noncompetitive antagonist of IL-1 receptor. *J. Immunol.* **2008**, *180*, 6977–6987. [CrossRef]
263. Gillingham, A.K.; Munro, S. The small G proteins of the Arf family and their regulators. *Annu. Rev. Cell Dev. Biol.* **2007**, *23*, 579–611. [CrossRef]
264. Singh, R.; Wang, B.; Shirvaikar, A.; Khan, S.; Kamat, S.; Schelling, J.R.; Konieczkowski, M.; Sedor, J.R. The IL-1 receptor and Rho directly associate to drive cell activation in inflammation. *J. Clin. Investig.* **1999**, *103*, 1561–1570. [CrossRef]
265. Thumkeo, D.; Watanabe, S.; Narumiya, S. Physiological roles of Rho and Rho effectors in mammals. *Eur. J. Cell Biol.* **2013**, *92*, 303–315. [CrossRef]
266. Quiniou, C.; Kooli, E.; Joyal, J.S.; Sapieha, P.; Sennlaub, F.; Lahaie, I.; Shao, Z.; Hou, X.; Hardy, P.; Lubell, W.; et al. Interleukin-1 and ischemic brain injury in the newborn: Development of a small molecule inhibitor of IL-1 receptor. *Semin. Perinatol.* **2008**, *32*, 325–333. [CrossRef]
267. Rivera, J.C.; Sitaras, N.; Noueihed, B.; Hamel, D.; Madaan, A.; Zhou, T.; Honore, J.C.; Quiniou, C.; Joyal, J.S.; Hardy, P.; et al. Microglia and interleukin-1beta in ischemic retinopathy elicit microvascular degeneration through neuronal semaphorin-3A. *Arterioscler. Thromb. Vasc. Biol.* **2013**, *33*, 1881–1891. [CrossRef]
268. Dabouz, R.; Cheng, C.W.H.; Abram, P.; Omri, S.; Cagnone, G.; Sawmy, K.V.; Joyal, J.S.; Desjarlais, M.; Olson, D.; Weil, A.G.; et al. An allosteric interleukin-1 receptor modulator mitigates inflammation and photoreceptor toxicity in a model of retinal degeneration. *J. Neuroinflamm.* **2020**, *17*, 359. [CrossRef]
269. Hamel, D.; Sanchez, M.; Duhamel, F.; Roy, O.; Honore, J.C.; Noueihed, B.; Zhou, T.; Nadeau-Vallee, M.; Hou, X.; Lavoie, J.C.; et al. G-Protein-Coupled Receptor 91 and Succinate Are Key Contributors in Neonatal Postcerebral Hypoxia-Ischemia Recovery. *Arterioscler. Thromb. Vasc. Biol.* **2013**. [CrossRef]
270. Honore, J.C.; Kooli, A.; Hamel, D.; Alquier, T.; Rivera, J.C.; Quiniou, C.; Hou, X.; Kermorvant-Duchemin, E.; Hardy, P.; Poitout, V.; et al. Fatty acid receptor Gpr40 mediates neuromicrovascular degeneration induced by transarachidonic acids in rodents. *Arterioscler. Thromb. Vasc. Biol.* **2013**, *33*, 954–961. [CrossRef]
271. Sirinyan, M.; Sennlaub, F.; Dorfman, A.; Sapieha, P.; Gobeil, F., Jr.; Hardy, P.; Lachapelle, P.; Chemtob, S. Hyperoxic exposure leads to nitrative stress and ensuing microvascular degeneration and diminished brain mass and function in the immature subject. *Stroke* **2006**, *37*, 2807–2815. [CrossRef]
272. Beaudry-Richard, A.; Nadeau-Vallee, M.; Prairie, E.; Maurice, N.; Heckel, E.; Nezhady, M.; Pundir, S.; Madaan, A.; Boudreault, A.; Hou, X.; et al. Author Correction: Antenatal IL-1-dependent inflammation persists postnatally and causes retinal and sub-retinal vasculopathy in progeny. *Sci. Rep.* **2020**, *10*, 6634. [CrossRef]
273. Saltzman, W.M.; Torchilin, V.P. Drug delivery systems. *AccessScience* **2018**. [CrossRef]
274. Refuerzo, J.S.; Alexander, J.F.; Leonard, F.; Leon, M.; Longo, M.; Godin, B. Liposomes: A nanoscale drug carrying system to prevent indomethacin passage to the fetus in a pregnant mouse model. *Am. J. Obstet. Gynecol.* **2015**, *212*, 508.e1–508.e7. [CrossRef]
275. Dutta, E.H.; Behnia, F.; Harirah, H.; Costantine, M.; Saade, G. Perinatal Outcomes after Short versus Prolonged Indomethacin for Tocolysis in Women with Preterm Labor. *Am. J. Perinatol.* **2016**, *33*, 844–848. [CrossRef]
276. Moise, K.J., Jr.; Ou, C.N.; Kirshon, B.; Cano, L.E.; Rognerud, C.; Carpenter, R.J., Jr. Placental transfer of indomethacin in the human pregnancy. *Am. J. Obstet. Gynecol.* **1990**, *162*, 549–554. [CrossRef]
277. Paul, J.; Hua, S.; Smith, R. A Targeted Drug Delivery System for the Uterus. *Reprod. Sci.* **2015**, *22*, 57A.

278. Fuchs, A.R.; Fuchs, F.; Husslein, P.; Soloff, M.S. Oxytocin receptors in the human uterus during pregnancy and parturition. *Am. J. Obstet. Gynecol.* **1984**, *150*, 734–741. [CrossRef]
279. Wathes, D.C.; Borwick, S.C.; Timmons, P.M.; Leung, S.T.; Thornton, S. Oxytocin receptor expression in human term and preterm gestational tissues prior to and following the onset of labour. *J. Endocrinol.* **1999**, *161*, 143–151. [CrossRef] [PubMed]
280. Parkington, H.C.; Stevenson, J.; Tonta, M.A.; Paul, J.; Butler, T.; Maiti, K.; Chan, E.C.; Sheehan, P.M.; Brennecke, S.P.; Coleman, H.A.; et al. Diminished hERG K+ channel activity facilitates strong human labour contractions but is dysregulated in obese women. *Nat. Commun.* **2014**, *5*, 4108. [CrossRef]
281. Paul, J.W.; Hua, S.; Ilicic, M.; Tolosa, J.M.; Butler, T.; Robertson, S.; Smith, R. Drug delivery to the human and mouse uterus using immunoliposomes targeted to the oxytocin receptor. *Am. J. Obstet. Gynecol.* **2017**, *216*, 283.e1–283.e14. [CrossRef]
282. Refuerzo, J.S.; Leonard, F.; Bulayeva, N.; Gorenstein, D.; Chiossi, G.; Ontiveros, A.; Longo, M.; Godin, B. Uterus-targeted liposomes for preterm labor management: Studies in pregnant mice. *Sci. Rep.* **2016**, *6*, 34710. [CrossRef]
283. Hua, S.; Vaughan, B. In vitro comparison of liposomal drug delivery systems targeting the oxytocin receptor: A potential novel treatment for obstetric complications. *Int. J. Nanomed.* **2019**, *14*, 2191–2206. [CrossRef]
284. De Ziegler, D.; Bulletti, C.; De Monstier, B.; Jääskeläinen, A.S. The first uterine pass effect. *Ann. N. Y. Acad. Sci.* **1997**, *828*, 291–299. [CrossRef]
285. Ensign, L.M.; Tang, B.C.; Wang, Y.Y.; Tse, T.A.; Hoen, T.; Cone, R.; Hanes, J. Mucus-penetrating nanoparticles for vaginal drug delivery protect against herpes simplex virus. *Sci. Transl. Med.* **2012**, *4*, 138ra179. [CrossRef]
286. Hoang, T.; Zierden, H.; Date, A.; Ortiz, J.; Gumber, S.; Anders, N.; He, P.; Segars, J.; Hanes, J.; Mahendroo, M.; et al. Development of a mucoinert progesterone nanosuspension for safer and more effective prevention of preterm birth. *J. Control. Release* **2019**, *295*, 74–86. [CrossRef]
287. Zierden, H.C.; Ortiz, J.I.; DeLong, K.; Yu, J.; Li, G.; Dimitrion, P.; Bensouda, S.; Laney, V.; Bailey, A.; Anders, N.M.; et al. Enhanced drug delivery to the reproductive tract using nanomedicine reveals therapeutic options for prevention of preterm birth. *Sci. Transl. Med.* **2021**, *13*. [CrossRef]
288. Vyas, V.; Ashby, C.R., Jr.; Olgun, N.S.; Sundaram, S.; Salami, O.; Munnangi, S.; Pekson, R.; Mahajan, P.; Reznik, S.E. Inhibition of sphingosine kinase prevents lipopolysaccharide-induced preterm birth and suppresses proinflammatory responses in a murine model. *Am. J. Pathol.* **2015**, *185*, 862–869. [CrossRef]
289. Giusto, K.; Patki, M.; Koya, J.; Ashby, C.R., Jr.; Munnangi, S.; Patel, K.; Reznik, S.E. A vaginal nanoformulation of a SphK inhibitor attenuates lipopolysaccharide-induced preterm birth in mice. *Nanomedicine* **2019**, *14*, 2835–2851. [CrossRef]
290. Rani, S.; Rana, R.; Saraogi, G.K.; Kumar, V.; Gupta, U. Self-Emulsifying Oral Lipid Drug Delivery Systems: Advances and Challenges. *AAPS PharmSciTech* **2019**, *20*, 129. [CrossRef]
291. Washington, H.A. *Medical Apartheid: The Dark History of Medical Experimentation on Black Americans from Colonial Times to the Present*; First Anchor Books: New York, NY, USA, 2006.
292. Turner, M.A.; Davis, J.M.; McCune, S.; Bax, R.; Portman, R.J.; Hudson, L.D. The International Neonatal Consortium: Collaborating to advance regulatory science for neonates. *Pediatr Res.* **2016**, *80*, 462–464. [CrossRef]

Systematic Review

A Systematic Review of the Safety of Blocking the IL-1 System in Human Pregnancy

Marie-Eve Brien [1], Virginie Gaudreault [1], Katia Hughes [1], Dexter J. L. Hayes [2], Alexander E. P. Heazell [2] and Sylvie Girard [3,4,*]

1. Ste-Justine Hospital Research Center, Montreal, QC H3T 1C5, Canada; marie-eve.brien.hsj@ssss.gouv.qc.ca (M.-E.B.); virginie.gaudreault7@gmail.com (V.G.); khugh049@uottawa.ca (K.H.)
2. Maternal and Fetal Health Research Centre, Faculty of Biology, Medicine and Health, University of Manchester, Manchester Academic Health Science Centre, Manchester M13 9PL, UK; dexter.hayes@manchester.ac.uk (D.J.L.H.); alexander.heazell@manchester.ac.uk (A.E.P.H.)
3. Department of Obstetrics and Gynecology, Universite de Montreal, Montreal, QC H3T 1J4, Canada
4. Department of Obstetrics and Gynecology, Department of Immunology, Mayo Clinic, Rochester, MN 55902, USA
* Correspondence: girard.sylvie@mayo.edu; Tel.: +1-507-284-0545

Abstract: Blockade of the interleukin-1 (IL-1) pathway has been used therapeutically in several inflammatory diseases including arthritis and cryopyrin-associated periodic syndrome (CAPS). These conditions frequently affect women of childbearing age and continued usage of IL-1 specific treatments throughout pregnancy has been reported. IL-1 is involved in pregnancy complications and its blockade could have therapeutic potential. We systematically reviewed all reported cases of IL-1 blockade in human pregnancy to assess safety and perinatal outcomes. We searched several databases to find reports of specific blockade of the IL-1 pathway at any stage of pregnancy, excluding broad spectrum or non-specific anti-inflammatory intervention. Our literature search generated 2439 references of which 22 studies included, following extensive review. From these, 88 different pregnancies were assessed. Most (64.8%) resulted in healthy term deliveries without any obstetrical/neonatal complications. Including pregnancy exposed to Anakinra or Canakinumab, 12 (15.0%) resulted in preterm birth and one stillbirth occurred. Regarding neonatal complications, 2 cases of renal agenesis (2.5%) were observed, and 6 infants were diagnosed with CAPS (7.5%). In conclusion, this systematic review describes that IL-1 blockade during pregnancy is not associated with increased adverse perinatal outcomes, considering that treated women all presented an inflammatory disease associated with elevated risk of pregnancy complications.

Keywords: IL-1 blockade; anakinra; canakinumab; pregnancy; human; inflammation

1. Introduction

Pregnancy complications are often associated with inflammation at the maternal-fetal interface. During pregnancy complication, such as preeclampsia (PE), preterm birth (PTB) and fetal growth restriction (FGR), inflammation can be found in the maternal circulation as well as in the placenta. Uncontrolled inflammation can negatively affect placental function [1–6]. Any alteration in placental function is associated with neonatal complications and altered child development particularly neurodevelopmental delay [7–10]. Therapeutically targeting inflammation in pregnancy has been challenging since inflammatory processes are also involved in physiological pregnancies, especially at the time of implantation and parturition [11–16] and a proinflammatory profile can be observed toward the end of uncomplicated pregnancy [16–18]. Therefore, there is a need to differentiate between physiological and pathological inflammation in order to develop and apply novel anti-inflammatory strategies in the clinical setting.

Inflammation has been observed at all stages of pregnancy [19–26]. Inflammation can occur in response to bacterial or viral infections (collectively referred to as pathogens-associated molecular patterns—PAMPs), as well as in response to sterile or endogenous mediators, termed damage-associated molecular pattern—DAMPs or alarmins, the latter increasingly associated with pathological pregnancies [27–32]. In order to mitigate the effects of dysregulated inflammation during pregnancy, multiple broad-spectrum anti-inflammatory therapies have been used and developed with interesting results [33,34]. Amongst these therapies, corticosteroids and nonsteroidal anti-inflammatory drugs (NSAIDs) are the most prevalent. However, studies have investigated the effect of corticosteroids during pregnancy and found an association between corticosteroid use and pregnancy/neonatal complications [35–38]. In a systematic review, Bandoli G. et al. found little to no association between corticosteroids and adverse pregnancy outcomes [35] whilst other groups reported concerns such as higher rate of cerebral palsy among children who had been exposed to repeated doses of corticosteroids or impaired growth of the lung parenchyma in cases of treatment without premature birth [36–38]. As for NSAIDs, acting through the inhibition of cyclooxygenase enzymes (COX-1 and COX-2), a study by Bérard A. et al., showed elevated risk of prematurity associated with the use of COX-2 inhibitors [39]. However, NSAIDs use during the first trimester of pregnancy was not associated with congenital malformations [40].

In case of pregnancies complicated with infections, antibiotics are often used. However, several studies have shown the detrimental effects of antibiotics on the development of the newborn. In the ORACLE series of clinical studies, the use of some antibiotics in pregnancy has been associated with elevated incidence of neurodevelopmental disorders [41,42]. Others have found increased risk of spontaneous miscarriage [43], without any association with congenital malformation [44]. All these drugs have benefits, but also major risk associated with their use. Since these are not specific and affect several inflammatory pathways at once, it is possible that pathways important in physiological pregnancy are impacted and responsible for the side effects observed. Targeting specific inflammatory mediators/pathways involved in pathological pregnancies could provide an efficient mean to mitigate the negative impact of inflammation, subsequently protecting the placenta and developing fetus, whilst having less deleterious effects.

The interleukin-1 (IL-1) system has been consistently associated with pregnancy complications such as preterm birth, including chorioamnionitis, FGR and PE [1,5,6,32,45–49] as well as high-risk pregnancies with reduced fetal movements [50]. The IL-1 system has been targeted in several animal models of pregnancy complications and blockade of this pathway appears to reduce the incidence of complications and protect the placenta as well as both fetal/neonatal development [4,51–58] and as reviewed previously by us, with emphasis on means of blocking the IL-1 pathway and their mechanisms of action with schematic representation [59]. Aside from studies in animal models, Il-1 blockers have been used for many years to help mitigate/resolve inflammatory conditions in humans [60–63]. The IL-1 receptor antagonist, IL-1Ra, is the most commonly used IL-1 system antagonist and is known under the generic name Anakinra (brand name Kineret). Anakinra has been approved for clinical use for over 20 years and has been commonly used for several chronic inflammatory conditions (such as arthritis and lupus) and in the pediatric population [60,64–68]. Canakinumab, brand name Ilaris, is a monoclonal antibody targeting IL-1β which has been approved for inflammatory condition such as cryopyrin-associated periodic syndromes (CAPS), since 2009 [69,70]. These inflammatory conditions commonly affect women of reproductive age and continued usage of Anakinra and/or Canakinumab during pregnancy has been reported [71–73]. Despite their wide range of beneficial effects, these drugs are not yet approved for use in pregnant women and are used solely when the benefit of continuing the treatment during the pregnancy outweigh the risk.

In light of the important need for targeted anti-inflammatory therapies during pregnancy, the evidence that the IL-1 system is central to both PAMPs and DAMPs-induced inflammation at the maternal-fetal interface, our objective was to perform a systematic review of all reports of any specific blockers of the IL-1 system being used during human pregnancy, to assess their potential impact on pregnancy outcome and neonatal health.

2. Materials and Methods

The systematic review is reported in accordance with Preferred Reporting Items for Systematic Reviews and Meta-Analyses (PRISMA) guidelines [74]. The review protocol was registered with the International Prospective Register of Systematic Reviews (PROSPERO) on 6 July 2020 (CRD42020197186).

2.1. Information Sources, Search Strategy and Eligibility Criteria

Literature searches were conducted in PubMed, EMBASE, MEDLINE, Cochrane Database of Systematic Reviews and Google Scholar. The search was not limited by dates but was limited to titles, abstracts and manuscripts written in English and French (for practical reasons). Reviews were excluded to ensure inclusion of original research only. Abstract from conferences were included as well, unless the same data was published and therefore only the final research article was included to avoid duplication of the same cases. Reference lists of included studies were checked for any other relevant papers. Manuscripts were identified with the search terms 'pregnancy' and 'IL-1 blockage' or 'IL-1 blockade' or 'IL-1 receptor agonist' or 'IL-1ra' or 'Anakinra' or 'Kineret' or 'Rilonacept' or 'Canakinumab' or 'Rytvela'. All searches were completed by 9 July 2021. An example search is included in Data S1.

We included cohort studies (prospective and retrospective), case series and case reports which reported the used of IL-1 blockage during pregnancy. We included all studies involving pregnant individuals who received IL-1 blockage at any stage during their pregnancy.

Our main objective was to document pregnancy outcomes related to treatment (i.e., IL-1 blockade) with IL-1 antagonists during pregnancy. The medical indication for the treatment, chronic inflammatory pathologies diagnosed prior to pregnancy in most cases, was also considered. Data regarding the rates of pregnancy complications (including: congenital anomalies, hypertensive disorders of pregnancy, preterm birth—delivery before 37 weeks of gestation, FGR, neonatal and maternal death) were extracted. We compared all these outcomes to the reported incidence in the general population and population of women with inflammatory pathologies.

2.2. Data Extraction

Duplicates were removed, and all citations were screened for relevance using the full abstract and indexing terms. Two out of three reviewers (MEB, VG or KH) had to agree that a study for it to be included, according to the pre-specified inclusion and exclusion criteria. When available, full-length manuscripts were obtained. Two reviewers (MEB and VG) made final inclusions decisions independently and a third reviewer (SG) was consulted to resolve any conflict when necessary.

2.3. Assessment of Risk of Bias and Methodological Quality

Included cohort studies were assessed using the Risk of Bias in Non-randomised Studies—of Interventions (ROBINS-I) with 7 domains, since all the studies included in this systematic review were observational. This method categorises each study by low, moderate, serious, critical risk of bias or no information [75]. If a study' risk of bias was categorised as serious or critical, the effect of removing this study was tested and the relevant outcome reported. Individual case reports were assessed using a specific tool to assess the methodological quality of case reports [76]. This assesses 8 characteristics in 4 domains of selection, ascertainment, causality and reporting.

2.4. Data Synthesis

Studies with continuous data (i.e., birthweight and gestational age) were taken to obtain overall means and standard deviations. It was intended to investigate effect of exposure to IL-1 blockade at different times of pregnancy, but data could not be stratified by trimester of exposure since too many data were missing.

3. Results

The search strategy (Figure 1) identified 2439 articles. After removing duplicates (n = 742), 1697 papers were screened based on their title and abstracts. 1569 papers were excluded based of irrelevant to the question, exposure not during pregnancy and IL-1 blockade effects were not reported. On this basis, resulting in 128 papers for which full text was evaluated. 106 studies were excluded as they were reviews, conference abstract with original article already included, missing information or reports of animal studies, meaning 22 papers were included in the final synthesis. The 22 included studies were 9 case reports, 13 cohort studies (6 retrospective and 7 prospective).

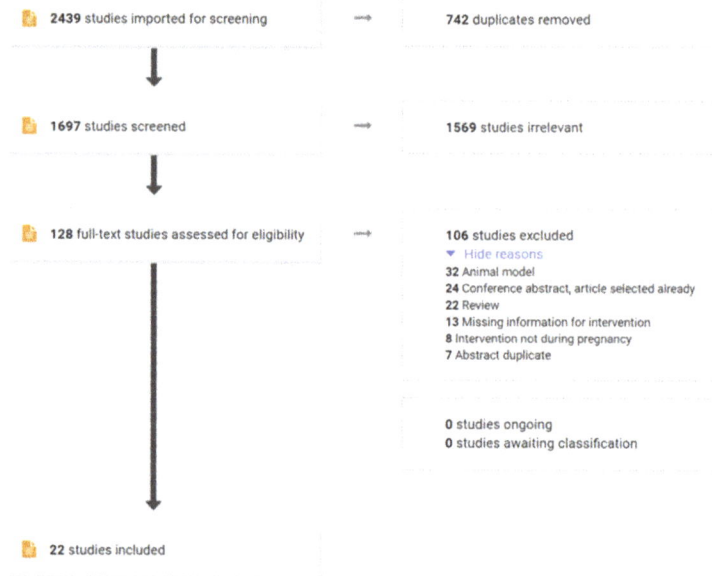

Figure 1. PRISMA flow chart of the systemic review of studies investigating the effect of IL-1 blockage during pregnancy.

3.1. Risk of Bias/Methodological Quality of Included Studies

The majority of studies included in this systematic review had a low risk of bias in the assessed domains as evaluated with the ROBINS-I tool. The majority of the case reports included adequate case ascertainment and follow-up, but there was limited data about the causal relationship between exposure to Anakinra and Canakinumab and adverse reactions (Table S1). It is important to note that almost half of the studies included in this systematic review were published conference abstracts and therefore provided limited data which could impact the results presented. Furthermore, five pregnancies were exposed to both Anakinra and Canakinumab which could affect the classification of the intervention and their outcomes.

3.2. Study Characteristics

Characteristics of each study and summary of findings are presented in Table 1. Within the 22 studies included, 88 individual pregnancies were reported. 75 pregnancies (85.2%) received Anakinra and 13 (14.8%) Canakinumab. Of these 88 pregnancies, 5.7% were exposed to both agents over the course of their pregnancy. The indications for these treatments were mostly cryopyrin-associated periodic syndrome—CAPS (34.1%), including familial cold autoinflammatory syndrome—FCAS, neonatal-onset multisystem inflammatory disorder—NOMID and Muckle-Wells syndrome—MWS; familial Mediterranean fever—FMF (33.0%); and adult-onset Still's disease—AOSD or systemic juvenile idiopathic arthritis—SJIA (20.4%). The remaining cases (11 women/12.5%) received treatment for the "TNF receptor associated periodic syndrome"—TRAPS (3.4%), haemophagocytic lymphohistiocytosis—HLH (2.3%) or other pathologies such as idiopathic pericarditis, Cogan syndrome or chronic inflammatory rheumatic disease (6.8%).

Table 1. Characteristics and summary from studies included.

Study	Study Design	Year of Publication	Population	Number of Pregnancies Included in This Study	Indication for Treatment	Treatment; Doses	Outcome	Notes
1	Case report	2009	1	1	AOSD	Anakinra; 100 mg/day	Healthy term baby	
2	Case report	2011	2	2	AOSD	Anakinra; 100 mg/day	Two healthy babies, one PTB 36 weeks	
3	Retrospective cohort study	2013	51	1	SOJIA	Anakinra; NA	Term baby	Big cohort of SOJIA patients but only one pregnant
4	Prospective cohort study	2014	9	9	FCAS (6) NOMID (1) MWS/NOMID (1)	Anakinra; mostly 100 mg/day but also 239–300 mg/day	All term babies, three with FCAS, one with MWS and one twin pregnancy resulted in one death at 30 weeks	
5	Prospective cohort study	2015	4	0	FMF	Anakinra; 100 mg/day	All healthy babies, one PTB 36 weeks	Data in another study already included
6	Prospective cohort study	2015	6	3	FMF	Anakinra; 100 mg/day or NA	All healthy babies, one PTB 36 weeks	Data in another study already included
7	Prospective cohort study	2015	79	1	Chronic inflammatory rheumatic disease	Anakinra; NA	Voluntary pregnancy termination	Big cohort of biological drug during pregnancy, only one took anakinra
8	Case report	2017	1	1	FMF	Anakinra; 100 mg/day	Healthy term baby	
9	Prospective cohort study	2018	5	5	AOSD (3) SOJIA (2)	Anakinra; 100 mg/day	All healthy term babies but one with right hydrocele, heart murmur and resolved low birthweight	
10	Retrospective cohort study	2018	4	4	FMF	Anakinra; 100 mg/day– 2 days	All healthy babies but one PTB at 33 weeks with hypotrophic, respiratory distress syndrome, hyperbilirubinemia and poor drinking	

Table 1. Cont.

Study	Study Design	Year of Publication	Population	Number of Pregnancies Included in This Study	Indication for Treatment	Treatment; Doses	Outcome	Notes
11	Prospective cohort study	2019	13	12	FMF	Anakinra; 100 mg/day or NA	One miscarriage, two PTB, one stillbirth but overall healthy babies	Two pregnancies still ongoing, no obstetrical information and two pregnancies with data in another study already included
12	Case report	2019	1	1	FMF	Anakinra; 100 mg/day	Term healthy baby	Cohort of four patients with FMF, only one pregnant
13	Prospective cohort study	2019	54	1	FMF	Anakinra; 100 mg/day	Obstetrical and neonatal information NA	Cohort of patient with FMF, only one pregnant
14	Case report	2019	1	1	HLH	Anakinra; 200 mg/twice daily	Healthy but had anaemia and marrow suppression	
15	Retrospective cohort study	2020	16	3	AOSD	Anakinra; NA	All healthy babies but one had PTB at 28 weeks	Cohort of child exposed to DMARDs, only 3 exposed to anakinra during pregnancy
16	Case report	2020	1	1	HLH	Anakinra; NA	PTB at 31 weeks and IUGR but overall healthy	
17	Case report	2017	1	1	MWS	Canakinumab; 150 mg/ 4–8 weeks	Healthy term baby	
18	Case report	2018	1	1	SOJIA	Canakinumab; NA	Healthy term baby	
19	Retrospective cohort study	2020	23	1	FMF	Canakinumab; 150 mg/ 6–8 weeks	One healthy term pregnancy and one without information	Cohort of patient with FMF, only 2 pregnant
20	Retrospective cohort study	2013	7	7	AOSD (1) CAPS (3) TRAPS (1) FMF (1) Idiopathic pericarditis (1)	Anakinra; NA (6), Canakinumab; NA (1)	All healthy babies, one PTB 36 weeks and one with unilateral reduced hearing at 6 weeks	Two pregnancies still ongoing, no obstetrical information
21	Case report	2015	1	1	MWS	Canakinumab; NA and Anakinra; NA	Healthy but with CAPS	
22	Retrospective cohort study	2017	43	31	AOSD (4) CAPS (16) Cogan syndrome (2) FMF (5) Idiopathic pericarditis (1) TRAPS (2) Un-SAID (1)	Anakinra; mostly 100 mg/day but also 50–300 mg/day Canakinumab; 150 mg/ 4–8 weeks	Two miscarriage (same women), two PTB, all healthy babies but one with left renal agenesis and ectopic neurohypophysis with hormone deficiency	43 pregnancies exposed to IL-1 inhibitor but 11 were male exposure

HLH: hemophagocytic lymphohistiocytosis, FMF: familial mediterranean fever, AOSD: adult-onset Still's disease, FCAS: familial cold autoinflammatory Syndrome, NOMID: neonatal-onset multisystem inflammatory disease, MWS: Muckle-Wells syndrome, sJIA: systemic juvenile idiopathic arthritis, CAPS: cryopyrin-associated autoinflammatory syndromes, NA: not available.

Of the 88 pregnancies, 4 women (4.5%) were still pregnant at the time of publication without any follow up available for their pregnancies. Of these women, three were within their first trimester and one in the second trimester, all without any complication reported to date. In the rest of pregnancies, three (3.4%) resulted in miscarriage during the first trimester (two exposed to Anakinra and one to Canakinumab). Two of these spontaneous miscarriages occurred in the same patient, the first whilst on Canakinumab and the second with Anakinra since she presented with refractory Cogan syndrome. Unfortunately, the patient only had a partial clinical and biochemical response of her underlying diseases despite dose escalation of both treatment regimens. Finally, one patient on Anakinra terminated her pregnancy electively. For the rest of the analysis, these patients were excluded due to the lack of information.

3.3. Duration of Exposure to Drugs during Pregnancy

In 48 cases (60.0%) of the remaining 80 pregnancies, the women were already taking the medication prior to getting pregnant; in 6 cases, this was unknown. In 50 cases (62.5%), the drug therapy was continued throughout pregnancy (when it was started either prior to or during the first trimester until birth). In nine cases, treatment was stopped after the first trimester and, in 2 cases, after the second trimester, due to the lack of data on safety of these drugs in pregnancy. In 13 cases, treatment was started either during the second half of pregnancy (10 patients) or during the third trimester (3 patients). Of these 13 cases, 4 were due to a lack of improvement with their previous treatment (i.e., colchicine or prednisone), 2 women were diagnosed with AOSD or HLH while pregnant and no information was given for the remaining seven women. Details of the treatment duration is shown in a flow chart (Figure 2). Information concerning each pregnancy separately are shown in Table 2.

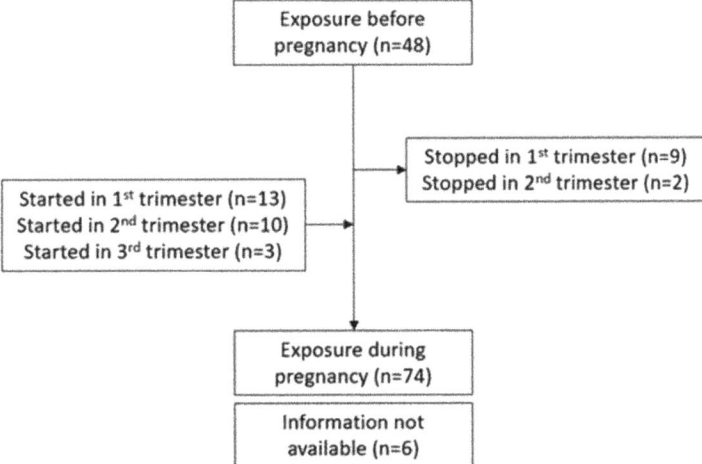

Figure 2. Flow chart of IL-1 blockade exposure during pregnancy (for the 11 pregnancies that stopped treatment during their 1st or 2nd trimester, treatment was initiated before conception and therefore they were included in the n = 48).

Table 2. Pregnancies details with maternal characteristic and neonatal outcomes.

Pregnancy ID	Pregnancy from Study	Indication for Treatment	Treatment	Doses	Exposure Time	Mode of Delivery	GA at Delivery (Weeks)	Birth Weight (g)	Obstetric Complication	Child Sex	Child Wellbeing	Breastfeeding
1	14	HLH	Anakinra	200 mg/twice daily	22 w–B	C-section	NA	NA	None	NA	Anaemia and bone marrow suppression	NA
2	19	FMF + amyloidosis	Canakinumab	150 mg/6 weeks	PC–8 w	NA	Term	NA	None	NA	Healthy	NA
3	19	FMF	Canakinumab	150 mg/8 weeks	PC–PPT	NA	NA	NA	NA	NA	NA	NA
4 *	7	Chronic inflammatory rheumatic disease	Anakinra	NA	NA	Vaginal	NA	NA	Voluntary abortion	NA	NA	NA
5	1	AOSD	Anakinra	100 mg/day	PC–B	Vaginal	40.7	2700	Placental retention requiring manual abruption	F	Healthy	Yes
6	4	FCAS	Anakinra	100 mg/day	PC–B	Vaginal	41.0	3742	None	NA	Healthy	No
7	4	FCAS	Anakinra	100 mg/day	PC–B	Vaginal	41.0	3629	None	NA	FCAS	No
8	4	FCAS	Anakinra	100 mg/day	PC–B	Vaginal	38.0	3402	None	NA	FCAS	Yes
9	4	FCAS	Anakinra	100 mg/day	PC–B	Vaginal	37.0	3459	None	NA	Healthy	No
10	4	FCAS	Anakinra	100 mg/day	PC–B	Vaginal	37.7	2977	None	NA	FCAS	No
11	4	FCAS	Anakinra	100 mg/day	PC–B	Vaginal	39.0	3345	None	NA	Healthy	No
12	4	NOMID	Anakinra	300 mg/day	PC–B	C-section	40.0	4139	Chronic hypertension	NA	Healthy	Yes
13	4	NOMID	Anakinra	239–300 mg/day	PC–B	Vaginal	A: 38.7 B: 30.0	A: 2637 B: NA	A: None B: PTB	NA	A: Healthy B: Renal agenesis (death)	A: Yes B: No

Table 2. Cont.

Pregnancy ID	Pregnancy from Study	Indication for Treatment	Treatment	Doses	Exposure Time	Mode of Delivery	GA at Delivery (Weeks)	Birth Weight (g)	Obstetric Complication	Child Sex	Child Wellbeing	Breastfeeding
14	4	MWS/NOMID	Anakinra	100 mg/day	PC–B	C-section	Term	3515	None	NA	MWS	No
15	15	AOSD	Anakinra	NA	PC–B	C-section	28.0	1175	PTB	F	Healthy	NA
16	15	AOSD	Anakinra	NA	PC–B	Vaginal	40.0	3480	None	M	Healthy	NA
17	15	AOSD	Anakinra	NA	PC–B	Vaginal	38.0	3450	None	M	Healthy	NA
19	12	FMF	Anakinra	100 mg/day	6 w–B	C-section	Term	3340	None	F	Healthy	Yes
20	17	MWS	Canakinumab	150 mg/8 weeks, then every 4–5 weeks	PC–34 w	C-section	39.0	2994	None	F	Healthy with NLRP3 mutation	NA
22	11	FMF	Anakinra	100 mg/day	PC–29 w + 33 w–B	C-section	38.0	NA	Incision site infection in postpartum	M	Healthy	NA
24	11	FMF	Anakinra	NA	16 w–B	C-section	31.0	NA	PTB	F-F twins	Healthy	NA
25	11	FMF	Anakinra	NA	23 w–B	C-section	37.0	NA	NA	F	Healthy	NA
26	11	FMF	Anakinra	NA	32 w–B	C-section	40.0	NA	NA	F	Healthy	NA
27	11	FMF	Anakinra	NA	PC–B with 1 month interruption	C-section	38.0	NA	NA	F	Healthy	NA
28	11	FMF	Anakinra	NA	34 w–B	Vaginal	37.0	NA	Stillbirth	M		NA
29	11	FMF	Anakinra	NA	6 w–B	C-section	36.0	NA	PTB	F	Healthy	NA
30	11	FMF	Anakinra	NA	NA	NA	NA	NA	NA	NA	NA	NA
31 *	11	FMF	Anakinra	NA	5 w–8 w (ongoing)	NA	NA	NA	NA	NA	NA	NA
32 *	11	FMF	Anakinra	NA	PC–8 w (ongoing)	NA	NA	NA	NA	NA	NA	NA

Table 2. Cont.

Pregnancy ID	Pregnancy from Study	Indication for Treatment	Treatment	Doses	Exposure Time	Mode of Delivery	GA at Delivery (Weeks)	Birth Weight (g)	Obstetric Complication	Child Sex	Child Wellbeing	Breastfeeding
33	2	AOSD	Anakinra	100 mg/day	PC–B	Vaginal	39.0	3100	None	M	Healthy	No
34	2	AOSD	Anakinra	NA	12 w–B	C-section	36.0	2800	PTB	M	Healthy	No
35	18	sJIA	Canakinumab	NA	PC–35 w	Vaginal	39.0	NA	Forceps + minor episiotomy wound infection	M	Healthy	NA
36	21	MWS	Canakinumab and Anakinra	NA	PC–B	NA	NA	NA	NA	M	Healthy with CAPS	Yes
37	8	FMF	Anakinra	100 mg/day	PC–B	C-section	38.0	2700	None	NA	Healthy	Yes
38 *	20	CAPS	Anakinra	NA	PC–NA (ongoing)	NA	NA	NA	NA	NA	NA	NA
39 *	20	CAPS	Canakinumab	NA	PC–8 w (ongoing)	NA	NA	NA	NA	NA	NA	NA
40	20	CAPS	Anakinra	NA	PC–B	Vaginal	NA	NA	None	M	Healthy	No
41	20	TRAPS	Anakinra	NA	PC–B	Vaginal	NA	NA	None	M	Unilateral reduced hearing at 6 weeks	No
42	20	FMF	Anakinra	100 mg/day	21 w–B	C-section	36.0	NA	Vaginal bleeding, PTB	M	Healthy	Yes
43	20	idiopathic pericarditis	Anakinra	NA	PC–B	Vaginal	NA	NA	None	M	Healthy	No
44	20	AOSD	Anakinra	NA	22 w–33 w	Vaginal	NA	NA	None	M	Healthy	No
50	6	FMF	Anakinra	100 mg/day	12 w–B	Vaginal	40.0	NA	None	F	Healthy	Yes

Table 2. *Cont.*

Pregnancy ID	Pregnancy from Study	Indication for Treatment	Treatment	Doses	Exposure Time	Mode of Delivery	GA at Delivery (Weeks)	Birth Weight (g)	Obstetric Complication	Child Sex	Child Wellbeing	Breastfeeding
52	6	FMF	Anakinra	NA	15 w–B	Vaginal	38.0	NA	None	M	Low thrombocyte count treated by IVIG	NA
54	3	sJIA	Anakinra	NA	P–B	NA	Term	NA	NA	NA	NA	NA
55	13	FMF	Anakinra	100 mg/day	P–B	NA	NA	NA	None	NA	NA	NA
56	9	sJIA	Anakinra	100 mg/day	PC–20.4 w	C-section	37.1	2419	Hypertension, oligohydramnios, breech presentation	M	Jaundice, right hydrocele and heart murmur	No
57	9	AOSD	Anakinra	100 mg/day	20 w–38.1 w	Vaginal	40.1	2940	None	M	Jaundice	NA
58	9	AOSD	Anakinra	100 mg/day	PC–16.6 w + 19.4 w–37.3 w	C-section	39.4	3632	None	M	Jaundice	Yes
59	9	AOSD	Anakinra	100 mg/day	PC–2 w + 9.6 w–36.7 w	Vaginal	38.7	3519	None	M	Tongue-tied	Yes
60	9	sJIA	Anakinra	100 mg/day	PC–37.3 w	Vaginal	39.4	2640	Oligohydramnios	F	Healthy	No
61	10	FMF	Anakinra	100 mg/day	P–B	C-section	40.6	4025	None	NA	Healthy	Yes
62	10	FMF	Anakinra	100 mg/day	2e trimester–B	C-section	33.7	3320	PTB	NA	Healthy, hypotrophic, respiratory distress syndrome, hyperbilirubinemia and poor drinking	No
63	10	FMF	Anakinra	100 mg/2 days	P–B	C-section	39.3	4030	Premature bleeding	NA	Healthy	NA

Table 2. *Cont.*

Pregnancy ID	Pregnancy from Study	Indication for Treatment	Treatment	Doses	Exposure Time	Mode of Delivery	GA at Delivery (Weeks)	Birth Weight (g)	Obstetric Complication	Child Sex	Child Wellbeing	Breastfeeding
64	10	FMF	Anakinra	100 mg/2 days	P–B	C-section	36.4	3320	PTB	NA	Healthy	NA
66	16	HLH	Anakinra	NA	22 w–B	C-section	31.7	NA	PTB, IUGR, abnormal umbilical artery Doppler and subsequent cardiotocography was abnormal	M	Neonatal unit briefly but healthy	NA
67	22	CAPS	Canakinumab	150 mg/8 weeks	PC–8 w	C-section	38.0	3540	Gestationnal diabetes	M	Healthy	No
68	22	CAPS	Canakinumab	150 mg/8 weeks	PC–12 w	Vaginal	40.0	4480	None	F	Healthy	Yes
69	22	CAPS	Canakinumab	150 mg/8 weeks	1 w–36 w	NA	40.0	3570	None	M	Healthy	NA
70	22	CAPS	Canakinumab	120 mg (single dose)	P	NA	38.0	3290	None	M	Healthy	Yes
71	22	Un-SAID	Canakinumab	300 mg/8 weeks	PC–B	Vaginal	39.0	NA	None	M	Healthy	NA
72	22	FMF	Canakinumab	150 mg/4 weeks	PC–B	C-section	37.0	3300	None	M	Healthy	Yes
73	22	FMF	Canakinumab	150 mg/8 weeks	PC–4 w	C-section	40.0	3300	None	F	Healthy	Yes
74 *	22	Cogan syndrome	Canakinumab	150 mg/4 weeks	PC–4 w	Vaginal	4.0	NA	Miscarriage	NA		NA
75	22	CAPS	Anakinra	50 mg/day	PC–B	Vaginal	39.0	3940	None	M	Healthy	No
76	22	CAPS	Anakinra	50 mg/day	PC–B	Vaginal	39.0	NA	None	F	Healthy	No
77	22	CAPS	Anakinra	100 mg/day	PC–B	Vaginal	41.1	3600	None	M	Healthy	Yes

Table 2. Cont.

Pregnancy ID	Pregnancy from Study	Indication for Treatment	Treatment	Doses	Exposure Time	Mode of Delivery	GA at Delivery (Weeks)	Birth Weight (g)	Obstetric Complication	Child Sex	Child Wellbeing	Breastfeeding
78	22	CAPS	Anakinra	100 mg/day	PPT–B	Vaginal	40.0	4480	None	F	Healthy	Yes
79	22	CAPS	Anakinra	100 mg/day	36 w–B	NA	40.0	3570	None	M	Healthy	NA
80	22	CAPS	Anakinra	100 mg/day	1 w–PPT	NA	36.9	2830	PTB	M	Healthy	No
81	22	CAPS	Anakinra	100 mg/day	PC–B	C-section	38.9	NA	C-section due to failure to progress	NA	Healthy	NA
82	22	CAPS	Anakinra	100 mg/day	PC–6 w	C-section	40.0	NA	None	M	Healthy	NA
83	22	CAPS	Anakinra	100 mg/day	PC–B	NA	NA	NA	None	M	Healthy	Yes
84	22	CAPS	Anakinra	100 mg/day	NA	NA	40.1	NA	None	F	Healthy	NA
85	22	CAPS	Anakinra	100 mg/day	NA	NA	NA	NA	None	F	Healthy	NA
86	22	CAPS	Anakinra	100 mg/day	NA	NA	NA	NA	None	F	Healthy	NA
87	22	FMF	Anakinra	100 mg/day	PC–B	C-section	36.1	2170	Vaginal bleeding, PTB	M	Healthy	Yes
88	22	FMF	Anakinra	100 mg/day	12 w–B	Vaginal	40.0	3170	None	F	Healthy	Yes
89	22	FMF	Anakinra	100 mg/day	PC–B	Vaginal	36.0	1600	PTB	F	Healthy	Yes
90	22	idiopathic pericarditis	Anakinra	100 mg/day	PC–PPT	Vaginal	38.3	2930	None	M	Healthy	No
91	22	AOSD	Anakinra	200–300 mg/day	PC–16 w	NA	37.0	2450	None	F	Healthy	No
92	22	AOSD	Anakinra	100 mg/day	22 w–33 w	NA	35.1	2020	PTB	M	Healthy	Yes
93	22	AOSD	Anakinra	100 mg/day	9 w–B	C-section	38.1	NA	None	M	Left renal agenesis	Yes

Table 2. *Cont.*

Pregnancy ID	Pregnancy from Study	Indication for Treatment	Treatment	Doses	Exposure Time	Mode of Delivery	GA at Delivery (Weeks)	Birth Weight (g)	Obstetric Complication	Child Sex	Child Wellbeing	Breastfeeding
94	22	AOSD	Anakinra	100 mg/day	NA	Vaginal	38.0	3060	None	F	Healthy	Yes
95	22	TRAPS	Anakinra	100 mg/day	PC–B	Vaginal	41.0	3230	None	M	Healthy	Yes
96	22	TRAPS	Anakinra	100 mg/day	PC–B	NA	NA	NA	None	F	Healthy	NA

HLH: hemophagocytic lymphohistiocytosis, FMF: familial mediterranean fever, AOSD: adult-onset Still's disease, FCAS: familial cold autoinflammatory Syndrome, NOMID: neonatal-onset multisystem inflammatory disease, MWS: Muckle-Wells syndrome, sJIA: systemic juvenile idiopathic arthritis, CAPS: cryopyrin-associated autoinflammatory syndromes, NA: not available, PC: prior to conception, B: birth, PPT: pregnancy positive test, P: pregnancy, GA: gestational age, PTB: preterm birth, IUGR: intra-uterine growth restriction, M: male, F: female, *: Excluded from further analysis since data missing.

3.4. Anakinra Use during Pregnancy and Maternal/Fetal Outcome

Women treated with Anakinra received doses ranging from 50 to 200 mg/daily, but the majority (59.4%) received 100 mg/day. In 20 cases (29.0%), this information was unavailable.

Of the 69 pregnancies exposed to Anakinra, 63.8% had term births, 17.4% were preterm (mean gestational age: 34.1 weeks (range: 28–36.9)) and for the rest (18.8%) this information was not given. Overall, the mean gestational age at delivery in the Anakinra exposed group was 37.9 (28.0–41.1) weeks. Within Anakinra-exposed pregnancies, 63.8% had no adverse obstetric outcome and 26.1% had complications with the most predominant being preterm birth (12/18) while the rest presented one or more of the following complication; vaginal bleeding, hypertension and/or oligohydramnios. One case ended in stillbirth, and the women received Anakinra for familial Mediterranean fever from 34 weeks of gestation to the time of stillbirth (37 weeks). No additional information was available about this event. It is also important to note that one twin dichorionic-diamniotic pregnancy occurred with the demise of one fetus due to bilateral renal agenesis at 30 weeks' gestation. However, the surviving twin had no abnormality and was born at 38.7 weeks. This pregnancy was treated from the first trimester with Anakinra for neonatal-onset multisystem inflammatory disorder. The obstetric data were not available in 10.1% of the cases.

As for the neonates, 86.4% were healthy whereas 13.6% presented some mild complications. Of these, five babies were diagnosed with CAPS whereas three presented with other problems such as hypotrophic, respiratory distress syndrome, renal agenesis, ectopic neurohypophysis, right hydrocele and/or heart murmur. Rates of breastfeeding were available for 42 pregnancies with half of them being breastfeed; however, it was not clear if the treatment was maintained during this time.

3.5. Canakinumab Use during Pregnancy and Maternal/Fetal Outcome

The women using Canakinumab received doses starting from a single 120 mg dose to 300 mg/8 weeks but 54.5% received 150 mg/8 weeks. Of the 11 pregnancies exposed to Canakinumab, 90.9% delivered at term and the mean gestational age in this population was 38.8 (37.0–40.0) weeks whilst for the remaining one case the information was unavailable. In this group, 90.0% had no adverse obstetrical outcome with only one woman developing gestational diabetes and one without any information.

All the babies exposed to Canakinumab were healthy with one presenting the same NLPR3 mutation as the mother. Rates of breastfeeding were available for 5 cases and 80.0% were breastfeed but again, no data on treatment during this period.

4. Discussion

This systematic review aimed to review the effects of IL-1 antagonists used during pregnancy in humans. We found 22 studies including 12 original articles and 10 conference abstracts published which were reporting at least one pregnancy exposed to IL-1 blockade. Of these 22 studies, data extraction was performed, and 88 different pregnancies were included in this systematic review. Furthermore, some pregnancies were reported more than once and therefore the extraction were combined to obtained complete information whilst avoiding duplicates.

Of the 88 pregnancies included, 85.2% of women received Anakinra whereas 14.8% received Canakinumab. This disparity could be due to the fact that Anakinra has been approved for therapeutic use for over 20 years as opposed to Canakinumab [65]. Furthermore, Canakinumab has a higher cost and is less widely used [77]. In a recent review by Soh and Moretto, the authors summarize the European League Against Rheumatism—EULAR and British Society on Rheumatology—BSR guidelines for biologic therapies used during pregnancy [61]. In the EULAR guidelines, Anakinra is tolerated in early pregnancy and can be continued during pregnancy if there are no other options. On the other hand, the BSR guidelines reports insufficient data to recommend the use of Anakinra during pregnancy, but stipulate that "unintentional use during first trimester is unlikely to cause harm". Furthermore, these guidelines states that it is "not recommended to continue the treatment during gestation". The data for Canakinumab are even more sparse. One case report measured its transplacental transfer and found a cord blood to maternal blood ratio of 2.11 [78] which needs to be further studied.

Autoimmune diseases often have negative impact on fertility and pregnancy outcomes [76,77]. Two factors can be considered to affect the course of pregnancy, the disease or the treatment for this disease. In the exposed pregnancies included in this review, the indications for treatment were CAPS (34.1%), Familial Mediterranean Fever (FMF-33%), and AOSD/SJIA (20.4%). There is only one report, to our knowledge, of CAPS during pregnancy treated with medication other than those targeting the IL-1 system [78]. This study reported a rate of miscarriage of 30% as compared to 10% for CAPS-patients treated with Anakinra [78]. Only two studies reported pregnancy with those pathologies all exposed to Anakinra or Canakinumab, therefore it is difficult to distinguish the treatment effect to that from the inflammatory pathology itself [75,78]. There is only one report of untreated pregnancies with different autoimmune disease that the one that are reported in this study making the evaluation of the pathologies themselves difficult. In this study, the authors compared pregnancy with or without all kind of DMARDs and healthy pregnancy. However, this study did not discriminate for different treatments and only three pregnancies were exposed to Anakinra [79]. Autoimmune diseases often have negative impact on fertility and pregnancy outcomes [79,80]. Two factors can be considered to affect the course of pregnancy, the disease or the treatment for this disease. In the exposed pregnancies included in this review, the indications for treatment were CAPS (34.1%), Familial Mediterranean Fever (FMF-33%), and AOSD/SJIA (20.4%). There is only one report, to our knowledge, of CAPS during pregnancy treated with medication other than those targeting the IL-1 system [81]. This study reported a rate of miscarriage of 30% as compared to 10% for CAPS-patients treated with Anakinra [81]. Only two studies reported pregnancy with those pathologies all exposed to Anakinra or Canakinumab, therefore it is difficult to distinguish the treatment effect to that from the inflammatory pathology itself [78,81]. There is only one report of untreated pregnancies with different autoimmune disease that the one that are reported in this study making the evaluation of the pathologies themselves difficult. In this study, the authors compared pregnancy with or without all kind of DMARDs and healthy pregnancy. However, this study did not discriminate for different treatments and only three pregnancies were exposed to Anakinra [82].

For patients with FMF, increased rates of miscarriage, premature rupture of membranes and low birth weight were observed compared to pregnant women without the disease [80]. In this study, 80% of women received Colchicine and none received anti-inflammatory treatment [80]. Furthermore, one retrospective study by Ben-Chetrit et al., reported an elevated rate of spontaneous abortion in untreated FMF as opposed to those treated with Colchicine [83]. Unfortunately, Colchicine resistance is often observed in FMF patients and Anakinra is increasingly used to prevent flare-ups of the disease [73]. As for AOSD, 5 case reports and 17 pregnancies were reviewed by [84]. In this cohort, most women were exposed to corticosteroid with several reported adverse outcomes such as spontaneous miscarriage observed (9.1%), premature delivery (18.2%) and FGR (9.1%). In the current systematic review, 3/14 pregnancies complicated with AOSD ended in premature delivery which is comparable to that reported by Mok et al. In a study by Garcia-Fernandez et al., on women with SJIA, 20% had preterm delivery [85], which is in contrast to the current work in which we observed no preterm delivery in SJIA with anti-IL-1 treatment. This difference could be explained by the treatment since most women in this systematic review received Anakinra as opposed to corticosteroid or other DMARDs.

We reported three miscarriages out of 88 pregnancies. All these losses occurred during the first trimester and two were exposed to Anakinra whereas one exposed to Canakinumab. This is in accordance with the literature that most miscarriages will occur during the first trimester; however, it is very difficult to measure the rate of miscarriages in the general population. Furthermore, in this cohort, two out of the three miscarriage occurs in the same women who had Cogan syndrome, a rare and severe autoimmune disease. In the literature, only eight cases of successful pregnancy with this disease have been reported [86–91]. Thus, it cannot be concluded that the therapy caused pregnancy loss in these women.

In the current work, the rate of preterm birth was 17.6% (all conditions combined) as opposed to a baseline of 11.1% [92]. However, the reported rate of preterm birth in a population with inflammatory disease is known to be higher; namely 13.6% in FMF [80], 18.1% in AOSD [84] and 20% in SJIA [85]. Although the rate of preterm birth are similar overall, it is important to keep in mind that there is no report of untreated pregnancies with those inflammatory pathologies. Only one study reported a preterm birth rate of 9% in pregnancy with inflammatory pathologies without DMARDs treatment. The maternal condition in this study were Sjögren syndrome, undifferentiated connective tissue disease (UTCD), systemic lupus erythematosus (SLE), antiphospholipid syndrome (APS) and others [82].

Our review reports neonatal complications in 13.6% of pregnancies exposed to Anakinra and 10.0% for those exposed to Canakinumab, totaling 13.2% who had complications overall. Of the 10 babies who had complications, six were diagnosed with CAPS whereas three had minor developmental delays or other problems and one died at 37 weeks (stillbirth). One baby of a FMF mother was hypotrophic, had respiratory distress syndrome and hyperbillirubilemia at birth; however, this baby was delivered prematurely at 33 + 5 weeks and was healthy at 12 months of age [93]. Baby born preterm has more neonatal complication then their counterpart born at 37 week and onwards [94,95]. Another baby born to a mother with SJIA had right hydrocele and heart murmur at birth but these complications could be due to maternal exacerbation of symptom such as oligohydramnios and hypertension. At the follow up, this baby had no major long-term complications nor malformations [96]. Finally, one baby born to a mother with active refractory AOSD had renal agenesis and ectopic neurohypophysis [97]. This is the second case of renal agenesis in Anakinra-exposed patient. The first case was in a mother diagnose with NOMID and it was a twin dichorionic-diamniotic pregnancy with fetal demise of one fetus with bilateral renal agenesis at 30 weeks. The surviving twin had no congenital abnormality and was born at 38.7 weeks. This case of congenital malformation could potentially be explained by the increased risk factor of renal tract abnormalities in twin birth as mentioned by the authors [97,98]. Furthermore, a study by Wiesel et al. reported that renal agenesis occurs in 58 of 709,030 live birth, significantly lower than 2 cases out of 88 pregnancies in this systematic review. One group has made a hypothesis that a link between uncontrolled maternal disease and renal abnormalities can occurs [96] but the potential link between renal malformation and IL-1 pathway should be the focus of future studies.

It is interesting to note that three studies, not included in the current systematic review, have evaluated 10 men who received IL-1 blockade prior to conception, resulting in 13 pregnancies. In those studies, six men had CAPS, two AOSD, one SJIA and one FMF. Seven received Anakinra (100 mg/day) and three were treated with Canakinumab (150 mg/8 weeks) at the time of conception. No adverse effect on the child wellbeing were reported after paternal exposure to IL-1 blockage [97,99,100].

This is the first systematic review to examine the effects of IL-1 blockade during pregnancy and we provide a summary of all pregnancies exposed to Anakinra or Canakinumab. Our study also highlighted the current lack of data and identified research gaps to be addressed, particularly the difference between the effects on pregnancy of the inflammatory pathology being treated as compared to the treatment itself. Our study was limited by the fact that abstracts from conferences were also included, in order to cover all exposed pregnancies, but some information were missing in relation to doses and outcomes in these abstracts.

5. Conclusions

In conclusion, this review summarizes all the pregnancy exposed to Il-1 blockage and no major obstetrical and neonatal complication was reported. Il-1 blockage during pregnancy could be safe and beneficial in cases of pregnancy with inflammatory conditions.

Supplementary Materials: The following are available online at https://www.mdpi.com/article/10.3390/jcm11010225/s1; Data S1: Search strategy used for this systematic review. Table S1: Search strategy used for this systematic review.

Author Contributions: Conceptualization and methodology, M.-E.B. and S.G.; data curation, M.-E.B., V.G., K.H. and S.G.; writing original draft preparation, M.-E.B. and S.G., writing review and editing, M.-E.B., D.J.L.H., A.E.P.H. and S.G.; supervision, S.G. All authors have read and agreed to the published version of the manuscript.

Funding: This research received no external funding.

Institutional Review Board Statement: Not applicable.

Informed Consent Statement: Not applicable.

Conflicts of Interest: The authors declare no conflict of interest.

References

1. Aye, I.L.; Jansson, T.; Powell, T.L. Interleukin-1beta inhibits insulin signaling and prevents insulin-stimulated system A amino acid transport in primary human trophoblasts. *Mol. Cell. Endocrinol.* **2013**, *381*, 46–55. [CrossRef] [PubMed]
2. Bainbridge, S.A.; Roberts, J.M.; von Versen-Hoynck, F.; Koch, J.; Edmunds, L.; Hubel, C.A. Uric acid attenuates trophoblast invasion and integration into endothelial cell monolayers. *Am. J. Physiol. Cell Physiol.* **2009**, *297*, C440–C450. [CrossRef] [PubMed]
3. Bainbridge, S.A.; von Versen-Höynck, F.; Roberts, J.M. Uric acid inhibits placental system A amino acid uptake. *Placenta* **2009**, *30*, 195–200. [CrossRef] [PubMed]
4. Lei, J.; Vermillion, M.S.; Jia, B.; Xie, H.; Xie, L.; McLane, M.W.; Sheffield, J.S.; Pekosz, A.; Brown, A.; Klein, S.L.; et al. IL-1 receptor antagonist therapy mitigates placental dysfunction and perinatal injury following Zika virus infection. *JCI Insight* **2019**, *4*, e122678. [CrossRef]
5. Mulla, M.J.; Myrtolli, K.; Potter, J.; Boeras, C.; Kavathas, P.B.; Sfakianaki, A.K.; Tadesse, S.; Norwitz, E.R.; Guller, S.; Abrahams, V.M. Uric acid induces trophoblast IL-1beta production via the inflammasome: Implications for the pathogenesis of preeclampsia. *Am. J. Reprod. Immunol.* **2011**, *65*, 542–548. [CrossRef]
6. Brien, M.E.; Duval, C.; Palacios, J.; Boufaied, I.; Hudon-Thibeault, A.A.; Nadeau-Vallee, M.; Vaillancourt, C.; Sibley, C.P.; Abrahams, V.M.; Jones, R.L.; et al. Uric Acid Crystals Induce Placental Inflammation and Alter Trophoblast Function via an IL-1-Dependent Pathway: Implications for Fetal Growth Restriction. *J. Immunol.* **2017**, *198*, 443–451. [CrossRef]
7. Depino, A.M. Perinatal inflammation and adult psychopathology: From preclinical models to humans. *Semin. Cell Dev. Biol.* **2018**, *77*, 104–114. [CrossRef]
8. Hagberg, H.; Gressens, P.; Mallard, C. Inflammation during fetal and neonatal life: Implications for neurologic and neuropsychiatric disease in children and adults. *Ann. Neurol.* **2012**, *71*, 444–457.
9. Van Vliet, E.O.; de Kieviet, J.F.; van der Voorn, J.P.; Been, J.V.; Oosterlaan, J.; van Elburg, R.M. Placental pathology and long-term neurodevelopment of very preterm infants. *Am. J. Obstet. Gynecol.* **2012**, *206*, e481–e487. [CrossRef]
10. Neiger, R. Long-Term Effects of Pregnancy Complications on Maternal Health: A Review. *J. Clin. Med.* **2017**, *6*, 76. [CrossRef]
11. Erlebacher, A. Immunology of the maternal-fetal interface. *Annu. Rev. Immunol.* **2013**, *31*, 387–411. [CrossRef]
12. Moffett, A.; Loke, C. Immunology of placentation in eutherian mammals. *Nat. Rev. Immunol.* **2006**, *6*, 584–594. [CrossRef]
13. Mor, G.; Cardenas, I.; Abrahams, V.; Guller, S. Inflammation and pregnancy: The role of the immune system at the implantation site. *Ann. N. Y. Acad. Sci.* **2011**, *1221*, 80–87. [CrossRef]
14. Menon, R.; Richardson, L.S.; Lappas, M. Fetal membrane architecture, aging and inflammation in pregnancy and parturition. *Placenta* **2019**, *79*, 40–45. [CrossRef]
15. Romero, R.; Espinoza, J.; Gonçalves, L.F.; Kusanovic, J.P.; Friel, L.A.; Nien, J.K. Inflammation in preterm and term labour and delivery. *Semin. Fetal Neonatal Med.* **2006**, *11*, 317–326. [CrossRef]
16. Brien, M.E.; Boufaied, I.; Bernard, N.; Forest, J.C.; Giguere, Y.; Girard, S. Specific inflammatory profile in each pregnancy complication: A comparative study. *Am. J. Reprod. Immunol.* **2020**, *84*, e13316. [CrossRef]
17. Salazar Garcia, M.D.; Mobley, Y.; Henson, J.; Davies, M.; Skariah, A.; Dambaeva, S.; Gilman-Sachs, A.; Beaman, K.; Lampley, C.; Kwak-Kim, J. Early pregnancy immune biomarkers in peripheral blood may predict preeclampsia. *J. Reprod. Immunol.* **2018**, *125*, 25–31. [CrossRef]
18. Freeman, D.J.; McManus, F.; Brown, E.A.; Cherry, L.; Norrie, J.; Ramsay, J.E.; Clark, P.; Walker, I.D.; Sattar, N.; Greer, I.A. Short- and long-term changes in plasma inflammatory markers associated with preeclampsia. *Hypertension* **2004**, *44*, 708–714. [CrossRef]

19. Ferguson, K.K.; Meeker, J.D.; McElrath, T.F.; Mukherjee, B.; Cantonwine, D.E. Repeated measures of inflammation and oxidative stress biomarkers in preeclamptic and normotensive pregnancies. *Am. J. Obstet. Gynecol.* **2017**, *216*, e521–e527. [CrossRef]
20. Redman, C.W.; Staff, A.C. Preeclampsia, biomarkers, syncytiotrophoblast stress, and placental capacity. *Am. J. Obstet. Gynecol.* **2015**, *213*, S9.e1–S9.e4. [CrossRef]
21. Taylor, B.D.; Ness, R.B.; Klebanoff, M.A.; Zoh, R.; Bass, D.; Hougaard, D.M.; Skogstrand, K.; Haggerty, C.L. First and second trimester immune biomarkers in preeclamptic and normotensive women. *Pregnancy Hypertens.* **2016**, *6*, 388–393. [CrossRef]
22. Taylor, B.D.; Tang, G.; Ness, R.B.; Olsen, J.; Hougaard, D.M.; Skogstrand, K.; Roberts, J.M.; Haggerty, C.L. Mid-pregnancy circulating immune biomarkers in women with preeclampsia and normotensive controls. *Pregnancy Hypertens.* **2016**, *6*, 72–78. [CrossRef]
23. Ronzoni, S.; Steckle, V.; D'Souza, R.; Murphy, K.E.; Lye, S.; Shynlova, O. Cytokine Changes in Maternal Peripheral Blood Correlate With Time-to-Delivery in Pregnancies Complicated by Premature Prelabor Rupture of the Membranes. *Reprod. Sci.* **2018**, *26*, 1266–1276. [CrossRef]
24. Giguere, Y.; Masse, J.; Theriault, S.; Bujold, E.; Lafond, J.; Rousseau, F.; Forest, J.C. Screening for pre-eclampsia early in pregnancy: Performance of a multivariable model combining clinical characteristics and biochemical markers. *BJOG* **2015**, *122*, 402–410. [CrossRef]
25. Kuc, S.; Wortelboer, E.J.; van Rijn, B.B.; Franx, A.; Visser, G.H.; Schielen, P.C. Evaluation of 7 serum biomarkers and uterine artery Doppler ultrasound for first-trimester prediction of preeclampsia: A systematic review. *Obstet. Gynecol. Surv.* **2011**, *66*, 225–239. [CrossRef]
26. Yu, N.; Cui, H.; Chen, X.; Chang, Y. First trimester maternal serum analytes and second trimester uterine artery Doppler in the prediction of preeclampsia and fetal growth restriction. *Taiwan J. Obstet. Gynecol.* **2017**, *56*, 358–361. [CrossRef]
27. Bianchi, M.E. DAMPs, PAMPs and alarmins: All we need to know about danger. *J. Leukoc. Biol.* **2007**, *81*, 1–5. [CrossRef]
28. Matzinger, P. The danger model: A renewed sense of self. *Science* **2002**, *296*, 301–305. [CrossRef]
29. Brien, M.E.; Baker, B.; Duval, C.; Gaudreault, V.; Jones, R.L.; Girard, S. Alarmins at the maternal-fetal interface: Involvement of inflammation in placental dysfunction and pregnancy complications (1). *Can. J. Physiol. Pharmacol.* **2019**, *97*, 206–212. [CrossRef]
30. Nadeau-Vallee, M.; Obari, D.; Palacios, J.; Brien, M.E.; Duval, C.; Chemtob, S.; Girard, S. Sterile inflammation and pregnancy complications: A review. *Reproduction* **2016**, *152*, R277–R292. [CrossRef]
31. Sharps, M.C.; Baker, B.C.; Guevara, T.; Bischof, H.; Jones, R.L.; Greenwood, S.L.; Heazell, A.E.P. Increased placental macrophages and a pro-inflammatory profile in placentas and maternal serum in infants with a decreased growth rate in the third trimester of pregnancy. *Am. J. Reprod. Immunol.* **2020**, *84*, e13265. [CrossRef] [PubMed]
32. Saji, F.; Samejima, Y.; Kamiura, S.; Sawai, K.; Shimoya, K.; Kimura, T. Cytokine production in chorioamnionitis. *J. Reprod. Immunol.* **2000**, *47*, 185–196. [CrossRef]
33. Russo, R.C.; Garcia, C.C.; Teixeira, M.M. Anti-inflammatory drug development: Broad or specific chemokine receptor antagonists? *Curr. Opin. Drug Discov. Dev.* **2010**, *13*, 414–427.
34. Grainger, D.J.; Reckless, J. Broad-spectrum chemokine inhibitors (BSCIs) and their anti-inflammatory effects in vivo. *Biochem. Pharmacol.* **2003**, *65*, 1027–1034. [CrossRef]
35. Bandoli, G.; Palmsten, K.; Forbess Smith, C.J.; Chambers, C.D. A Review of Systemic Corticosteroid Use in Pregnancy and the Risk of Select Pregnancy and Birth Outcomes. *Rheum. Dis. Clin. N. Am.* **2017**, *43*, 489–502. [CrossRef]
36. Shanks, A.L.; Grasch, J.L.; Quinney, S.K.; Haas, D.M. Controversies in antenatal corticosteroids. *Semin. Fetal Neonatal Med.* **2019**, *24*, 182–188. [CrossRef]
37. Wapner, R.J.; Sorokin, Y.; Mele, L.; Johnson, F.; Dudley, D.J.; Spong, C.Y.; Peaceman, A.M.; Leveno, K.J.; Malone, F.; Caritis, S.N.; et al. Long-term outcomes after repeat doses of antenatal corticosteroids. *N. Engl. J. Med.* **2007**, *357*, 1190–1198. [CrossRef]
38. Bandyopadhyay, A.; Slaven, J.E.; Evrard, C.; Tiller, C.; Haas, D.M.; Tepper, R.S. Antenatal corticosteroids decrease forced vital capacity in infants born fullterm. *Pediatr. Pulmonol.* **2020**, *55*, 2630–2634. [CrossRef]
39. Bérard, A.; Sheehy, O.; Girard, S.; Zhao, J.P.; Bernatsky, S. Risk of preterm birth following late pregnancy exposure to NSAIDs or COX-2 inhibitors. *Pain* **2018**, *159*, 948–955. [CrossRef]
40. Daniel, S.; Matok, I.; Gorodischer, R.; Koren, G.; Uziel, E.; Wiznitzer, A.; Levy, A. Major malformations following exposure to nonsteroidal antiinflammatory drugs during the first trimester of pregnancy. *J. Rheumatol.* **2012**, *39*, 2163–2169. [CrossRef]
41. Kenyon, S.; Pike, K.; Jones, D.R.; Brocklehurst, P.; Marlow, N.; Salt, A.; Taylor, D.J. Childhood outcomes after prescription of antibiotics to pregnant women with spontaneous preterm labour: 7-year follow-up of the ORACLE II trial. *Lancet* **2008**, *372*, 1319–1327. [CrossRef]
42. Kenyon, S.; Pike, K.; Jones, D.R.; Brocklehurst, P.; Marlow, N.; Salt, A.; Taylor, D.J. Childhood outcomes after prescription of antibiotics to pregnant women with preterm rupture of the membranes: 7-year follow-up of the ORACLE I trial. *Lancet* **2008**, *372*, 1310–1318. [CrossRef]
43. Muanda, F.T.; Sheehy, O.; Bérard, A. Use of antibiotics during pregnancy and risk of spontaneous abortion. *CMAJ* **2017**, *189*, E625–E633. [CrossRef]
44. Muanda, F.T.; Sheehy, O.; Bérard, A. Use of antibiotics during pregnancy and the risk of major congenital malformations: A population based cohort study. *Br. J. Clin. Pharmacol.* **2017**, *83*, 2557–2571. [CrossRef]

45. Reis, A.S.; Barboza, R.; Murillo, O.; Barateiro, A.; Peixoto, E.P.M.; Lima, F.A.; Gomes, V.M.; Dombrowski, J.G.; Leal, V.N.C.; Araujo, F.; et al. Inflammasome activation and IL-1 signaling during placental malaria induce poor pregnancy outcomes. *Sci. Adv.* **2020**, *6*, eaax6346. [CrossRef]
46. Equils, O.; Kellogg, C.; McGregor, J.; Gravett, M.; Neal-Perry, G.; Gabay, C. The role of the IL-1 system in pregnancy and the use of IL-1 system markers to identify women at risk for pregnancy complications. *Biol. Reprod.* **2020**, *103*, 684–694. [CrossRef]
47. Southcombe, J.H.; Redman, C.W.; Sargent, I.L.; Granne, I. Interleukin-1 family cytokines and their regulatory proteins in normal pregnancy and pre-eclampsia. *Clin. Exp. Immunol.* **2015**, *181*, 480–490. [CrossRef]
48. Licini, C.; Tossetta, G.; Avellini, C.; Ciarmela, P.; Lorenzi, T.; Toti, P.; Gesuita, R.; Voltolini, C.; Petraglia, F.; Castellucci, M.; et al. Analysis of cell-cell junctions in human amnion and chorionic plate affected by chorioamnionitis. *Histol. Histopathol.* **2016**, *31*, 759–767.
49. Tossetta, G.; Paolinelli, F.; Avellini, C.; Salvolini, E.; Ciarmela, P.; Lorenzi, T.; Emanuelli, M.; Toti, P.; Giuliante, R.; Gesuita, R.; et al. IL-1β and TGF-β weaken the placental barrier through destruction of tight junctions: An in vivo and in vitro study. *Placenta* **2014**, *35*, 509–516. [CrossRef]
50. Girard, S.; Heazell, A.E.; Derricott, H.; Allan, S.M.; Sibley, C.P.; Abrahams, V.M.; Jones, R.L. Circulating cytokines and alarmins associated with placental inflammation in high-risk pregnancies. *Am. J. Reprod. Immunol.* **2014**, *72*, 422–434. [CrossRef]
51. Girard, S.; Sébire, H.; Brochu, M.E.; Briota, S.; Sarret, P.; Sébire, G. Postnatal administration of IL-1Ra exerts neuroprotective effects following perinatal inflammation and/or hypoxic-ischemic injuries. *Brain Behav. Immun.* **2012**, *26*, 1331–1339. [CrossRef]
52. Girard, S.; Tremblay, L.; Lepage, M.; Sebire, G. IL-1 receptor antagonist protects against placental and neurodevelopmental defects induced by maternal inflammation. *J. Immunol.* **2010**, *184*, 3997–4005. [CrossRef]
53. Leitner, K.; Al Shammary, M.; McLane, M.; Johnston, M.V.; Elovitz, M.A.; Burd, I. IL-1 receptor blockade prevents fetal cortical brain injury but not preterm birth in a mouse model of inflammation-induced preterm birth and perinatal brain injury. *Am. J. Reprod. Immunol.* **2014**, *71*, 418–426. [CrossRef]
54. Nadeau-Vallee, M.; Chin, P.Y.; Belarbi, L.; Brien, M.E.; Pundir, S.; Berryer, M.H.; Beaudry-Richard, A.; Madaan, A.; Sharkey, D.J.; Lupien-Meilleur, A.; et al. Antenatal Suppression of IL-1 Protects against Inflammation-Induced Fetal Injury and Improves Neonatal and Developmental Outcomes in Mice. *J. Immunol.* **2017**, *198*, 2047–2062. [CrossRef]
55. Nadeau-Vallee, M.; Quiniou, C.; Palacios, J.; Hou, X.; Erfani, A.; Madaan, A.; Sanchez, M.; Leimert, K.; Boudreault, A.; Duhamel, F.; et al. Novel Noncompetitive IL-1 Receptor-Biased Ligand Prevents Infection- and Inflammation-Induced Preterm Birth. *J. Immunol.* **2015**, *195*, 3402–3415. [CrossRef]
56. McDuffie, R.S., Jr.; Davies, J.K.; Leslie, K.K.; Lee, S.; Sherman, M.P.; Gibbs, R.S. A randomized controlled trial of interleukin-1 receptor antagonist in a rabbit model of ascending infection in pregnancy. *Infect. Dis. Obstet. Gynecol.* **2001**, *9*, 233–237. [CrossRef]
57. Presicce, P.; Park, C.W.; Senthamaraikannan, P.; Bhattacharyya, S.; Jackson, C.; Kong, F.; Rueda, C.M.; DeFranco, E.; Miller, L.A.; Hildeman, D.A.; et al. IL-1 signaling mediates intrauterine inflammation and chorio-decidua neutrophil recruitment and activation. *JCI Insight* **2018**, *3*, e98306. [CrossRef]
58. Karisnan, K.; Bakker, A.J.; Song, Y.; Noble, P.B.; Pillow, J.J.; Pinniger, G.J. Interleukin-1 receptor antagonist protects against lipopolysaccharide induced diaphragm weakness in preterm lambs. *PLoS ONE* **2015**, *10*, e0124390.
59. Nadeau-Vallee, M.; Obari, D.; Quiniou, C.; Lubell, W.D.; Olson, D.M.; Girard, S.; Chemtob, S. A critical role of interleukin-1 in preterm labor. *Cytokine Growth Factor Rev.* **2016**, *28*, 37–51. [CrossRef]
60. Prieto-Peña, D.; Dasgupta, B. Biologic agents and small-molecule inhibitors in systemic autoimmune conditions: An update. *Pol. Arch. Intern. Med.* **2020**, *131*, 171–181. [CrossRef]
61. Soh, M.C.; Moretto, M. The use of biologics for autoimmune rheumatic diseases in fertility and pregnancy. *Obstet. Med.* **2020**, *13*, 5–13. [CrossRef] [PubMed]
62. Götestam Skorpen, C.; Hoeltzenbein, M.; Tincani, A.; Fischer-Betz, R.; Elefant, E.; Chambers, C.; da Silva, J.; Nelson-Piercy, C.; Cetin, I.; Costedoat-Chalumeau, N.; et al. The EULAR points to consider for use of antirheumatic drugs before pregnancy, and during pregnancy and lactation. *Ann. Rheum. Dis.* **2016**, *75*, 795–810. [CrossRef] [PubMed]
63. Nuki, G.; Bresnihan, B.; Bear, M.B.; McCabe, D. Long-term safety and maintenance of clinical improvement following treatment with anakinra (recombinant human interleukin-1 receptor antagonist) in patients with rheumatoid arthritis: Extension phase of a randomized, double-blind, placebo-controlled trial. *Arthritis Rheum.* **2002**, *46*, 2838–2846. [CrossRef] [PubMed]
64. Buckley, L.F.; Viscusi, M.M.; Van Tassell, B.W.; Abbate, A. Interleukin-1 blockade for the treatment of pericarditis. *Eur. Heart J. Cardiovasc. Pharmacother.* **2018**, *4*, 46–53. [CrossRef]
65. Kary, S.; Burmester, G.R. Anakinra: The first interleukin-1 inhibitor in the treatment of rheumatoid arthritis. *Int. J. Clin. Pract.* **2003**, *57*, 231–234.
66. Ramírez, J.; Cañete, J.D. Anakinra for the treatment of rheumatoid arthritis: A safety evaluation. *Expert Opin. Drug Saf.* **2018**, *17*, 727–732. [CrossRef]
67. Dinarello, C.A.; van der Meer, J.W. Treating inflammation by blocking interleukin-1 in humans. *Semin. Immunol.* **2013**, *25*, 469–484. [CrossRef]
68. Vastert, S.J.; Jamilloux, Y.; Quartier, P.; Ohlman, S.; Osterling Koskinen, L.; Kullenberg, T.; Franck-Larsson, K.; Fautrel, B.; de Benedetti, F. Anakinra in children and adults with Still's disease. *Rheumatology* **2019**, *58*, vi9–vi22. [CrossRef]
69. Church, L.D.; McDermott, M.F. Canakinumab, a fully-human mAb against IL-1beta for the potential treatment of inflammatory disorders. *Curr. Opin. Mol. Ther.* **2009**, *11*, 81–89.

70. Savic, S.; McDermott, M.F. Inflammation: Canakinumab for the cryopyrin-associated periodic syndromes. *Nat. Rev. Rheumatol.* **2009**, *5*, 529–530. [CrossRef]
71. Ortona, E.; Pierdominici, M.; Maselli, A.; Veroni, C.; Aloisi, F.; Shoenfeld, Y. Sex-based differences in autoimmune diseases. *Ann. Ist. Super. Sanita* **2016**, *52*, 205–212.
72. Fischer-Betz, R.; Specker, C. Pregnancy in systemic lupus erythematosus and antiphospholipid syndrome. *Best Pract. Res. Clin. Rheumatol.* **2017**, *31*, 397–414. [CrossRef]
73. Ugurlu, S.; Ergezen, B.; Egeli, B.H.; Selvi, O.; Ozdogan, H. Anakinra treatment in patients with familial Mediterranean fever: A single-centre experience. *Rheumatology* **2021**, *60*, 2327–2332. [CrossRef]
74. Moher, D.; Liberati, A.; Tetzlaff, J.; Altman, D.G. Preferred reporting items for systematic reviews and meta-analyses: The PRISMA statement. *PLoS Med.* **2009**, *6*, e1000097. [CrossRef]
75. Sterne, J.A.; Hernán, M.A.; Reeves, B.C.; Savović, J.; Berkman, N.D.; Viswanathan, M.; Henry, D.; Altman, D.G.; Ansari, M.T.; Boutron, I.; et al. ROBINS-I: A tool for assessing risk of bias in non-randomised studies of interventions. *BMJ* **2016**, *355*, i4919. [CrossRef]
76. Murad, M.H.; Sultan, S.; Haffar, S.; Bazerbachi, F. Methodological quality and synthesis of case series and case reports. *BMJ Evid.-Based Med.* **2018**, *23*, 60–63. [CrossRef]
77. Sfriso, P.; Bindoli, S.; Doria, A.; Feist, E.; Galozzi, P. Canakinumab for the treatment of adult-onset Still's disease. *Expert Rev. Clin. Immunol.* **2020**, *16*, 129–138. [CrossRef]
78. Egawa, M.; Imai, K.; Mori, M.; Miyasaka, N.; Kubota, T. Placental Transfer of Canakinumab in a Patient with Muckle-Wells Syndrome. *J. Clin. Immunol.* **2017**, *37*, 339–341. [CrossRef]
79. Mijatovic, V.; Hompes, P.G.; Wouters, M.G. Familial Mediterranean fever and its implications for fertility and pregnancy. *Eur. J. Obstet. Gynecol. Reprod. Biol.* **2003**, *108*, 171–176. [CrossRef]
80. Yasar, O.; Iskender, C.; Kaymak, O.; Taflan Yaman, S.; Uygur, D.; Danisman, N. Retrospective evaluation of pregnancy outcomes in women with familial Mediterranean fever. *J. Matern. Fetal Neonatal Med.* **2014**, *27*, 733–736. [CrossRef]
81. Chang, Z.; Spong, C.Y.; Jesus, A.A.; Davis, M.A.; Plass, N.; Stone, D.L.; Chapelle, D.; Hoffmann, P.; Kastner, D.L.; Barron, K.; et al. Anakinra use during pregnancy in patients with cryopyrin-associated periodic syndromes (CAPS). *Arthritis Rheum.* **2014**, *66*, 3227–3232. [CrossRef]
82. De Lorenzo, R.; Ramirez, G.A.; Punzo, D.; Lorioli, L.; Rovelli, R.; Canti, V.; Barera, G.; Rovere-Querini, P. Neonatal outcomes of children born to mothers on biological agents during pregnancy: State of the art and perspectives. *Pharmacol. Res.* **2020**, *152*, 104583. [CrossRef]
83. Ben-Chetrit, E.; Ben-Chetrit, A.; Berkun, Y.; Ben-Chetrit, E. Pregnancy outcomes in women with familial Mediterranean fever receiving colchicine: Is amniocentesis justified? *Arthritis Care Res.* **2010**, *62*, 143–148. [CrossRef]
84. Mok, M.Y.; Lo, Y.; Leung, P.Y.; Lau, C.S. Pregnancy outcome in patients with adult onset Still's disease. *J. Rheumatol.* **2004**, *31*, 2307–2309.
85. García-Fernández, A.; Gerardi, M.C.; Crisafulli, F.; Filippini, M.; Fredi, M.; Gorla, R.; Lazzaroni, M.G.; Lojacono, A.; Nalli, C.; Ramazzotto, F.; et al. Disease course and obstetric outcomes of pregnancies in juvenile idiopathic arthritis: Are there any differences among disease subtypes? A single-centre retrospective study of prospectively followed pregnancies in a dedicated pregnancy clinic. *Clin. Rheum.* **2021**, *40*, 239–244. [CrossRef]
86. Bakalianou, K.; Salakos, N.; Iavazzo, C.; Danilidou, K.; Papadias, K.; Kondi-Pafiti, A. A rare case of uneventful pregnancy in a woman with Cogan's syndrome. *Clin. Exp. Obstet. Gynecol.* **2008**, *35*, 301–302.
87. Currie, C.; Wax, J.R.; Pinette, M.G.; Blackstone, J.; Cartin, A. Cogan's syndrome complicating pregnancy. *J. Matern. Fetal Neonatal Med.* **2009**, *22*, 928–930. [CrossRef]
88. Deliveliotou, A.; Moustakarias, T.; Argeitis, J.; Vaggos, G.; Vitoratos, N.; Hassiakos, D. Successful full-term pregnancy in a woman with Cogan's syndrome: A case report. *Clin. Rheum.* **2007**, *26*, 2181–2183. [CrossRef]
89. Riboni, F.; Cosma, S.; Perini, P.G.; Benedetto, C. Successful Pregnancy in a Patient with Atypical Cogan's Syndrome. *Isr. Med. Assoc. J.* **2016**, *18*, 495–496.
90. Tarney, C.M.; Wilson, K.; Sewell, M.F. Cogan syndrome in pregnancy. *Obstet. Gynecol.* **2014**, *124*, 428–431. [CrossRef]
91. Venhoff, N.; Thiel, J.; Schramm, M.A.; Jandova, I.; Voll, R.E.; Glaser, C. Case Report: Effective and Safe Treatment with Certolizumab Pegol in Pregnant Patients With Cogan's Syndrome: A Report of Three Pregnancies in Two Patients. *Front. Immunol.* **2020**, *11*, 616992. [CrossRef] [PubMed]
92. Blencowe, H.; Cousens, S.; Chou, D.; Oestergaard, M.; Say, L.; Moller, A.B.; Kinney, M.; Lawn, J. Born too soon: The global epidemiology of 15 million preterm births. *Reprod. Health* **2013**, *10* (Suppl. 1), S2. [CrossRef] [PubMed]
93. Venhoff, N.; Voll, R.E.; Glaser, C.; Thiel, J. IL-1-blockade with Anakinra during pregnancy: Retrospective analysis of efficacy and safety in female patients with familial Mediterranean fever. *Z. Rheum.* **2018**, *77*, 127–134. [CrossRef] [PubMed]
94. Romero, R.; Dey, S.K.; Fisher, S.J. Preterm labor: One syndrome, many causes. *Science* **2014**, *345*, 760–765. [CrossRef]
95. Saigal, S.; Doyle, L.W. An overview of mortality and sequelae of preterm birth from infancy to adulthood. *Lancet* **2008**, *371*, 261–269. [CrossRef]
96. Smith, C.J.F.; Chambers, C.D. Five successful pregnancies with antenatal anakinra exposure. *Rheumatology* **2018**, *57*, 1271–1275. [CrossRef]

97. Youngstein, T.; Hoffmann, P.; Gül, A.; Lane, T.; Williams, R.; Rowczenio, D.M.; Ozdogan, H.; Ugurlu, S.; Ryan, J.; Harty, L.; et al. International multi-centre study of pregnancy outcomes with interleukin-1 inhibitors. *Rheumatology* **2017**, *56*, 2102–2108. [CrossRef]
98. Rider, R.A.; Stevenson, D.A.; Rinsky, J.E.; Feldkamp, M.L. Association of twinning and maternal age with major structural birth defects in Utah, 1999 to 2008. *Birth Defects Res. A Clin. Mol. Teratol.* **2013**, *97*, 554–563. [CrossRef]
99. Viktil, K.K.; Engeland, A.; Furu, K. Use of antirheumatic drugs in mothers and fathers before and during pregnancy-a population-based cohort study. *Pharmacoepidemiol. Drug Saf.* **2009**, *18*, 737–742. [CrossRef]
100. Drechsel, P.; Stüdemann, K.; Niewerth, M.; Horneff, G.; Fischer-Betz, R.; Seipelt, E.; Spähtling-Mestekemper, S.; Aries, P.; Zink, A.; Klotsche, J.; et al. Pregnancy outcomes in DMARD-exposed patients with juvenile idiopathic arthritis-results from a JIA biologic registry. *Rheumatology* **2020**, *59*, 603–612. [CrossRef]

MDPI
St. Alban-Anlage 66
4052 Basel
Switzerland
Tel. +41 61 683 77 34
Fax +41 61 302 89 18
www.mdpi.com

Journal of Clinical Medicine Editorial Office
E-mail: jcm@mdpi.com
www.mdpi.com/journal/jcm

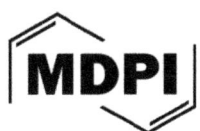

www.ingramcontent.com/pod-product-compliance
Lightning Source LLC
LaVergne TN
LVHW070411100526
838202LV00014B/1440